Sensors for
Human Activity Recognition

Sensors for
Human Activity Recognition

Editors

Hui Liu
Hugo Gamboa
Tanja Schultz

MDPI • Basel • Beijing • Wuhan • Barcelona • Belgrade • Manchester • Tokyo • Cluj • Tianjin

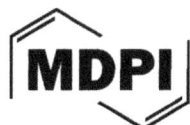

Editors

Hui Liu
University of Bremen,
Bremen, Germany

Hugo Gamboa
NOVA University Lisbon,
Lisbon, Portugal

Tanja Schultz
University of Bremen,
Bremen, Germany

Editorial Office
MDPI
St. Alban-Anlage 66
4052 Basel, Switzerland

This is a reprint of articles from the Special Issue published online in the open access journal *Sensors* (ISSN 1424-8220) (available at: https://www.mdpi.com/journal/sensors/special_issues/ Sensors_Human_Activity_Recognition).

For citation purposes, cite each article independently as indicated on the article page online and as indicated below:

LastName, A.A.; LastName, B.B.; LastName, C.C. Article Title. *Journal Name* **Year**, *Volume Number*, Page Range.

ISBN 978-3-0365-7554-4 (Hbk)
ISBN 978-3-0365-7555-1 (PDF)

Contents

About the Editors

Hui Liu

Hui Liu, Dr.-Ing. is a researcher at the Cognitive Systems Lab, University of Bremen (since 2016), focusing on biosignal processing, activity recognition, virtual reality, and information retrieval. He studied electrical engineering at the Technical University of Berlin (Dipl.-Ing., 2009) and information and communication systems at Shanghai Jiao Tong University (M. Sc., 2011). He received his Ph.D. from the University of Bremen (2021). He is co-responsible for the multi-partner projects Arthrokinemat (intelligent knee bandage, finished 2019), ETAP (AI-based movement monitoring for long-term care assistance), and IntEL4CoRo (interactive learning for cognitive robotics). He developed the first wearable-based system for knee bandage that recognizes users' activities in real-time (Best Paper Award (Student Author), BIODEVICES 2019). Meanwhile, he proposed Motion Units, an activity modeling method with interpretability, generalizability, and expandability, rationalizing knowledge from kinesiology and speech recognition into activity research (2021). A 19-channel, 22-activity, 20-subject human activity dataset CSL-SHARE was collected and shared by him, on which six-hour data of an 11.52-h recording are well segmented, annotated, and post-verified (2021). His two papers on high-level feature design (co-author) and music signal processing (first author), respectively, were the Best Paper Finalists (BIOSIGNALS 2022 and SIGMAP 2022). He received the YERUN Research Mobility Award and the CAMPUSiDEEN Public Choice Award for his advanced technology study of biosignal processing and activity recognition (2022).

Hugo Gamboa

Hugo Gamboa, Prof. Dr. received his Ph.D. degree in electrical and computer engineering from the Instituto Superior Técnico of University of Lisbon (IST UL), in 2007. He is a Co-Founder and the President of PLUX, a company that develops bio-signals monitoring wearable technology. He is currently a Researcher at the Laboratory for Instrumentation, Biomedical Engineering and Radiation Physics (LIBPhys), Faculdade de Ciências e Tecnologia of NOVA University of Lisbon (FCT NOVA), where he is also an Associate Professor with Habilitation at the Physics Department. Since 2014, he has been a Senior Researcher at the Fraunhofer Center for Assistive Information and Communication Solutions (AICOS). His research interests include bio-signals processing and instrumentation.

Tanja Schultz

Tanja Schultz, Prof. Dr.-Ing. received her doctoral and diploma degree in Informatics from University of Karlsruhe, Germany in 2000 and 1995 respectively and successfully passed the German state examination for teachers of Mathematics, Sports, and Educational Science at Heidelberg University, in 1990. In 2000 she joined Carnegie Mellon University in Pittsburgh, Pennsylvania where she holds a position as Research Professor at the Language Technologies Institute. From 2007 to 2015 she was a Full Professor at the Department of Informatics of the Karlsruhe Institute of Technology (KIT) in Germany before she accepted an offer from the University of Bremen in April 2015. Since 2007, Tanja Schultz directs the Cognitive Systems Lab, where her research activities focus on human-machine communication with a particular emphasis on multilingual speech processing and human-machine interfaces. Together with her team, she investigates the processing, recognition and interpretation of biosignals, i.e., human signals resulting from physical and mental activities, to enable human interaction with machines in a natural way. Tanja Schultz received several awards for her work, such as the FZI award for an outstanding Ph.D. thesis (2001), the Allen Newell Medal for

Research Excellence from Carnegie Mellon (2002), the ISCA best journal award for her publication on language independent acoustic modeling (2002) and on Silent Speech Interfaces (2015), the Plux Wireless award (2011) for the development of Airwriting, the Alcatel-Lucent Research Award for Technical Communication (2012), the Otto-Haxel Award (2013), a Google Research Award (2013 and 2020) as well as several best paper awards. She is the author of more than 450 articles published in books, journals, and proceedings, and is regularly invited as panelist and keynote speaker. Tanja Schultz serves as a member for numerous conference committees, as Associate Editor of IEEE Transactions (2002–2004), as an Associate Editor for ACM TALLIP (since 2013), as editorial board member of Speech Communication (since 2001), and served as board member and elected president of the International Speech Communication Association ISCA from 2007–2015.

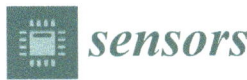

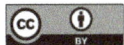
MDPI

Editorial

Sensor-Based Human Activity and Behavior Research: Where Advanced Sensing and Recognition Technologies Meet

Hui Liu [1,2,*], Hugo Gamboa [2] and Tanja Schultz [1]

1   Cognitive Systems Lab, University of Bremen, Enrique-Schmidt-Str. 5, 28359 Bremen, Germany
2   LIBPhys (Laboratory for Instrumentation, Biomedical Engineering and Radiation Physics), NOVA School of Science and Technology (Campus de Caparica), 2829-516 Caparica, Portugal
*   Correspondence: hui.liu@uni-bremen.com

Citation: Liu, H.; Gamboa, H.; Schultz, T. Sensor-Based Human Activity and Behavior Research: Where Advanced Sensing and Recognition Technologies Meet. *Sensors* **2023**, *23*, 125. https://doi.org/10.3390/s23010125

Received: 10 December 2022
Accepted: 13 December 2022
Published: 23 December 2022

1. Introduction

Human activity recognition (HAR) and human behavior recognition (HBR) have been playing increasingly important roles in the digital age. High-quality sensory observations applicable to recognizing users' activities and behaviors, including electrical, magnetic, mechanical (kinetic), optical, acoustic, thermal, and chemical biosignals, are inseparable from sensors' sophisticated design and appropriate application.

Traditional sensors suitable for HAR and HBR, including external sensors for smart homes, optical sensors such as cameras for capturing video signals, and bioelectrical, biomagnetic, and biomechanical sensors for wearable applications, have been studied and verified adequately. They continue to be researched in-depth for more effective and efficient usage, and brand new areas facilitated by sensor-based HAR/HBR are emerging, such as interactive edutainment [1], single motion duration analysis [2], time series information retrieval [3], handcrafted and high-level feature design [4–6], and fall detection [7]. Meanwhile, innovative sensor research for HAR or HBR is also very active in the academic community, including new sensors appropriate for HAR/HBR, new designs and applications of the above-mentioned traditional sensors, and the usage of non-traditional HAR/HBR-related sensor types, among others.

This Special Issue aims to provide researchers in related fields with a platform to demonstrate their unique insights and late-breaking achievements.

2. Overview of the Contributions

Ten high-quality representative articles, including eight research papers and two surveys, have undergone a rigorous selection and review process to be published in this Special Issue. Although it cannot be said that they cover all aspects of the topic "sensors for human activity recognition," they reflect the latest developments in the field in a high-profile manner.

We follow the sequence of tasks indicated by the state-of-the-art HAR research pipeline [8,9] to organize and introduce these contributions. Therefore, it should be emphasized that the order in which the articles appear does not correlate with their academic value.

2.1. Hardware Preparation: Sensing Technologies and Camera Calibration Technologies

As the hardware cornerstone of all relevant research areas, sensing technology is a topic that cannot be jumped. We are delighted to have such an opening article in this Special Issue [10], which presented a thorough, in-depth survey on the state-of-the-art sensing modalities in HAR tasks to supply a solid understanding of the variant sensing principles for younger researchers of the community. The HAR-related sensing modalities are reasonably categorized into five classes: mechanical kinematic sensing, field-based sensing, wave-based sensing, physiological sensing, and hybrid/others, with the strengths and weaknesses of each modality across the categorization compared and discussed to provide newcomers with a better overview and references.

Equipped with advanced knowledge of sensing technology, researchers step into the door of sensor-based HAR to select appropriate high-quality sensors for their research scenarios. Afterward, preparatory work is required to acquire continuous, high-quality biosignals. For example, the calibration task is essential for video camera-based HAR, where high-precision distortion calibration is a prerequisite for perfect activity recognition with external sensing. Conventional approaches sometimes need hundreds or thousands of images to optimize the camera model. Jin et al. put forward an innovative point-to-point distortion calibration procedure that requires only dozens of images to obtain a dense distortion rectification map, contributing to a 28.5% enhancement to the reprojection error over the polynomial distortion model [11]. It is worthy of academic focus that although the authors emphasized the application of the new method in HAR, we find that the applicability is not limited to HAR and deserves a more extensive scope of attention.

2.2. Signal Processing: Traditional Feature Extraction versus Deep Neural Representations

After the aspects of devices have been adequately studied, sensor signals will be acquired, archived, and analyzed. Digital signal processing (DSP) techniques are widely used in the subsequent stage, among which feature extraction serves as the bridge that connects the raw data with machine learning. Traditional machine learning for HAR generally employs conventional features in statistical, temporal, and frequency domains to execute experiments such as combination, selection, stacking, and dimensionality reduction. In contrast, deep learning requires deep neural representations. It is a very arresting academic work to compare the two through a new and rational approach [12]. The work analyzes both approaches in multiple domains utilizing homogenized public datasets, verifying that even though deep learning initially outperforms handcrafted features, the situation is reversed as the distance from the training distribution increases, which supports the hypothesis that handcrafted features may generalize better across specific domains.

2.3. Recognition and Localization on Human Activities or Behaviors: Deep Learning versus No Training

The vast majority of sensor-based HAR tasks rely on machine learning. Despite the irreplaceable advantages of traditional feature-based machine learning suggested in Section 2.2, deep learning is increasingly demonstrating its powerful adaptive capabilities. Besides [12], this Special Issue contains three more articles on deep learning [13–15], offering us multiple dimensions of thinking:

- The training of HAR models requires a large amount of annotated data corpus. Most current models are not robust when facing anonymized data from new users; meanwhile, capturing each new subject's data is usually not possible. Yang et al. described semi-supervised adversarial learning using the long-short term memory (LSTM) approach for HAR [13], which trains labeled and anonymous data by adapting the semi-supervised learning paradigms on which adversarial learning capitalizes to enhance the learning capabilities handling errors.

- The device-free, privacy-protected, and light-insensitive characteristics have pushed WIFI-based HAR technology into the limelight. Evolving machine learning techniques have significantly improved sensing accuracy with existing methods. To improve the performance of the challenging multi-location recognition, researchers in [14] proposed an amplitude- and phase-enhanced deep complex network (AP-DCN) for multi-location HAR to exploit the amplitude and phase information synchronously and thus retrieve richer information from limited samples. A perception method based on a deep complex network-transfer learning (DCN-TL) structure was practiced to effectively achieve knowledge sharing among multiple locations, aiming to address the imbalance in sample numbers.

- Sensor-based indoor localization is also relevant to this Special Issue's scope by using acceleration signals to represent human behavior to be useful additional information on GPS signals for modeling and learning. Sensor-based indoor localization is also relevant to this Special Issue by using acceleration signals to represent human behavior to be useful additional information on GPS signals for modeling and learning. Study [15] exhibited a pedestrian dead reckoning-based indoor localization system on a smartphone, where accelerometer and GPS data were used as input and labels to estimate moving speed through deep learning. A distance error of approximately 3 to 5 m in the experiments within a 240 m-long horseshoe-shaped building is a welcome level of accuracy.

Model training for machine learning, or, furthermore, deep learning, is not the sole path to reaching human activity or behavior recognition. We have a research piece that seeks to achieve behavioral recognition without training [16]. The convenience store is a daily business form worldwide; for Japanese society, its transliteration abbreviation "Kombini" goes beyond shopping, representing a unique cultural and emotional sustenance. Recognizing customer behaviors in monitoring videos can supply analytical material for business management in smart retail solutions. Therefore, the scientists from Japan put the analysis of human behavior in the convenience store scene, which is an appropriate and attractive setting. Unlike previous approaches based on model training, customer behavior in this research is combined with primitives to achieve flexibility, where a primitive is a unit describing an object's motion or multiple objects' relationships.

2.4. Evaluating the Experimental Results: Also an Essential Research Topic

Besides the machine learning task for HAR, what research can be further executed before practical applications? In [17], the authors proposed explainable methods to understand the performance of mobile HAR mobile systems according to the chosen validation strategies. A novel approach, SHAP (Shapley additive explanations), was used to discover potential bias problems of accuracy overestimation based on the inappropriate choice of validation methodology. We believe this study is academically significant and of guiding value for practice.

2.5. More Referential Topics Linked to Body Sensor Networks and Human Physiological Signals

As an academic expansion, we have also selected two articles about wearable sensors combined with human physiological signal applications to benefit our readers. They provide sensor-based human activity/behavior researchers with references and inspirations for the device and experimental design.

Authors of [18] successfully modeled subjects' psychological stress in different states through electrocardiogram (ECG) signals during a virtual reality high-altitude experiment. Participants wore in-house-designed smart T-shirts with embedded multiple sensors to complete different tasks. A deep, gated recurrent unit (GRU) neural network was developed to capture the mapping between subjects' ECG and stress represented by heart rate variability (HRV) features.

The ankle joint, one of the body's most important joints for maintaining the ability to walk, can be damaged due to stroke or osteoarthritis, which will cause gait disturbances. Ankle-foot orthoses have been widely applied to help patients regain their natural gait. Article [19] reviewed the development of ankle-foot orthoses and prospected combining ankle-foot orthoses with rehabilitation techniques, such as myoelectric stimulation, to reduce the energy expenditure of patients in walking.

3. Conclusions, Outlook, and Acknowledgments

Having attracted many contributions from outstanding world scientists, this Special Issue has become thriving and full of academic tensions. Given the enthusiasm of the submissions, the second volume of this Special Issue has been launched, and we look forward to more scholars publishing their admiring contributions.

We pay special tribute and appreciation to all 51 authors of the articles, as well as all professional and diligent reviewers.

Conflicts of Interest: The authors declare no conflict of interes.

References

1. Hartmann, Y.; Liu, H.; Schultz, T. Interactive and Interpretable Online Human Activity Recognition. In Proceedings of the 2022 IEEE International Conference on Pervasive Computing and Communications Workshops and other Affiliated Events (PerCom Workshops), Pisa, Italy, 21–25 March 2022; pp. 109–111. [CrossRef]
2. Liu, H.; Schultz, T. How Long Are Various Types of Daily Activities? Statistical Analysis of a Multimodal Wearable Sensor-based Human Activity Dataset. In Proceedings of the 15th International Joint Conference on Biomedical Engineering Systems and Technologies-HEALTHINF, INSTICC, Online, 8–10 February 2022; pp. 680–688. [CrossRef]
3. Folgado, D.; Barandas, M.; Antunes, M.; Nunes, M.L.; Liu, H.; Hartmann, Y.; Schultz, T.; Gamboa, H. TSSEARCH: Time Series Subsequence Search Library. *SoftwareX* **2022**, *18*, 101049. [CrossRef]
4. Hartmann, Y.; Liu, H.; Schultz, T. Feature Space Reduction for Multimodal Human Activity Recognition. In Proceedings of the 13th International Joint Conference on Biomedical Engineering Systems and Technologies-BIOSIGNALS, INSTICC, Valletta, Malta, 20–24 February 2020; pp. 135–140. [CrossRef]
5. Hartmann, Y.; Liu, H.; Schultz, T. Feature Space Reduction for Human Activity Recognition based on Multi-channel Biosignals. In Proceedings of the 14th International Joint Conference on Biomedical Engineering Systems and Technologies-BIOSIGNALS, INSTICC, Online, 11–13 February 2021; pp. 215–222. [CrossRef]
6. Hartmann, Y.; Liu, H.; Schultz, T. Interpretable High-level Features for Human Activity Recognition. In Proceedings of the 15th International Joint Conference on Biomedical Engineering Systems and Technologies-BIOSIGNALS, INSTICC, Online, 9–11 February 2022; pp. 40–49. [CrossRef]
7. Xue, T.; Liu, H. Hidden Markov Model and Its Application in Human Activity Recognition and Fall Detection: A Review. In Proceedings of the Communications, Signal Processing, and Systems, Changbaishan, China, 22–23 October 2022; Springer: Singapore, 2022; pp. 863–869. [CrossRef]
8. Liu, H.; Hartmann, Y.; Schultz, T. A Practical Wearable Sensor-Based Human Activity Recognition Research Pipeline. In Proceedings of the 15th International Joint Conference on Biomedical Engineering Systems and Technologies-HEALTHINF, INSTICC, Online, 9–11 February 2022; pp. 847–856. [CrossRef]
9. Liu, H. Biosignal Processing and Activity Modeling for Multimodal Human Activity Recognition. Ph.D. Thesis, University of Bremen, Bremen, Germany, 2021. [CrossRef]
10. Bian, S.; Liu, M.; Zhou, B.; Lukowicz, P. The State-of-the-Art Sensing Techniques in Human Activity Recognition: A Survey. *Sensors* **2022**, *22*, 4596. [CrossRef] [PubMed]
11. Jin, Z.; Li, Z.; Gan, T.; Fu, Z.; Zhang, C.; He, Z.; Zhang, H.; Wang, P.; Liu, J.; Ye, X. A Novel Central Camera Calibration Method Recording Point-to-Point Distortion for Vision-Based Human Activity Recognition. *Sensors* **2022**, *22*, 3524. [CrossRef] [PubMed]
12. Bento, N.; Rebelo, J.; Barandas, M.; Carreiro, A.V.; Campagner, A.; Cabitza, F.; Gamboa, H. Comparing Handcrafted Features and Deep Neural Representations for Domain Generalization in Human Activity Recognition. *Sensors* **2022**, *22*, 7324. [CrossRef] [PubMed]
13. Yang, S.H.; Baek, D.G.; Thapa, K. Semi-Supervised Adversarial Learning Using LSTM for Human Activity Recognition. *Sensors* **2022**, *22*, 4755. [CrossRef] [PubMed]
14. Ding, X.; Hu, C.; Xie, W.; Zhong, Y.; Yang, J.; Jiang, T. Device-Free Multi-Location Human Activity Recognition Using Deep Complex Network. *Sensors* **2022**, *22*, 6178. [CrossRef] [PubMed]
15. Yoon, J.; Kim, S. Practical and Accurate Indoor Localization System Using Deep Learning. *Sensors* **2022**, *22*, 6764. [CrossRef] [PubMed]
16. Wen, J.; Abe, T.; Suganuma, T. A Customer Behavior Recognition Method for Flexibly Adapting to Target Changes in Retail Stores. *Sensors* **2022**, *22*, 6740. [CrossRef] [PubMed]
17. Bragança, H.; Colonna, J.G.; Oliveira, H.A.B.F.; Souto, E. How Validation Methodology Influences Human Activity Recognition Mobile Systems. *Sensors* **2022**, *22*, 2360. [CrossRef] [PubMed]
18. Zhong, J.; Liu, Y.; Cheng, X.; Cai, L.; Cui, W.; Hai, D. Gated Recurrent Unit Network for Psychological Stress Classification Using Electrocardiograms from Wearable Devices. *Sensors* **2022**, *22*, 8664. [CrossRef] [PubMed]
19. Zhou, C.; Yang, Z.; Li, K.; Ye, X. Research and Development of Ankle–Foot Orthoses: A Review. *Sensors* **2022**, *22*, 6596. [CrossRef] [PubMed]

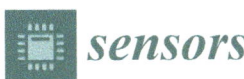

MDPI

Article

The State-of-the-Art Sensing Techniques in Human Activity Recognition: A Survey

Sizhen Bian *, Mengxi Liu, Bo Zhou and Paul Lukowicz

German Research Centre for Artificial Intelligence (DFKI), 67663 Kaiserslautern, Germany;
mengxi.liu@dfki.de (M.L.); bo.zhou@dfki.de (B.Z.); paul.lukowicz@dfki.de (P.L.)
* Correspondence: sizhen.bian@dfki.de

Abstract: Human activity recognition (HAR) has become an intensive research topic in the past decade because of the pervasive user scenarios and the overwhelming development of advanced algorithms and novel sensing approaches. Previous HAR-related sensing surveys were primarily focused on either a specific branch such as wearable sensing and video-based sensing or a full-stack presentation of both sensing and data processing techniques, resulting in weak focus on HAR-related sensing techniques. This work tries to present a thorough, in-depth survey on the state-of-the-art sensing modalities in HAR tasks to supply a solid understanding of the variant sensing principles for younger researchers of the community. First, we categorized the HAR-related sensing modalities into five classes: mechanical kinematic sensing, field-based sensing, wave-based sensing, physiological sensing, and hybrid/others. Specific sensing modalities are then presented in each category, and a thorough description of the sensing tricks and the latest related works were given. We also discussed the strengths and weaknesses of each modality across the categorization so that newcomers could have a better overview of the characteristics of each sensing modality for HAR tasks and choose the proper approaches for their specific application. Finally, we summarized the presented sensing techniques with a comparison concerning selected performance metrics and proposed a few outlooks on the future sensing techniques used for HAR tasks.

Keywords: human activity recognition; sensing technique

Citation: Bian, S.; Liu, M.; Zhou, B.; Lukowicz, P. The State-of-the-Art Sensing Techniques in Human Activity Recognition: A Survey. *Sensors* **2022**, *22*, 4596. https://doi.org/10.3390/s22124596

Academic Editors: Tanja Schultz, Hui Liu and Hugo Gamboa

Received: 13 May 2022
Accepted: 16 June 2022
Published: 17 June 2022

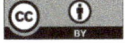
1. Introduction

A better understanding of human behavior benefits individuals on a large scale, including healthcare, well-being, social interaction, life assistance, etc. Thus human activity recognition (HAR) has been tremendously explored in recent years, driven by the enormous technical advances in sensing, computation, and immense human-centric user scenarios. The explosive advancement in machine learning and hardware architecture has dramatically improved the accuracy and robustness of HAR tasks and enabled the technique to be deployed at the far edge near the body. Besides the computational ability, the sensing technique plays a fundamental and critical role in HAR tasks. Therefore, a broader range of sensing modalities has been explored in recent years, aiming to boost the development of reliable body activity digitalized recording. The proposed sensing modalities range from traditional motion sensing methods such as accelerometers, to novel TOF-based sensing such as mmWave, from neural network-aided image processing for activity abstraction to very straightforward proximity detection approaches such as RF-tags.

To acquire a comprehensive overview of the state-of-the-art sensing modalities in human activity recognition, categorization of the adopted sensors is an efficient approach for a deeper understanding of the sensing medium. Researchers have already categorized related sensors into different classes, such as active and passive sensors depending on the need for external excitation [1], or intrusive and non-intrusive sensors depending on the interference of the sensors in the process flow [2,3]. With a further step, we elaborately categorized the HAR-related sensing modalities into five classes depending on the following sensing principles: kinematic sensing, field-based sensing, wave-based sensing, physiological sensing, and hybrid or other approaches, as Figure 1 presents. We enumerated most of the sensing modalities within each class with an in-depth description of the sensing tricks in the HAR tasks.

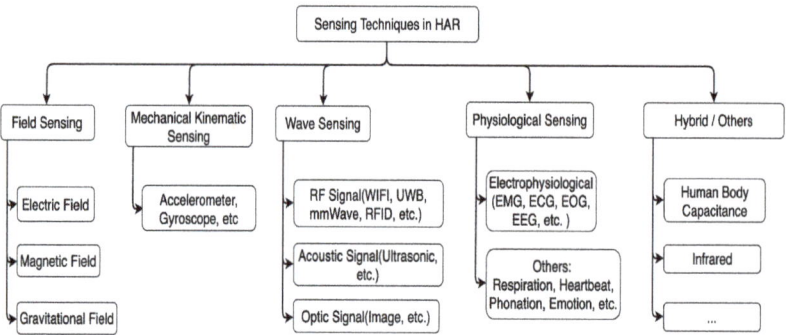

Figure 1. Sensing techniques in human activity recognition.

1.1. Relevant Surveys

Despite the enormous scope of sensing modalities in HAR tasks, related survey works are limited. The existing surveys on HAR sensing are primarily focused either on a specific scenario (such as wearable sensing or video-based sensing) or on full-stack presentation of both sensing and data processing techniques, which results in a weak focus on HAR-related sensing techniques. Table 1 lists the latest HAR sensing-related surveys in recent years from the literature. Those high-related surveys (as well as other references listed in this paper) are first searched using keywords such as human activity recognition, survey, overview, and sensing technique, from platforms including Google Scholar, IEEE Xplore, Microsoft Academic, etc. Second, the survey papers cited in the searched surveys were also considered. As can be seen, nearly all the exiting surveys only focused on a specific domain of HAR sensing techniques, such as device-free sensors [4], smartphone sensors [5], radar sensors [6], etc. Such surveys could supply a detailed research result on the particular sensing domain but lack focus on the adopted sensors in HAR. In contrast, there are only a few surveys [7,8] that supply thorough sensor modalities. However, an in-depth introduction and comparison of the sensing tricks is still lacking.

Table 1. Surveys on HAR sensing techniques.

Focused Subject	Ref	Year	Contribution
Device-free sensors	[4]	2020	• Categorized sensors into wearable, object-tagged, device-free, etc. • Focused on device-free sensing approaches for 10 kinds of activities. • Extensive analysis based on 10 important metrics of each sensing approach.
Full-stack (sensors and algorithms)	[7]	2020	• Categorized sensors into wearable, object, environmental, and video-based. • Focused on data processing approaches.
Overall sensors	[8]	2020	• Categorized sensors by physical principles (acoustic, optical, etc.). • Summarized publicly available databases and common evaluation metrics to evaluate and compare the performance of the developed algorithms and systems.
Smartphone sensors	[5]	2019	• Enumeration and description of embedded sensors. • Data labeling, processing, etc.
Surveillance video	[9]	2019	• Summarized the general process of human action recognition in video processing domain. • Surveyed different features and models used in video surveillance, and the related datasets.

Table 1. *Cont.*

Focused Subject	Ref	Year	Contribution
Radar sensors	[6]	2019	• Overview of various radar systems adopted to recognize human activities. • Overview of DL techniques applied to radar-based HAR tasks.
Bespoke sensors in smart home	[10]	2017	• Highlighted that smart home intelligence involved sensing technology. • Highlighted the multi-resident activity recognition including concurrent, interleave, and cooperative interaction activity.
Vision-based	[11]	2017	• Comprehensive survey of different phases of vision-based HAR (image segmentation, feature extraction, activity classification).
WiFi-based	[12]	2016	• Survey of the WiFi-based contactless HAR from four aspects including historical overview, theories and models, and key techniques for applications.
Non-invasive sensors	[13]	2016	• Survey of technologies that are close to entering the commercial market or have only recently become available.
Vision-based	[14]	2015	• Proposed categorization of human activities into unimodal and multimodal according to the nature of sensor data they employ. • Reviewed various human activity recognition methods and analyzed the strengths and weaknesses of each category separately.
Wearable sensors	[15]	2014	• Reviewed the latest reported systems on activity monitoring of humans based on wearable sensors. • Forecasted the light-weight physiological sensors that lead to comfortable wearable devices to tackle the challenges.

1.2. Paper Aims and Contribution

This work tries to fill the gap by presenting an extensive and in-depth survey on the state-of-the-art sensing modalities in HAR tasks, aiming to supply a solid understanding of most sensing modalities for researchers in the community. Overall, we provide the following contributions in this survey:

1. For a clear overview of the multifaceted nature of HAR tasks, we firstly sorted the human activities into three types: body position-related services ("where"), body action-related services ("what"), and body status-related services ("how"). Such sorting coarsely but briefly introduces the final objective of the utilized sensing technique, which supplies the readers with an elementary step for the sensing concept.

2. We then categorized the sensing techniques in HAR tasks into five classes based on the underlying physical principle: mechanical kinematic sensing, wave-based sensing, field-based sensing, physiological sensing, and hybrid or others. We enumerated broadly the adopted sensing modalities within each category and supplied an in-depth description of the underlying technical tricks. Such a sensor-oriented categorization supplies the readers a further understanding of the distinct HAR tasks.

3. We gave each sensing modality an in/cross-class comparison with eight metrics to better understand each modality's limitation and dominant properties and its typical applications in HAR. Finally, we provided a few insights regarding its future development.

This survey is constructed as follows: in Section 1, we briefly stated the motivation of this survey considering the existing works and the development of the state-of-the-art HAR sensing techniques. We then summarized and categorized all human activities in the research scope according to the activity attribute in Section 2, followed by a brief description of the general process of the HAR task. Section 3 showed our categorization of the current HAR sensing techniques and gave an in-depth and extensive description of each sensing modality, followed by a summary regarding eight critical sensing performance metrics. Sections 4 and 5 presented a few outlooks into the future development of the HAR-related sensing techniques and the conclusion of our work.

2. Background

2.1. Object of Human Activities Recognition (HAR)

Human activities refer to human behaviors concerning the body or the environment. The recognition of human activity aims to capture the action/status of the agents from a series of observations. A successful recognition could provide personalized support in plenty of human-centric applications [16,17]. Since the HAR tasks cover a wide range of activities, it is necessary to sort the related topics in an impressive and compact way. Most research works assort the task into a few levels according to the activity complexity [4,7] (from gestures to actions), followed by human object/human interaction. Group activities [18,19] are the most complicated ones, requiring multiple people and essentially composed of series of gestures, actions, and interactions. In this work, we sorted the human activity recognition into three problems (Figure 2) according to the attributes of the targeted task: body position-related problem, body action-related problem, and body status-related problem corresponding to the questions of "where", "what", and "how", respectively. The"where" problem addresses the position-related recognition, such as indoor positioning [20], tracking [21], proximity [22], etc. The "what" problem deals with the action-related recognition, which belongs to the most widely researched section under the HAR task. Examples are fall detection [23], gait analysis [24], ADL (activity of daily life) [25], etc. The last one is the "how" problem, inferring the body status-related research, such as emotion-sensing [26], respiration/heartrate sensing [27], healthcare [28], etc. This task-oriented categorization aims to supply a basic concept of the objectives of human activity recognition. As can be seen, HAR is a multifaceted topic covering almost all human-related activities and needs interdisciplinary knowledge to understand the behaviors and provide assistance properly.

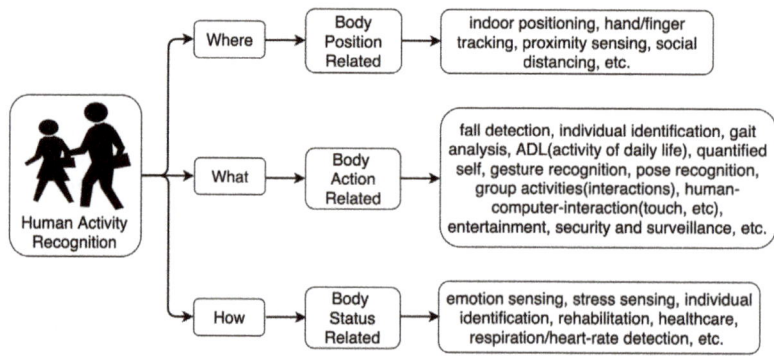

Figure 2. Categorization of human activities.

2.2. General Process of Human Activity Recognition

Human activity recognition explains comprehensive body behaviors aiming to supply ethical-respect assistance. A complete recognition task is generally composed of three steps (Figure 3): sensing, data processing, and decision making. Sensing techniques play a fundamental role in the procedure, trying to perceive as much contextual knowledge as possible so that a reliable recognition becomes possible. A successful HAR task depends firstly on the data quality perceived from the applied sensors and secondly on the processing skills of the acquired data. With the developments in physics, electronics, and other fundamental subjects, novel sensors and devices are emerging to supply more efficient signal patterns for human activity recognition [29–31]. The revolution of the ToF camera, as an example, has enabled the camera to move from simply capturing the streamed images to providing additional depth information to the images, thus provoking a wide range of recognition tasks such as hand gestures [32] and facial expressions [33]. Recently, significant advances in detection accuracy and range, and the power consumption of the ToF sensor, have continued to boost novel applications in both industrial automation [34] and consumer electronics [35]. Diverse sensing techniques have been utilized for specific HAR scenarios and have provided outperforming recognition performance, which motivated us to write this survey focusing on those state-of-the-art sensing techniques with in-depth exploration and extensive analysis. After getting the knowledge from the sensing approaches, the second step is to process the data. According to the data quality and the deployed algorithms, a pre-processing step such as normalization or calibration might be needed. For small volume data such as single-dimensional ECG data or RSSI-based positioning data, a rule-based [36] or multi-lateration [37] algorithm will supply good results. For extensive volume data such as image and speech, the algorithms deployed on the pre-processed data have been dominated by deep neural network-based models [38] with a training process due to its cutting-edge recognition performance compared with traditional approaches [39], such as feature descriptors in object detection. Currently, a large amount of HAR tasks are conducted based on the image streams captured from different kinds of cameras. Those works were focused on spatio-temporal relations of the individuals in the scene. Traditionally, researchers handcraft the features [40] to deduce the target activity, but such approaches firstly heavily rely on the individual experience for the selection of high-relative features; secondly, the handcrafted features might be inefficient and lack generalization in dynamic and environments. The last decade's exploration of machine learning has impressively influenced the processing pipeline in HAR applications. Network models based on convolutional computing [41] or attentional mechanisms [42] for feature abstraction have dominated the approaches for data processing and presented the state-of-the-art recognition performance. The corresponding general framework comprises steps including data acquisition from the applied sensing technique, feature abstraction with distinct network models, and target decision-making based on the inference result of the network model [43,44]. After the patterns of the activities are acquired from the data in the processing step, a decision on the activity recognition could be concluded as a final step. This survey will, however, not cover the recognition algorithms adopted in the data processing step and the final inference step based on the network models. The aim of this survey is to supply a detailed explanation of the physical principles under the applied sensing techniques in HAR tasks and discuss the differences between them so that researchers can choose the right one for their applications. As the first component in the pipeline of the HAR application, the sensing techniques transform human physical activities into numerical information that could be further processed. The following section will extensively present the related HAR-targeted sensing approaches and the behind.

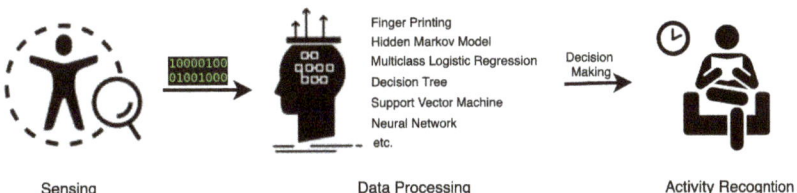

Figure 3. The general process of an HAR task.

3. Sensing Techniques

As Figure 1 depicts, we categorized the sensing techniques into five classes according to the sensing principles: mechanical kinematic sensing, field sensing, wave sensing, physiological sensing, and the hybrid or others. Compared with other categorization approaches such as the deployment approach (wearable, object, environmental, etc.), the principle-based categorization gives a better understanding of the sensing technique's physical background. In the following subsections, we will enumerate the leading sensing modalities in each class with their sensing tricks and related state-of-the-art research works. After the enumeration, we also provide an evaluation and comparison of the sensing modalities with the following performance metrics:

- Cost . Low: less than 10 USD. High: hundreds to thousands of USD.
- Power efficiency. Low: level of mW. High: level of W.
- Signal source. Active or passive according to the source of the measured physical characteristics (naturally or emitted by the sensing system).
- Robustness. The ability to tolerate perturbations that might affect the performance of the sensor.
- Privacy concern. If the sensing approach records individual information beyond the need of interest.
- Computational load. The demand of the hardware resources for successful decision making.
- Typical application. A list of HAR tasks being addressed by the sensing approach.
- Other criterion. Such as installing/maintaining complexity, environmental dependency (line of sight, etc.), accuracy and sensitivity, etc.

3.1. Mechanical Kinematic Sensing

Mechanical sensing refers to mechanical mobility and deformation when a force is deployed on/from the target. The mobility and deformation are perceived by the mechanical sensors, which transform the mechanical variation into electric signals. Mechanical sensors have been widely used to monitor body activity such as the kinematic senors.

In physics and maths, kinematics is a field of study exploring geometrical motion. Kinematics sensing in HAR is based on the human body-related motion properties such as velocity, acceleration, rotation, etc. Since the recognition of body motion activities is the most related object of HAR tasks compared to other objects such as positioning, status monitoring, etc., kinematic sensors have become the dominant sensing approach in scientific research and industry application. The most popular deployed sensors are inertial ones such as accelerometers and gyroscopes. Another reason for the massive usage of inertial sensors is the power effectiveness and small size, enabling a pervasive embedding of the sensing unit into personal assistant devices such as smartphones and wearable devices such as fitness bands.

Nearly all of the current commercial wearable devices are embedded with inertial sensors that deliver motion signals of a distinct body part without much concern about power consumption and comfort. Both academic and industrial researchers have developed plenty of works with inertial-sensor-embedded wearable applications. For example, Hristijan et al. [45] explored a weighted ensemble learning algorithm with data from head-mounted inertial sensors to recognize eight everyday activities. Tobias et al. [46] proposed a respiration rate monitoring using an in-ear headphone inertial sensor. Wrist-, hand-, finger-worn inertial sensors are primarily used for gesture recognition as a means of human–machine interface [47–49]. Related wearables are smart gloves, smart watches, smart rings, wristbands, etc. Another popular motion-recognition-enabled wearable modality is the smart garment. Kang et al. [50] designed an IMU and conductive-yarn-integrated clothes to prevent spinal disease by continuous posture monitoring. Zhang [51] evaluated an innovative full-body wearable garment system based on IMUs for motion analysis during different exercises. Wang et al. [52] evaluated stroke patients' acceptance of an IMU-embedded smart garment for supporting upper extremity rehabilitation and received positive responses in a clinical setting. Besides the wearable electric devices and smart garments, inertial sensors could also be integrated into shoes and soles for foot- and leg-related motion-based research, such as gait analysis [53], indoor pedestrian navigation [54], workout recognition [55], injury prevention [56], etc.

Besides the advantage in wearability (power consumption, small size, low cost, pervasiveness), inertial sensors also outperform in data quality regarding sensitivity and accuracy. A high-resolution accelerometer could sense minor vibrations on bodies. Cesareo et al. [57] assessed breathing parameters using the IMU-based system. With the proposed algorithm, they reconstructed respiration-induced movement and precisely perceived the respiratory rate through an automatic method. Huang et al. [58] demonstrated a novel method for

3D pose reconstruction with six IMUs, which outperformed the camera-based methods in situations such as heavy occlusions and fast motion.

Regarding the above-listed advantages, inertial sensors currently play the most critical role in HAR tasks, even in the unique cases of commercial wearable targeting motion-related applications [59]. However, inertial sensors need to be mounted on the target part to sense the part motion pattern, which might be annoying regarding the user habit when long-term continuous motion monitoring is demanded and might cause burden and discomfort for users. For highly accurate motion reconstruction, the inertial sensor also faces the challenge of accumulated errors, which need to addressed by constant recalibration.

3.2. Wave Sensing

Wave sensing is a non-contact sensing technique based on the propagation properties of waves. Three kinds of wave sensing approaches are mainly used for HAR tasks. The first is the RF signals such as WiFi, BT, mmWave, etc., referring to a wireless electromagnetic signal with identified radio frequencies ranging from 3 kHz to 300 GHz. The propagation of the wireless electromagnetic wave is based on the electric and magnetic fields that are orthogonal to each other. The second wave signal is the acoustic signal, a mechanical wave that includes vibration, sound, ultrasound, and infrasound. The third is the optical signal, an electromagnetic signal with the typical extremely high frequency in THz order. In HAR, those wave sensing approaches have been explored widely and deeply. For example, image-based activity recognition analyzes the target actions in the images from the video and can supply recognition with high accuracy. Since video information is captured by a camera that takes all light rays and focuses it via the lens onto a grid of tiny light-sensitive photosites, it is essentially optic-enabled sensing. RF and acoustic signals, as ambient sensors, offer advantages in both privacy protection and reducing the extra burden of objects.

Two kinds of sensing methods exist in wave-based human-centric sensing: active and passive sensing. Figure 4 shows the essential difference between the two methods. Active sensing requires an external source of energy. The source emits waves to the measured object and receives the wave's reflection, transmission, and absorption. Features abstracted from the received information are then utilized for object description. On the other hand, passive sensing does not need an active wave source and perceives the object variables by receiving a measured wave signal from the object.

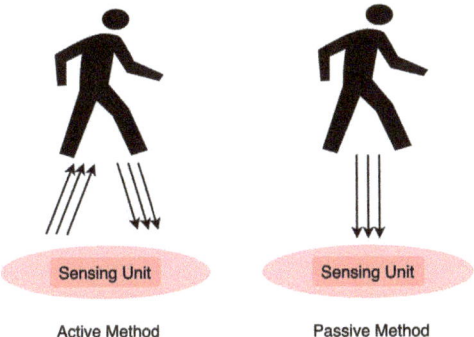

Figure 4. Wave-based human-centric sensing in two methods: active and passive.

(A) RF Signal

RF-based HAR is a non-intrusive approach that can bypass the burden and discomfort caused by wearable activity monitoring sensors. The basic principle of the RF-based HAR system is that the propagation path of the RF wave will be affected by the intrusiveness of the human body. The resulting variations in the received wave can then be used as features to deduce different activities.

A series of RF signals were explored for HAR tasks, such as WiFi, UWB, mmWave, etc. Among them, WiFi is the most popular due to its pervasiveness in the indoor environment. The critical intuition of WiFi-based HAR is that motions of the human body introduce different multipath distortions in WiFi signals and generate different patterns in the time series of channel state information. Li et al. [60] proposed a system named Wi-Motion, being able to jointly leverage the amplitude and phase information extracted from the channel state information sequence, and to achieve a mean accuracy of 96.6% in the line-of-sight environment and 92% in not line-of-sight environment regarding five predefined typical human activities (bend, half squat, step, stretch leg, and jump). Liu et al. [61] designed a WiFi-based sleep monitoring system to abstract fine-grained sleep information such as a person's respiration, sleeping postures and rollovers by continuously collecting the fine-grained wireless channel state information. Besides the activity recognition, the WiFi signal can be leveraged for indoor location tasks. An example work is from Wang et al. [62] where the authors proposed a dual-task residual convolutional neural network with one-dimensional convolutional layers for the joint task of activity recognition and indoor localization. Bluetooth technology is another RF approach to perform HAR tasks. However, compared with the WiFi signal, the Bluetooth signal is relatively weak [63]. Thus the accuracy and reaching range is limited. However, it enjoys advantages in cost and ease of use. Therefore, Bluetooth technology is mainly used for indoor locations by deploying plenty of small form-factor, power-saving, cost-efficient tags with high density [64].

Besides the WiFi and BT wave signal, the mmWave technology, which operates in the frequency range of 30 GHz and 300 GHz, recently exhibited high attraction to researchers. Since a higher frequency means a smaller antenna size, thus the mmWave radar is compact in form factor. Many antennas could be packaged into a small space to enable highly directional beams. Moreover, the mmWave signal enjoys a larger bandwidth than WiFi signals and higher range resolution. Recent advances in small and low-cost single-chip consumer radar systems operating at mmWave frequencies have opened up many new applications, such as automotive radar, health monitoring, etc. HAR has also been explored with mmWave-based approaches and has received outstanding results with fine-grained classifiers. Zhang et al. [65] predicted the target behavior by using the micro-Doppler effect (induced by micromotion dynamics of a target or its structure) from mmWave radar [65]. Using a neural network work-based classifier, they got 95.19% accuracy of bulk motion of the body and the micromotions from arms and legs. Zhao et al. [66] proposed a system named mBeats, where a robot mounted with mmWave radar system is used to provide periodic heart rate measurements under different user poses. A fall-detection system based on mmWave radar was also presented by Sun et al. [67] with the support of a recurrent neural network with long short-term memory units. Li et al. [68] designed another interesting mmWave radar-enabled system called ThuMouse, which regressively tracks the position of a finger aided by a deep neural network. MmWave-related exploration is still at an early stage and will have an explosive growth period in the following years triggered by its unusual behavior compared to WiFi, BT, and the large-scale chip-level commercialization.

Another greatly promising and widely used RF wave signal is the ultra wide band (UWB), which is a decades-old wireless technology used for short-range, high-bandwidth communication with a high data rate. Now it is also as a standard for high-accuracy location services. According to FiRa, a consortium founded by the dominating companies for UWB standards, the reborn UWB will mainly be focused on three use cases: hands-free access control, location-based services, and peer-to-peer communication, which will be complementary to current dominant wireless solutions. Recently, UWB support has started to appear in high-end smartphones. There is no question that the UWB will boost another wave on related applications. Figure 5 shows the wide spectrum of UWB compared with others, allowing UWB to operate at a shallow power state and build stable connectivity with other devices in a crowded radio environment. Thanks to the higher base frequency, UWB devices can provide higher accuracy in position with the level of around 10 cm [69], which is highly dominant compared with WiFi or BT-based positioning with accuracy of meter-level [70]. Another key feature is that UWB is resistive to the multipath effect, a common issue for most RF-based wave sensing technology. The multipath effect refers to the received radio signal from more than one path because of the reflection of retraction caused by objects near the main signal path. The large bandwidth of UWB provides frequency diversity that can make the time-modulated ultra-wideband (TM-UWB) signal resistant to the multipath effects [71]. Researchers have explored plentiful HAR-related applications with UWB, such as activity recognition in smart homes [72], gesture recognition [73], sleep postural transition recognition [74], healthcare monitoring [75], etc. With the popularization of low-cost UWB chips in wearable devices, there will be more short distance-based novel applications based on the UWB technique, such as swarm intelligence, social distancing, etc. However, despite the above-described advantages of UWB, there will still be some time for a wide deployment of UWB, considering its higher cost. Moreover, regarding the data streaming rate, UWB is not a good option for large data interaction between devices compared with other narrowband radio systems.

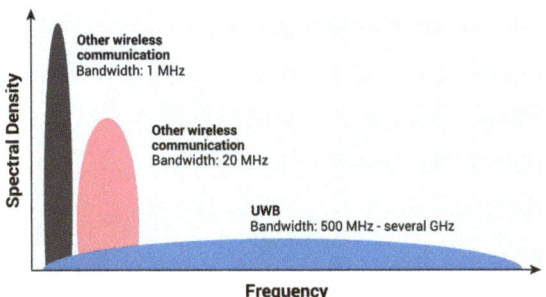

Figure 5. The wide UWB power spectrum results in a low power consumption compared to other technologies. (Source: FiRa Consortium).

(B) Acoustic Signal

An acoustic signal is a mechanical wave resulting from an oscillation of pressure and travels through the solid, liquid, or gas in the form of a wave. A clear, well-known acoustic signal is the audible sound from a speaker by the vibration of vocal folds. The vibration travels through air and reaches the outer ear and the eardrum. There are two kinds of sound outside the range of audible sound frequency (20–20 Khz): infrasound and ultrasound. An example of infrasound is the atmospheric infrasound caused by the earthquake when the earth's surface near the epicenter and surrounding regions oscillates in a low frequency. Ultrasound is an acoustic signal with a higher frequency than the upper audible limit of human hearings. A widely used example of ultrasound is medical imaging, where the ultrasound waves travel through the body and create a sonogram of organs, tissues, etc.

As an ambient sensor, ultrasound could firstly supply mm level positioning accuracy indoors based on the time of flight [76,77]. Such a positioning system is based on several wireless ultrasonic beacons with fixed and known coordination under an indoor environment, and receives or emits ultrasonic signals which are finally used for position deduction. The wireless module (WiFi, Bluetooth, or others) is used for data interaction and time synchronization. Finger motion recognition is another application based on ultrasound by leveraging the characteristic of detected morphological changes of deep muscles and tendons. Yang et al. [78] had obtained an accuracy of 95.4% for real-time finger motion recognition. Mokhtari et al. [79] proposed a resident identification system as an innovative home platform by using ultrasound arrays to detect the height of the moving resident and other sensors such as pyroelectric infrared to detect the moving direction. Wang et al. proposed a novel contactless respiration monitoring approach using ultrasound signals with off-the-shelf audio devices. Unlike other works based on chest displacement where false detection may often occur, they monitor the respiration by directly sensing the exhaled airflow from breathing. The principle is that the exhaled airflow from breathing can be regarded as air turbulence, scattering the sound wave and resulting in the doppler effect. The experiment's results showed an accuracy of 0.3 breaths/min (2%), and it was concluded that the ambient noise and the variation of respiration rate, respiration style, sensing distance, and transmitted signal frequency have little effect on respiration monitoring accuracy of the system.

Previous works on sound (captured by the microphone on a smartphone) are mainly focused on the following application cases: environment assessment [80,81], proximity sensing [82,83], or indoor positioning [84,85]. The sources of sound are either from fine-tuned tags or from the surroundings. In the work of Benjamin et al. [82], an algorithm using inaudible sound patterns was explored to accurately detect whether two mobile phones are within a few meters from each other. The method can be implemented as a standard smartphone application with real-time inferencing, enabling smartphone-based collaborative activity detection and other embedded sensors.

Overall, acoustic signals provide an alternative and competitive approach for highly accurate human or robot positioning and distance-related activity recognition. The method is non-intrusive, thus reducing users' extra burden and protecting privacy security. However, it still suffers from the computational load and is limited by complex environmental acoustic sources. For example, the accuracy and robustness of ultrasound-based indoor positioning enormously decrease when a collision-like sound occurs, or when a significant barrier between tags exists.

(C) Optic Signal

Optical signals for HAR tasks mainly refer to deep learning-enabled image processing with the images captured by the photosensitive elements in cameras. Most related works focused on spatio-temporal relations among the objects in the scene. Those works involved tracking multi-agents spots, evaluating their appearance, aggregating independent and joint features, segmenting their movements, extracting their actions, and then perceiving their activities. Image-based systems could cover almost every HAR task and achieve very high recognition accuracy because of the complete view of data captured in the scene. The covered tasks include positioning, navigation, body-part monitoring, full-body monitoring, individual activity recognition, group activity recognition, etc. Sathyamoorthy et al. [86] designed a system named COVID-robot for social distancing monitoring in crowded scenarios. With the help of an RGB-D camera and a 2-D Lidar, the mobile robot can avoid collision in a crowd and estimate distance between all detected individuals among the camera view during self-navigating. Lee et al. [87] presented a innovative wearable navigation system based on an RGBD camera to help the visually impaired. A glass-mounted RGBD camera collected the environment information, which is as a input to their navigation algorithm of real-time 6-DOF feature-based visual odometry. Kim et al. [88] proposed a hand gesture control system based on the tactile feedback to the user's hand. Amit et al. [89] proposed an approach to analyze a user's body posture during a workout and compare it to a professional's reference workout, thus getting visual feedback while performing a workout. The system aims to assist people in completing the exercises independently and prevent incorrectly performed motions that may eventually cause severe long-term injuries. Meng et al. [90] addressed the problem of recognizing person–person interaction by depth cameras providing multi-view data. They divided each person–person interaction into body part interactions at first. Then the pairwise features of these body part interactions were used to analyze the person–person interaction. The method was demonstrated in three public datasets. As can be seen, the image-based HAR tasks are profoundly dependent on the neural-network-based algorithms. Most of the researcher's effort in this field is in the advanced algorithm exploration to reach the state of the art.

Undoubtedly, camera-based HAR systems have succeeded in different scenarios, including indoor monitoring and outdoor surveillance. However, the problem is that the approach might not be well accepted due to severe privacy concerns. This is one reason that sensor-based HAR is still prevalent in research communities and has led to many research contributions recently. Another significant disadvantage of an image-based solution is located in the computation load. Since the image-based HAR needs strong hardware support (GPU, CPU, memory, bus) for running the millions of parameters (weights and activations) from the trained deep neural network, the cost of hardware resources, power, and maintenance is enormous. Additionally, since this is an optic sensing solution, the performance is deeply influenced by environmental conditions such as light, temperature, air quality, etc.

3.3. Physiological Sensing

The term "physiological sensing" refers to both the natural physiological signals and the kinematic signals activated from the organism. Physiological variables have been widely used in diagnosis, drug discovery, healthcare monitoring, etc. In human activity recognition, the human body, a compound of biochemistry, has a rich set of electrophysiological and kinematic variables that could be measured on the body to indicate the status and action of the object. Figure 6 summarizes the biological variables used in the task of HAR.

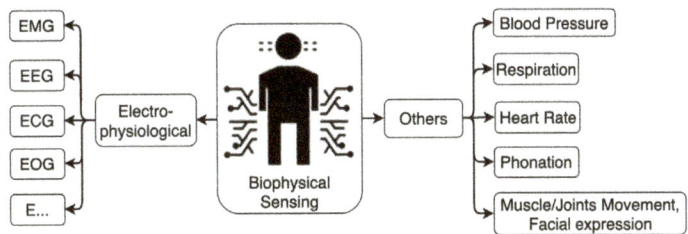

Figure 6. Physiological sensing modalities for HAR.

(A) Electrophysiological Signals

Electrophysiology focuses on the electrical properties of the neurons, molecular and cellular, of living beings. The behavior of neurons is essentially based on the electrical and chemical signals inside the physical body. A series of high-level expressions and actions could be interpreted by monitoring those signals. EMG (electromyography), ECG (electrocardiogram), EEG (electroencephalogram), and EOG (electrooculography) are commonly monitored electrophysiological signals in clinical scenarios. Research works in the last decade showed a significant contribution of electrophysiological signals in human behavior interpretation. For example, electromyography is a diagnostic procedure that monitors the electrical signals of muscles and motor neurons. Pancholi et al. [91] developed a low-cost EMG sensing system to recognize the arm activities such as hand open/close or wrist extension/flexion. Srikanth et al. [92] focused on the recognition of complex construction activities with wearable EMG and IMU sensors in a neural network-based way. Similar work has been explored for hand gesture recognition [93,94], human–computer interaction [95,96], etc. ECG records the electrical signal during the heartbeat. With up to twelve electrodes, ECG signals are commonly used to check different heart conditions. The ECG signal is also a popular explored signal for HAR and commonly combined with other inertial sensors [97,98]. Since the cells in the brain communicate through fast electrical impulses, researchers developed EEG equipment to record the brain's electrical activity by using small metal electrodes attached to the scalp [99]. The signal was also explored in HAR such as eyes open/close [100], emotion recognition [101], etc. EOG is a technique for recording the capitalization on the eyes' cornea–retina potential difference. Typical basic applications of EOG signals are ophthalmological diagnosis and eye movement recording. However, researchers have already explored the potential of EOG signals in HAR [102]. Lu et al. [103] also proposed a dual model to achieve EOG-based human activity recognition with an average recognition accuracy of 88.15% according to three types of activities (i.e., reading, writing, and resting). Besides the above-listed commonly used electrophysiological signals, many other related signals describing various electrical body-related variables could be explored for HAR tasks. Electrophysiological signals need more effort for activity interpretation compared with other sensing approaches because of the complexity of body anatomy and are used mostly as an auxiliary role. However, they have advantages such as ubiquity and the on-body measurement, indicating the potential of wearables in the implementation stage.

(B)   Other physiological signals

An example is from Paolo Palatini's study [104] exploring the relation between sports and blood pressure. One of the conclusions is that both systolic and diastolic blood pressure increase significantly during weight lifting, which is a solid support to the current belief that people with hypertension should not take isometric sports. Besides the blood pressure observation, monitoring kinematic signals such as respiration and heart rate plays a critical role in sleep studies, sports training, patient monitoring, etc. Lu et al. [105] designed a wearable sensor system with the fusion of heart rate, respiration, and motion measurement sensors to enhance the energy expenditure estimation. Their study shows that the fusion design supplies more stable estimation than existing systems. Brouwer et al. [106] improved real-life emotion estimates based on heart rate. Li et al. [107] proposed a sleep and wake classification model with heart rate and respiration signals for long-term sleep studies and reached 88% classification accuracy. Plenty of research work utilized the two sensing modalities in wearable configuration to monitor medicine and health state [108,109]. Phonation is when the vocal folds produce certain sounds through vibration, which has also been explored to help disabled and unhealthy individuals for a better expression or understanding. Lee et al. [110] developed a lip-reading algorithm using optical flow and properties of articulatory phonation for hearing-impaired people, supplying them with continuous feedback on their pronunciation and phonation through lip-reading training, aiming for more effective communication with people without hearing disabilities. Gomez et al. [111] proposed a monitoring approach of Parkinson's disease leveraging biomechanical instability of phonation for the frequent evaluation at a distance. Muscle (either on facial or other body parts) and joint movement monitoring is a more straightforward way for human activity recognition. The movement can be perceived by a series of sensors such as fabric stretch sensors, capacitive sensors, laser doppler vibrometry, etc. Applications based on muscle/joint movement monitoring include hand gesture recognition [112], physical stress [113], gait cycle estimation [114], chronic pain level recognition [115], etc. As electrophysiological sensing, kinematic biological sensing is an on-body approach that the monitoring can be placed near the body, enabling continuous observation and remote feedback, especially for healthcare, diagnosis, and rehabilitation applications.

3.4. Field Sensing

The field is a concept in physics, inferring a region in which each point will be affected by force. For example, electric charges will form an electric field. When another charged particle is placed in the electric field, it will bear an electric force that either repels or attracts it. A magnet will generate a magnetic field surrounding it, and a paper clip in the range of the field will be pulled towards the magnet. Two like magnetic poles will also repel each other when they are close enough to be in the range of either magnetic field. Any object with a quality on Earth will fall to the ground because of its gravity, as it is affected by the force of Earth's gravitational field.

The field strength means the magnitude of a vector-valued field. For example, in the electric field, the strength is represented by the unit of volts per meter (V/m). In the magnetic field, the field is represented by Oersted*Ampere/meter (Oe*A/m). Moreover, when the flux density defines the strength, the Gaus (G) units or Tesla (T) are used. The gravitational field strength is measured in meters per second squared (m/s^2) or Newtons per kilogram (N/kg). All the units used to represent the field strength are vector-valued.

Another approach to know the field strength is to look at the field contour lines. The closer the lines are, the stronger the forces in that part of the field are, and the stronger the field strength is.

Figures 7–9 show an electric field of a parallel plate capacitor, a magnetic field activated by a Helmholtz coil, and the gravitational field of the Earth, respectively. Field-based sensing is based either on the field strength measurement (such as magnetic field strength) or the strength variation caused by characteristics indirectly (such as the potential change of the capacitor, the pressure of object caused by the gravity).

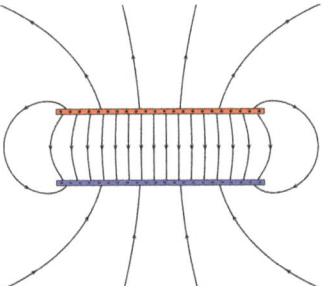

Figure 7. Eletric field (parallel plate capacitor).

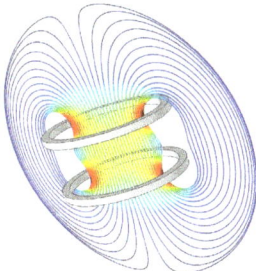

Figure 8. Magnetic field (Helmholtz coils).

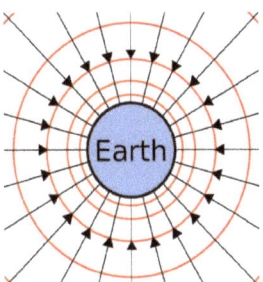

Figure 9. Gravitational field of Earth.

(A) Electric Field

The electric field is ubiquitous in our environment since any potential difference will construct an electric field. Either powered objects (such as appliances, walled power cables, etc.) or non-powered conductive items (such as metal frames near the power cable in a building, the human body, etc.) will activate an electric field to near objects that have a different potential level (especially the ground). The potential difference is essentially a difference in charge distribution. A typical example is that people sometimes feel mildly shocked when touching an appliance, even when the appliance is powered off. This is because there is a possibility of residual charge remaining inside the capacitors of the electronic circuits, which takes a little time to discharge. When the appliance is not appropriately grounded, touching it will cause a mild shock as the charge is transferred to the neutral body.

There are mainly two kinds of electric field-based HAR applications—active or passive—depending on the emitter of the field. An active electric field-based HAR application delivers the field variation as a signal source when the field is emitted from the environment and the human acts as an intruder. A passive one delivers the field variation when considering the electric field emitted from the body itself to the ground since the human body is a perfect conductor and can store the charges. The passive electric field describes a biological signal of the body, the human body capacitance, which will be introduced in the following subsection of the hybrid sensing technique in HAR. Here we firstly focused on the active electric field-based HAR application.

A very representative work is from Zhang et al. [116], where they introduced room-scale interactive and context-aware applications with a system named Wall++, which is a low-cost sensing technique that turns ordinary walls into smart infrastructures. The system can first track users' touch and gestures and estimate body pose when close with the principle of active mutual capacitance sensing, which measures the capacitance between two electrodes (namely the electric field strength between the electrodes). When a body part is near a transmitter–receiver pair, it interferes with the projected electric field, reducing the received current, which can be measured for inferencing. On the other hand, if the user's body touches an electrode, it dramatically increases the capacitance and the received current. Secondly, the system could also work in a passive airborne electromagnetic sensing mode to detect and track the active appliances and users when wearing an electromagnetic emitter. Another typical work is from Cheng et al. [117], where the authors used conductive textile-based electrodes that are easy to be integrated into garments to measure changes in the electric field strength (in capacitance) inside the human body. Since those changes are related to motions and shape changes of muscle, skin, and other tissue, the authors thus abstracted high-level knowledge from the changes and inferenced a broad range of activities and physiological parameters. For example, they embedded the prototype into a collar and performed quantitative evaluations of the recognition accuracy of actions such as chewing, swallowing, speaking, sighing (taking a deep breath), and different head motions and positions. There are other similar works based on active electric field sensing, such as touch detection [118], body tracking based on smart floor [119], respiration, heart rate, stereotyped motor behavior recording [120], hand gesture recognition [121], etc.

Active electric field sensing is non-intrusive, low-cost, has low power consumption, and has excellent potential for pervasive privacy-respecting environmental sensing. However, it is still more complex in hardware construction compared with the passive electric field sensing mode. Furthermore, it can be affected by electromagnetic interference. Thus its reliable operation has a demand in environmental conditions.

(B) Magnetic Field

Magnetic field sensing is an active approach for distance-based motion sensing. There are mainly two magnetic field-based motion-sensing systems depending on whether the magnetic field was generated by the direct current (DC) or alternative (AC) current.

In DC magnetic field motion sensing systems, electromagnets or permanent magnets are often used to generate the magnetic field. A magnetic sensor (magnetometer) senses the magnetic field strength. Since the magnetometer is widely embedded into wearable devices, the DC motion sensing system has been extensively explored for finger/hand tracking to enable a novel machine input approach. Chen et al. [122] designed a system named uTrack, which converts the thumb and fingers into a 3D input system using magnetic field sensing. A permanent magnet was affixed to the back of the thumb, and a pair of magnetometers were worn on the back of the fingers. A continuous data stream was obtained by moving the thumb across the fingers and was used for 3D pointing. The system shows a tracking accuracy of 4.84 mm in 3D space. Similar works [123,124] were conducted using a permanent magnet as the field generator for motion tracking.

In contrast, AC magnetic field sensing is mostly composed of oscillation-based magnetic field transmitters and receivers. The transmitter mostly uses coils to generate an alternating magnetic field. The receiver is also integrated with a coil to sense the strength of the magnetic field at different distances from the transmitter coil. This principle is that the oscillating magnetic flux through the receiver coils will induce an oscillating voltage with the same frequency. The voltage is later used for distance or pose estimation. Oscillating magnetic field has been explored in a variety of HAR tasks, such as indoor location [125], finger tracking [126], human–computer-interaction [127], wearable social distance monitoring [128–130], etc. It could also be implemented for underwater positioning to enable the tracking or navigation of underwater-unmanned vehicles or divers [131].

The advantage of the DC magnetic field motion sensing system is that the magnet used for field generating is easy to access. The sensing unit is at the chip level, thus enjoying the pervasiveness regarding the wide use of smart wearable devices. Moreover, the tracking accuracy can reach up to mm level. The disadvantage of such a system is located in the short sensing range. Since the field attenuates quickly, the detection range is limited to several centimeters. The AC magnetic field sensing's performance in range and accuracy mainly depends on coil design. The detection range could reach up to ten meters with a larger transmitter coil. Ordinary everyday used furniture made of wood and textile will not deform the distribution of the activated field. However, the drawback is that the metallic objects will cause magnetic field distortions. Fortunately, researchers have tried to address this issue by a secondary calibration (either with a look-up table or with neural network-based calibration) step and achieved outstanding results [132].

(C) Gravitational Field

A gravitational field explains gravitational phenomena when a massive body produces a force on another massive body. Earth's gravity is denoted by g, describing the net acceleration imparted to the physical objects caused by the combined effect of gravitation (caused by the mass distribution within Earth) and the centrifugal force (caused by Earth's rotation). On Earth, gravity gives weight to physical objects. The weight is calculated by multiplying the gravitational acceleration by the mass. Gravitational field-based HAR tasks mainly utilize the pressure sensed by pressure sensors caused by the body's weight. Different pressure sensors are presented for HAR tasks, such as the commercially available force-sensitive resistor (FSR), resistive textile, etc. By analyzing the pressure patterns caused by the motion of the body, extensive HAR applications are explored, such as gait analysis [133], workout recognition and user identification [134], indoor location [135], smart furniture [136], rehabilitation [137], etc. The textile-resistive pressure sensor is composed of a matrix of resistive units. By sensing the pressure of each unit from the matrix, the user motion patterns can be delivered. For a small number of resistive units, such as a few FSR units integrated into the insole, a one-dimensional data stream is used for action recognition. For a large number resistive units such as would be found on a mat-like surface, the data stream is usually converted to pressure images as two-dimensional arrays, which can be processed by a neural network-based algorithm used in computer version tasks for more accurate activity recognition.

One of the advantages of a pressure-based sensor is that the sensing component can be customized to any shape and size. Thus it is suitable for a large scale of surface types that needs to be sensed. The sensing precision could also be adjusted by arranging the density of the sensing units. Cheap, commercially available layer-wise films commonly construct the sensing unit. Thus the overall system is affordable to build. However, the cost comes into the system's deployment in a large area (such as floors for location and tracking) since the sensing only occurs during contact, which is a drawback compared with other sensing modalities such as RF-based sensing with no limitation of contact. In summary, gravitational field-based HAR is a non-intrusive and straightforward motion action monitoring and analysis method. It can be extensively deployed for intelligent ambient sensing but is limited by the contact constraints and cost of deployment in a large area.

3.5. Hybrid / Others

(A)   Human Body Capacitance

Human body capacitance (HBC) is essentially a biological variable describing the capacitance between the human body and the environment, mainly the ground. It is also a passive electric field-based sensing approach since the capacitance model comprises two conductive plates that store charges (corresponding to body and environment in the human electric field model) and a dielectric medium (corresponding to the air between body and ground). Figure 10 depicts the human body capacitance in a living room, where multiple electric fields exist, for example, the field between the appliance and the ground, between the metal frames of the window/door to the ground, as well as the human body capacitance between the body and the environment. person–person is a ubiquitous biological parameter that could be explored for a wide range of human-centric motion-related applications based on its sensitivity to both the body's motion and the variation of the environment.

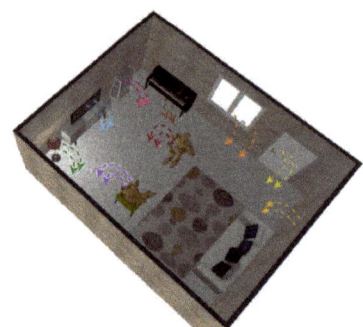

Figure 10. Human body capacitance: the static electric field between the body and the environment.

Unlike other biological features, such as ECG, EMG, etc., HBC is a feature that interacts with surroundings, especially the ground. Being insulated by the wearing, the body and the surroundings form a natural capacitor. HBC is used to describe the charges stored in the body. A series of studies [138–141] indicate a value of 100–400 pF of the body capacitance. The value varies with respect to skin state [142,143], garment [144], body postures [145], etc. Researchers have explored applications such as communication [146], cooperation perceiving [147], motion monitoring [117,148,149], etc., based on the concept, which has continued attracting the attention of researchers recently. Since HBC is a passive signal, the sensing units were mostly designed in a small form factor with small power consumption [149,150]. Wilmsdorff et al. [151] explored this passive capacitive sensing technique with a wide range of applications indoors and outdoors. In [152], the authors presented an HBC-based capacitive sensor for full-body gym exercise recognition and counting; by sensing the local potential variation of the body, different kinds of body actions could be classified. Besides motion sensing, HBC could also be used for proximity and joint activity recognition [147] by exploring the human body capacitance variation caused by the proximity and motion of an intruder.

As a passive motion-sensing approach, the systems based on human body capacitance enjoy the advantage of low cost, low power consumption, portability, and full-body sensing ability. However, although the sensitivity in motion and environmental variation forms the potential ability of this variable, at the same time they also limit the development of it, since any action, either from the body or from the environment, will induce an efficient signal, and there is difficulty in recognizing the source of the signal.

(B) Infrared

Infrared is electromagnetic radiation with wavelengths longer than visible light. The heat energy from the objects with a temperature above absolute zero is emitted as electromagnetic radiation, which is caused by the constant motion of molecules embodying heat. The electrons jump to higher energy band when they absorb energy by colliding with another. They can also release energy in the form of photons when falling to a lower energy band again. A hot molecule moves fast and generates higher frequencies (shorter wavelengths) of electromagnetic waves. Usually, the human eye cannot sense this radiation with infrared wavelengths, which can be measured by specific electronic sensors. Sensing the human body's infrared could deliver information such as body temperature, motion trajectory, etc. Two kinds of sensors are commonly utilized for this purpose: the passive infrared sensor (PIR) and the thermographic camera.

The electronic sensor PIR is designed to measure infrared (IR) light from objects. The term passive indicates that this sensor does not emit energy during the detection process. Instead, it detects the energy of infrared radiation from objects. It is widely used from motion detection to automatic lighting applications. In the field of HAR, PIR has been widely explored in the application of indoor positioning [153,154], device-free activity recognition [155,156], etc. The sensor is widely available in the market with low cost and low power consumption. The built system is privacy-secure and easy to deploy and maintain. However, a PIR sensor only detects general movement. It does not give information on who or what moved. For that purpose, a thermographic camera for imaging IR is required.

A thermographic camera generates an image by infrared radiation, which is different from a common camera sensing visible light. The objects with a temperature above absolute zero can be detected by the thermographic camera, and an object with higher temperature emits more radiation. Thus from the thermography, the temperature variations are also visible. For example, humans and other warm-blooded animals stand out very well against the environment, regardless of whether it is day or night. Thermography has been widely used in medical diagnosis, in the military, etc. In HAR applications, it has also been developed with image-processing algorithms for activity detection in residential spaces [157,158], muscle activity evaluation [159], respiration monitoring [160,161], etc. For detection in dark lighting conditions, namely in the work performed by Uddin et al. [162], the authors used the OpenPose framework for thermal images to check the possibility of body skeleton extraction. Their result shows that the thermal images can monitor humans in dark environments where the other typical RGB cameras fail. Although thermographic sensing could supply more detailed information on body action than the PIR approach, it suffers lightly from the cost and the computing load.

3.6. Summary

Depending on the targeted application, researchers have explored different sensing modalities to accomplish their tasks in HAR. Table 2 summarized the mainstream of the sensing modalities and compared them with aspects of cost, power consumption level, working type (active or passive), privacy concern, computing load, typical applications, and their critical advantages and shortcomings. We also supplied some of the publicly available datasets of each sensing modality for HAR tasks in the table, so that readers can check and have a better understanding of the data properties of each sensing technique, or try their own mining approach on the dataset. The cost and power consumption express the practicability of a sensing modality, such as the IMU as a low-cost and low-power-consumption approach, which is the most widely explored aspect of HAR tasks. The compute load and robustness, ranging from high to low, were ranked with specific references. Computations that require large memory (over hundreds of megabytes) and complex instruction (such as multiplication of float point data) are regarded as having a high compute load. A low compute load needs simply a few instructions for one inference on weak devices such as the micro-controller. High robustness indicates that the signal could hardly be interfered with by surroundings, such as the gravitational field. Bluetooth signal strength, as an example, could be easily affected by a variation in the nearby environment. The typical application lists the activities coarsely at a high level, such as the activity of daily living (ADL), which includes all fundamental actions of a human in everyday life, such as sleeping, eating, dressing, etc. The positioning includes the location of the whole body and the body part such as the hand and finger. Gesture Recognition implies gestures performed by hand, finger, arm, etc. Active/passive sensors indicate the complexity of the sensing modality because of the existence of the signal sources. A privacy-respect sensor does not abstract identity-sensitive messages from users, thus being more acceptable. The computing load and robustness show the sensor's working performance and are categorized into three levels: "low", "medium", and "high". Depending on the usage scenarios, each sensing modality could be deployed targeting different tasks among "where", "what", and "how". A passive electric field, as an example, can be used for both positioning and action sensing.

IMU sensor and optic approaches (mainly video-based) are the two most popular sensing modalities in the community, since the IMU sensor is pervasively deployed in smart devices and outperforms in power consumption, cost, size, and the visual modality can supply high accuracy for activity recognition benefiting from the advanced deep neural network models for feature abstraction. They both are utilized to target a much wider range of human activity recognition tasks than other sensors. However, there are still certain limitations, such as that they both suffer from computational load. Especially for the vision-based approach, which deals with 2D or 3D high resolution and high frame data stream with hundreds of thousands of conventional operations challenging the hardware resources, the computational load is high compared with other sensing modalities. Since the images from a video capture massive identity messages, the privacy issues need to be considered. The IMU sensors face accumulated errors, which results in the configuration demand for each new start for positioning applications with the demand of high accuracy.

Wave-based sensing modalities (RF waves and acoustic waves) are active approaches demanding signal sources from the sensing system and are mainly used for ambient intelligence. The corresponding systems are generally weak in robustness since the wave signal could be affected by the multipath effect (except for the UWB) and environmental noises. However, they are particularly efficient in privacy-respect scenarios since no other information beyond the wave property is collected. The cost and power consumption of such systems are much higher than the IMU-based solution, but still lower than the visual approach.

The electrophysiological signals (ExG) are perceived mostly by devices with high-resolution analog-to-digital chips for healthy monitoring such as mental state, stress level, sports quality evaluation, etc. The cost of such a system is relatively high compared with IMU and most field-based approaches. Since the signal sensing units are mainly at the chip-level design, the power consumption is an obvious advantage of those approaches. Depending on the channel numbers, the computational load of electrophysiological signals is distinct. The ECG signal, as an example, a simple rule-based approach that needs only a few computer instructions, can be used to detect the critical features from it efficiently. The EEG signal, on the other hand, requires a more complex algorithm to abstract the features from multiple channels to uncover the messages behind it.

Pressure sensing is versatile since the sensing unit (mainly composed of conductive layers) is highly customizable. Since the weight signal perceived from such a sensing system is quite straightforward, the detection accuracy of a certain human actions is high. However, maintaining such systems is costly because of the deployment complexity and the limited lifetime caused by the long-term stressful contact.

Table 2. Sensing techniques in HAR tasks.

Modality	Cost (USD)	Power Level	Active/ Passive	Privacy	Compute Load	Robustness	Target	Typical Application	Comment	Accessible Dataset
WiFi	tens	≈tens Watt	active	no	medium	low	where, what	positioning, ADL, ambient intelligence	pervasiveness, environmental sensitivity	[163,164]
UWB	tens	≈mW	active	no	low	low	where, what	positioning, proximity, ADL, gesture recognition, ambient intelligence	multi-path resistive, high accuracy, costly for massive consumer usage	[165–167]
mmWave	tens	≈W	active	no	medium	low	where, what, how	positioning, proximity, ADL, gesture recognition, health monitoring, ambient intelligence	high accuracy, low power efficiency for massive consumer usage	[168,169]
Ultrasonic	hundreds	≈mW to W	active	no	low	low	where, what	positioning, proximity, ambient intelligence	high accuracy, weak robustness	-
Optic	tens of hundreds	≈W and above	passive	yes	high	medium	where, what, how	positioning, proximity, ADL, gait analysis, gesture recognition, surveillance	comprehensive approach, high resource consumption	[170–172]
ExG	hundreds	≈tens mW	passive	no	medium	high	how, what	sports, healthcare monitoring, ADL	high resolution, noise sensitive	[173]
IMU	a few	≈mW	passive	no	high	medium	where, what	positioning, ADL, gesture recognition, healthcare monitoring, gait analysis, sports	dominant sensing modality, accumulated bias	[174,175]
Magnetic Field(AC)	tens	≈hundreds mW	active	no	low	high	where, what	positioning, proximity,	high robustness, limited detection range	-
Magnetic Field(DC)	a few	≈mW	passive	no	low	high	what	proximity, gesture recognition	high accuracy, short detection range	[176]
Electric Field(active)	tens	≈mW	active	no	low	low	where, what	positioning, proximity, ambient intelligence	high sensitivity, noise sensitive	-
Electric Field(Passive)	a few	≈sub-mW	passive	no	low	low	where, what	positioning, proximity, sports, gait analysis, ambient intelligence	high sensitivity, noise sensitive	[177]
Gravitational Field	tens of hundreds	area dependent	passive	no	depends	high	where, what	positioning, sports, gait analysis, ambient intelligence	versatility/customizability, costly maintenance	[178,179]

A magnetic field is a robust distance-based approach that can deliver reliable distance information with a lower computational load. The approach is low-cost and wearable (after minimizing), without limitation of multipath and line-of-sight. More importantly, it can be used for positioning in the underwater environment, which blocks most of the positioning techniques because of the quick attenuation of the adopted medium (such as RF-signal) in water. However, the detection range is limited by a few meters with the active magnetic field and a few decimeters with the passive magnetic field.

The electric field has recently become a novel sensing approach for HAR tasks, distinguished by its ability in full-body motion sensing and environmental electric sensing. It also enjoys the advantages of low power consumption and wearability. Since electrons exist anywhere in the environment where people live, including the human body, the body's motion will deform the distribution of the electric field. Therefore, human activity could be deduced by perceiving the electric field variation, either on the environmental side or on the body side. However, the environmental noise is a big challenge for electric field-based sensing and is hard to overcome because of the pervasiveness of the surrounding objects acting as noise sources.

4. Outlooks

HAR relates to a wide range of tasks that deal with daily life with digitalization, aiming to assist people to have a better quality of life. As the keystone, sensing skills for HAR tasks are still under intensive development. Based on the surveyed most prominent sensing techniques in this manuscript, we further conclude some outlooks on the development of sensing skills for HAR tasks.

- **Sensor fusion**: The sensor fusion method has great potential to improve sensing robustness by fusing different sensor data. Each sensor modality has inherent strengths and weaknesses. By merging data from various sensor modalities, a robust data model can be generated. For example, the long-term positioning tasks with a high-rate IMU sensor will be disturbed by the integration errors, which could be addressed by a lower rate sensor that provides absolute anchor points (such as visual features). Some classic and efficient algorithms could be designed for sensor fusing, such as Kalman Filter [180]. As another example, the electric field sensors can perceive the straightforward proximity information of an individual. Meanwhile, they are sensitive to environmental variation, resulting in multi-source issues. By deploying motion sensors such as IMU on both individuals and the environment, the electric field signal source could be recognized. Such fusion approaches could not only address the weakness of a particular sensing modality but also provide a more holistic appreciation of the system being monitored.

- **Smart sensors**: Driven by the pervasive practical user scenarios and power-efficient data processing techniques, as well as the chip manufacturing technology, there is an apparent trend that sensors are becoming smarter with the ability to process the signal data locally. Compared to conventional sensor systems, smart sensors take advantage of emerging machine learning algorithms and modern computer hardware to create sophisticated, intelligent systems tailored to specific sensing applications. In recent years, many smart sensors have been proposed for HAR tasks such as the pedometer integrated IMUs (BMI270), gesture recognition integrated sensors (PAJ7620), etc. All the recognition, classification, and decision processes are executed on the smart sensor system locally instead of uploading the raw data to the cloud for inferencing. Thus, the user's privacy is well protected, and the computing load of the central processing unit is significantly reduced.

- **Novel sensors**: With the development of materials and fabrication technology, novel sensing techniques and devices emerge to provide a broader perceiving ability towards the body and environment where people live. Novel sensors for HAR offer an alternative or complementary approach to existing solutions. More importantly, they supply a new method for body or environment knowledge collection that the current sensing technique cannot supply. An example is a microelectrode-based biosensor, which has been proposed for long-term monitoring of sweat glucose levels [181]. The multi-function microelectrode-based biosensor is fabricated on a flexible substrate, which offers greater wearing comfort than rigid sensors, thus providing long-term on-skin healthy monitoring.

Besides that, sensors are becoming more compact and power-efficient to provide always-on monitoring, or the sensors will be only in an active state triggered by a specific event. The energy harvesting techniques also provide ambient energy for sensors to extend the power life. With the growing number of wearable devices, the health monitoring sensors [182] are being deployed more near the body for continuous and real-time analysis of sweat, blood, etc., such as EEG monitoring by smart watches, or stress sensing by the Fitbit smart band, which uses an electrodermal activity skin response sensor to obtain a reading when the palm of user's hand is pressing the metal outer rim, and then the corresponding app will analyze the overall stress.

5. Conclusions

This work focused on the mainstream sensing techniques for HAR tasks, aiming to supply a concrete understanding of the variant sensing principles for younger community researchers. We categorized the human activities into three classes: where, what, and how, for body position-related, body action-related, and body status-related services. This task-oriented categorization aims to supply a basic concept of the objectives of human activity recognition. We also categorized the HAR-related sensing modalities into five classes: mechanical kinematic sensing, field-based sensing, wave-based sensing, physiological sensing, and hybrid/others, based on the properties of the sensing medium, aiming to give a better understanding of the sensing technique's physical background. Specific sensing modalities were presented in each category with state-of-the-art publications and a discussion of the modality's advantages and limitations. A summary and an outlook of the sensing techniques were also discussed. We hope this survey can help newcomers have a better overview of the characteristics of each sensing modality for HAR tasks and choose the proper approaches for their specific applications.

Author Contributions: Manuscript writing: S.B., M.L.; project administration: P.L. Formal analysis: B.Z. All authors have read and agreed to the published version of the manuscript.

Funding: This work was supported by the European Union project HUMANE-AI-NET (H2020-ICT-2019-3 #952026).

Institutional Review Board Statement: Not applicable.

Informed Consent Statement: Not applicable.

Data Availability Statement: Not applicable.

Conflicts of Interest: The authors declare no conflict of interest.

Abbreviations

The following abbreviations are used in this manuscript:

ToF	Time of Flight
RSS	Received Signal Strength
LiDAR	Light and Radar
UWB	Ultra-wideband
RF	Radio Frequency
ID	Identification
MAE	Mean Absolute Error
IMU	Inertial Measurement Unit
PWM	Pulse-Width Modulation
AUV	Autonomous Underwater Vehicles
SLAM	Simultaneous Localization and Mapping

References

1. Sigg, S.; Shi, S.; Buesching, F.; Ji, Y.; Wolf, L. Leveraging RF-channel fluctuation for activity recognition: Active and passive systems, continuous and RSSI-based signal features. In Proceedings of the International Conference on Advances in Mobile Computing & Multimedia, Vienna, Austria, 2–4 December 2013; pp. 43–52.
2. Ramos, R.G.; Domingo, J.D.; Zalama, E.; Gómez-García-Bermejo, J. Daily Human Activity Recognition Using Non-Intrusive Sensors. *Sensors* **2021**, *21*, 5270. [CrossRef] [PubMed]
3. Samadi, M.R.H.; Cooke, N. EEG signal processing for eye tracking. In Proceedings of the 2014 22nd European Signal Processing Conference (EUSIPCO), Lisbon, Portugal, 1–5 September 2014; pp. 2030–2034.
4. Hussain, Z.; Sheng, Q.Z.; Zhang, W.E. A review and categorization of techniques on device-free human activity recognition. *J. Netw. Comput. Appl.* **2020**, *167*, 102738. [CrossRef]
5. Yuan, G.; Wang, Z.; Meng, F.; Yan, Q.; Xia, S. An overview of human activity recognition based on smartphone. *Sens. Rev.* **2019**, *39*, 288–306. [CrossRef]
6. Li, Y.; Wang, S.; Jin, C.; Zhang, Y.; Jiang, T. A survey of underwater magnetic induction communications: Fundamental issues, recent advances, and challenges. *IEEE Commun. Surv. Tutor.* **2019**, *21*, 2466–2487. [CrossRef]
7. Dang, L.M.; Min, K.; Wang, H.; Piran, M.J.; Lee, C.H.; Moon, H. Sensor-based and vision-based human activity recognition: A comprehensive survey. *Pattern Recognit.* **2020**, *108*, 107561. [CrossRef]
8. Fu, B.; Damer, N.; Kirchbuchner, F.; Kuijper, A. Sensing technology for human activity recognition: A comprehensive survey. *IEEE Access* **2020**, *8*, 83791–83820. [CrossRef]
9. Raval, R.M.; Prajapati, H.B.; Dabhi, V.K. Survey and analysis of human activity recognition in surveillance videos. *Intell. Decis. Technol.* **2019**, *13*, 271–294. [CrossRef]
10. Mohamed, R.; Perumal, T.; Sulaiman, M.N.; Mustapha, N. Multi resident complex activity recognition in smart home: A literature review. *Int. J. Smart Home* **2017**, *11*, 21–32. [CrossRef]
11. Bux, A.; Angelov, P.; Habib, Z. Vision based human activity recognition: A review. *Adv. Comput. Intell. Syst.* **2017**, 341–371.
12. Ma, J.; Wang, H.; Zhang, D.; Wang, Y.; Wang, Y. A survey on wi-fi based contactless activity recognition. In Proceedings of the International Conference on Ubiquitous Intelligence & Computing, Advanced and Trusted Computing, Scalable Computing and Communications, Cloud and Big Data Computing, Internet of People, and Smart World Congress (UIC/ATC/ScalCom/CBDCom/IoP/SmartWorld), Toulouse, France, 18–21 July 2016; pp. 1086–1091.
13. Lioulemes, A.; Papakostas, M.; Gieser, S.N.; Toutountzi, T.; Abujelala, M.; Gupta, S.; Collander, C.; Mcmurrough, C.D.; Makedon, F. A survey of sensing modalities for human activity, behavior, and physiological monitoring. In Proceedings of the PETRA '16: 9th ACM International Conference on PErvasive Technologies Related to Assistive Environments, Corfu Island, Greece, 29 June 2016–1 July 2016; pp. 1–8.
14. Vrigkas, M.; Nikou, C.; Kakadiaris, I.A. A review of human activity recognition methods. *Front. Robot. AI* **2015**, *2*, 28. [CrossRef]
15. Mukhopadhyay, S.C. Wearable sensors for human activity monitoring: A review. *IEEE Sens. J.* **2014**, *15*, 1321–1330. [CrossRef]
16. Jalal, A.; Sarif, N.; Kim, J.T.; Kim, T.S. Human activity recognition via recognized body parts of human depth silhouettes for residents monitoring services at smart home. *Indoor Built Environ.* **2013**, *22*, 271–279. [CrossRef]
17. Javed, A.R.; Faheem, R.; Asim, M.; Baker, T.; Beg, M.O. A smartphone sensors-based personalized human activity recognition system for sustainable smart cities. *Sustain. Cities Soc.* **2021**, *71*, 102970. [CrossRef]
18. Li, R.; Chellappa, R.; Zhou, S.K. Learning multi-modal densities on discriminative temporal interaction manifold for group activity recognition. In Proceedings of the 2009 IEEE Conference on Computer Vision and Pattern Recognition, Miami, FL, USA, 20–25 June 2009; pp. 2450–2457.
19. Cho, N.G.; Kim, Y.J.; Park, U.; Park, J.S.; Lee, S.W. Group activity recognition with group interaction zone based on relative distance between human objects. *Int. J. Pattern Recognit. Artif. Intell.* **2015**, *29*, 1555007. [CrossRef]
20. Brena, R.F.; García-Vázquez, J.P.; Galván-Tejada, C.E.; Muñoz-Rodriguez, D.; Vargas-Rosales, C.; Fangmeyer, J. Evolution of indoor positioning technologies: A survey. *J. Sens.* **2017**, *2017*, 2630413 . [CrossRef]
21. Fuchs, C.; Aschenbruck, N.; Martini, P.; Wieneke, M. Indoor tracking for mission critical scenarios: A survey. *Pervasive Mob. Comput.* **2011**, *7*, 1–15. [CrossRef]
22. Navarro, S.E.; Mühlbacher-Karrer, S.; Alagi, H.; Zangl, H.; Koyama, K.; Hein, B.; Duriez, C.; Smith, J.R. Proximity perception in human-centered robotics: A survey on sensing systems and applications. *IEEE Trans. Robot.* **2021**, *38*, 1599–1620. [CrossRef]
23. Mubashir, M.; Shao, L.; Seed, L. A survey on fall detection: Principles and approaches. *Neurocomputing* **2013**, *100*, 144–152. [CrossRef]
24. Akhtaruzzaman, M.; Shafie, A.A.; Khan, M.R. Gait analysis: Systems, technologies, and importance. *J. Mech. Med. Biol.* **2016**, *16*, 1630003. [CrossRef]
25. Verbunt, J.A.; Huijnen, I.P.; Köke, A. Assessment of physical activity in daily life in patients with musculoskeletal pain. *Eur. J. Pain* **2009**, *13*, 231–242. [CrossRef] [PubMed]
26. Wang, Z.; Ho, S.B.; Cambria, E. A review of emotion sensing: Categorization models and algorithms. *Multimed. Tools Appl.* **2020**, *79*, 35553–35582. [CrossRef]
27. Arakawa, T. A Review of Heartbeat Detection Systems for Automotive Applications. *Sensors* **2021**, *21*, 6112. [CrossRef] [PubMed]

28. Alemdar, H.; Ersoy, C. Wireless sensor networks for healthcare: A survey. *Comput. Netw.* **2010**, *54*, 2688–2710. [CrossRef]

29. Oguntala, G.A.; Abd-Alhameed, R.A.; Ali, N.T.; Hu, Y.F.; Noras, J.M.; Eya, N.N.; Elfergani, I.; Rodriguez, J. SmartWall: Novel RFID-enabled ambient human activity recognition using machine learning for unobtrusive health monitoring. *IEEE Access* **2019**, *7*, 68022–68033. [CrossRef]

30. Gaglio, S.; Re, G.L.; Morana, M. Human activity recognition process using 3-D posture data. *IEEE Trans. Hum.-Mach. Syst.* **2014**, *45*, 586–597. [CrossRef]

31. Jiang, S.; Gao, Q.; Liu, H.; Shull, P.B. A novel, co-located EMG-FMG-sensing wearable armband for hand gesture recognition. *Sens. Actuators A Phys.* **2020**, *301*, 111738. [CrossRef]

32. Elniema Abdrahman Abdalla, H. Hand Gesture Recognition Based on Time-of-Flight Sensors. Ph.D Thesis, Politecnico di Torino, Turlin, Italy, 2021.

33. Nahler, C.; Plank, H.; Steger, C.; Druml, N. Resource-Constrained Human Presence Detection for Indirect Time-of-Flight Sensors. In Proceedings of the 2021 Digital Image Computing: Techniques and Applications (DICTA), Gold Coast, Australia, 29 November–1 December 2021; pp. 1–5.

34. Hossen, M.A.; Zahir, E.; Ata-E-Rabbi, H.; Azam, M.A.; Rahman, M.H. Developing a Mobile Automated Medical Assistant for Hospitals in Bangladesh. In Proceedings of the 2021 IEEE World AI IoT Congress (AIIoT), Seattle, WA, USA, 10–13 May 2021; pp. 366–372.

35. Lin, J.T.; Newquist, C.; Harnett, C. Multitouch Pressure Sensing with Soft Optical Time-of-Flight Sensors. *IEEE Trans. Instrum. Meas.* **2022**, *71*, 7000708. [CrossRef]

36. Bortolan, G.; Christov, I.; Simova, I. Potential of Rule-Based Methods and Deep Learning Architectures for ECG Diagnostics. *Diagnostics* **2021**, *11*, 1678. [CrossRef] [PubMed]

37. Ismail, M.I.M.; Dzyauddin, R.A.; Samsul, S.; Azmi, N.A.; Yamada, Y.; Yakub, M.F.M.; Salleh, N.A.B.A. An RSSI-based Wireless Sensor Node Localisation using Trilateration and Multilateration Methods for Outdoor Environment. *arXiv* **2019**, arXiv:1912.07801.

38. Chen, K.; Zhang, D.; Yao, L.; Guo, B.; Yu, Z.; Liu, Y. Deep learning for sensor-based human activity recognition: Overview, challenges, and opportunities. *ACM Comput. Surv. (CSUR)* **2021**, *54*, 1–40. [CrossRef]

39. Aggarwal, J.K.; Cai, Q. Human motion analysis: A review. *Comput. Vis. Image Underst.* **1999**, *73*, 428–440. [CrossRef]

40. Kellokumpu, V.; Pietikäinen, M.; Heikkilä, J. Human activity recognition using sequences of postures. In Proceedings of the MVA, Tsukuba, Japan, 16–18 May 2005; pp. 570–573.

41. Münzner, S.; Schmidt, P.; Reiss, A.; Hanselmann, M.; Stiefelhagen, R.; Dürichen, R. CNN-based sensor fusion techniques for multimodal human activity recognition. In Proceedings of the 2017 ACM International Symposium on Wearable Computers, Maui, HI, USA, 11–15 September 2017; pp. 158–165.

42. Yang, X.; Cao, R.; Zhou, M.; Xie, L. Temporal-frequency attention-based human activity recognition using commercial WiFi devices. *IEEE Access* **2020**, *8*, 137758–137769. [CrossRef]

43. Köping, L.; Shirahama, K.; Grzegorzek, M. A general framework for sensor-based human activity recognition. *Comput. Biol. Med.* **2018**, *95*, 248–260. [CrossRef] [PubMed]

44. Bustoni, I.A.; Hidayatulloh, I.; Ningtyas, A.; Purwaningsih, A.; Azhari, S. Classification methods performance on human activity recognition. *J. Phys. Conf. Ser.* **2020**, *1456*, 012027. [CrossRef]

45. Gjoreski, H.; Kiprijanovska, I.; Stankoski, S.; Kalabakov, S.; Broulidakis, J.; Nduka, C.; Gjoreski, M. Head-AR: Human Activity Recognition with Head-Mounted IMU Using Weighted Ensemble Learning. In *Activity and Behavior Computing*; Springer: Singapore, 2021; pp. 153–167.

46. Röddiger, T.; Wolffram, D.; Laubenstein, D.; Budde, M.; Beigl, M. Towards respiration rate monitoring using an in-ear headphone inertial measurement unit. In Proceedings of the 1st International Workshop on Earable Computing, London, UK, 9 September 2019; pp. 48–53.

47. Kim, M.; Cho, J.; Lee, S.; Jung, Y. IMU sensor-based hand gesture recognition for human-machine interfaces. *Sensors* **2019**, *19*, 3827. [CrossRef] [PubMed]

48. Georgi, M.; Amma, C.; Schultz, T. Recognizing Hand and Finger Gestures with IMU based Motion and EMG based Muscle Activity Sensing. In *Biosignals*; Citeseer: Princeton, NJ, USA, 2015; pp. 99–108.

49. Mummadi, C.K.; Leo, F.P.P.; Verma, K.D.; Kasireddy, S.; Scholl, P.M.; Kempfle, J.; Laerhoven, K.V. Real-time and embedded detection of hand gestures with an IMU-based glove. *Informatics* **2018**, *5*, 28. [CrossRef]

50. Kang, S.W.; Choi, H.; Park, H.I.; Choi, B.G.; Im, H.; Shin, D.; Jung, Y.G.; Lee, J.Y.; Park, H.W.; Park, S.; et al. The development of an IMU integrated clothes for postural monitoring using conductive yarn and interconnecting technology. *Sensors* **2017**, *17*, 2560. [CrossRef] [PubMed]

51. Zhang, Q. Evaluation of a Wearable System for Motion Analysis during Different Exercises. Master's Thesis. ING School of Industrial and Information Engineering, Milano, Italy, 2019. Available online: https://www.politesi.polimi.it/handle/10589/149029 (accessed on 30 April 2022).

52. Wang, Q.; Timmermans, A.; Chen, W.; Jia, J.; Ding, L.; Xiong, L.; Rong, J.; Markopoulos, P. Stroke patients' acceptance of a smart garment for supporting upper extremity rehabilitation. *IEEE J. Transl. Eng. Health Med.* **2018**, *6*, 1–9. [CrossRef] [PubMed]

53. Kim, H.; Kang, Y.; Valencia, D.R.; Kim, D. An Integrated System for Gait Analysis Using FSRs and an IMU. In Proceedings of the 2018 Second IEEE International Conference on Robotic Computing (IRC), Laguna Hills, CA, USA, 31 January–2 February 2018; pp. 347–351.

54. Abdulrahim, K.; Hide, C.; Moore, T.; Hill, C. Aiding MEMS IMU with building heading for indoor pedestrian navigation. In Proceedings of the 2010 Ubiquitous Positioning Indoor Navigation and Location Based Service, Kirkkonummi, Finland, 14–15 October 2010; pp. 1–6.
55. Wahjudi, F.; Lin, F.J. IMU-Based Walking Workouts Recognition. In Proceedings of the 2019 IEEE 5th World Forum on Internet of Things (WF-IoT), Limerick, Ireland, 15–18 April 2019; pp. 251–256.
56. Nagano, H.; Begg, R.K. Shoe-insole technology for injury prevention in walking. *Sensors* **2018**, *18*, 1468. [CrossRef] [PubMed]
57. Cesareo, A.; Previtali, Y.; Biffi, E.; Aliverti, A. Assessment of breathing parameters using an inertial measurement unit (IMU)-based system. *Sensors* **2019**, *19*, 88. [CrossRef]
58. Huang, Y.; Kaufmann, M.; Aksan, E.; Black, M.J.; Hilliges, O.; Pons-Moll, G. Deep inertial poser: Learning to reconstruct human pose from sparse inertial measurements in real time. *ACM Trans. Graph. (TOG)* **2018**, *37*, 1–15. [CrossRef]
59. Younas, J.; Margarito, H.; Bian, S.; Lukowicz, P. Finger Air Writing-Movement Reconstruction with Low-cost IMU Sensor. In Proceedings of the MobiQuitous 2020—17th EAI International Conference on Mobile and Ubiquitous Systems: Computing, Networking and Services, Online, 7–9 December 2020; pp. 69–75.
60. Li, H.; He, X.; Chen, X.; Fang, Y.; Fang, Q. Wi-motion: A robust human activity recognition using WiFi signals. *IEEE Access* **2019**, *7*, 153287–153299. [CrossRef]
61. Liu, X.; Cao, J.; Tang, S.; Wen, J. Wi-sleep: Contactless sleep monitoring via wifi signals. In Proceedings of the 2014 IEEE Real-Time Systems Symposium, Rome, Italy, 2–5 December 2014; pp. 346–355.
62. Wang, F.; Feng, J.; Zhao, Y.; Zhang, X.; Zhang, S.; Han, J. Joint activity recognition and indoor localization with WiFi fingerprints. *IEEE Access* **2019**, *7*, 80058–80068. [CrossRef]
63. Bahle, G.; Fortes Rey, V.; Bian, S.; Bello, H.; Lukowicz, P. Using privacy respecting sound analysis to improve bluetooth based proximity detection for COVID-19 exposure tracing and social distancing. *Sensors* **2021**, *21*, 5604. [CrossRef]
64. Hossain, A.M.; Soh, W.S. A comprehensive study of bluetooth signal parameters for localization. In Proceedings of the 2007 IEEE 18th International Symposium on Personal, Indoor and Mobile Radio Communications, Athens, Greece, 3–7 September 2007; pp. 1–5.
65. Zhang, R.; Cao, S. Real-time human motion behavior detection via CNN using mmWave radar. *IEEE Sens. Lett.* **2018**, *3*, 1–4. [CrossRef]
66. Zhao, P.; Lu, C.X.; Wang, B.; Chen, C.; Xie, L.; Wang, M.; Trigoni, N.; Markham, A. Heart rate sensing with a robot mounted mmwave radar. In Proceedings of the 2020 IEEE International Conference on Robotics and Automation (ICRA), Paris, France, 31 May–31 August 2020; pp. 2812–2818.
67. Sun, Y.; Hang, R.; Li, Z.; Jin, M.; Xu, K. Privacy-Preserving Fall Detection with Deep Learning on mmWave Radar Signal. In Proceedings of the 2019 IEEE Visual Communications and Image Processing (VCIP), Sydney, Australia, 1–4 December 2019; pp. 1–4.
68. Li, Z.; Lei, Z.; Yan, A.; Solovey, E.; Pahlavan, K. ThuMouse: A micro-gesture cursor input through mmWave radar-based interaction. In Proceedings of the 2020 IEEE International Conference on Consumer Electronics (ICCE), Las Vegas, NV, USA, 4–6 January 2020; pp. 1–9.
69. Cheng, Y.; Zhou, T. UWB indoor positioning algorithm based on TDOA technology. In Proceedings of the 2019 10th International Conference on Information Technology in Medicine and Education (ITME), Qingdao, China, 23–25 August 2019; pp. 777–782.
70. Lee, S.; Kim, J.; Moon, N. Random forest and WiFi fingerprint-based indoor location recognition system using smart watch. *Hum.-Centric Comput. Inf. Sci.* **2019**, *9*, 1–14. [CrossRef]
71. Porcino, D.; Hirt, W. Ultra-wideband radio technology: Potential and challenges ahead. *IEEE Commun. Mag.* **2003**, *41*, 66–74. [CrossRef]
72. Bouchard, K.; Maitre, J.; Bertuglia, C.; Gaboury, S. Activity recognition in smart homes using UWB radars. *Procedia Comput. Sci.* **2020**, *170*, 10–17. [CrossRef]
73. Ren, N.; Quan, X.; Cho, S.H. Algorithm for gesture recognition using an IR-UWB radar sensor. *J. Comput. Commun.* **2016**, *4*, 95–100. [CrossRef]
74. Piriyajitakonkij, M.; Warin, P.; Lakhan, P.; Leelaarporn, P.; Kumchaiseemak, N.; Suwajanakorn, S.; Pianpanit, T.; Niparnan, N.; Mukhopadhyay, S.C.; Wilaiprasitporn, T. SleepPoseNet: Multi-view learning for sleep postural transition recognition using UWB. *IEEE J. Biomed. Health Inform.* **2020**, *25*, 1305–1314. [CrossRef]
75. Bharadwaj, R.; Parini, C.; Koul, S.K.; Alomainy, A. Effect of Limb Movements on Compact UWB Wearable Antenna Radiation Performance for Healthcare Monitoring. *Prog. Electromagn. Res.* **2019**, *91*, 15–26. [CrossRef]
76. Qi, J.; Liu, G.P. A robust high-accuracy ultrasound indoor positioning system based on a wireless sensor network. *Sensors* **2017**, *17*, 2554. [CrossRef] [PubMed]
77. Hoeflinger, F.; Saphala, A.; Schott, D.J.; Reindl, L.M.; Schindelhauer, C. Passive indoor-localization using echoes of ultrasound signals. In Proceedings of the 2019 International Conference on Advanced Information Technologies (ICAIT), Yangon, Myanmar, 6–7 November 2019; pp. 60–65.
78. Yang, X.; Sun, X.; Zhou, D.; Li, Y.; Liu, H. Towards wearable A-mode ultrasound sensing for real-time finger motion recognition. *IEEE Trans. Neural Syst. Rehabil. Eng.* **2018**, *26*, 1199–1208. [CrossRef]

79. Mokhtari, G.; Zhang, Q.; Nourbakhsh, G.; Ball, S.; Karunanithi, M. BLUESOUND: A new resident identification sensor—Using ultrasound array and BLE technology for smart home platform. *IEEE Sens. J.* **2017**, *17*, 1503–1512. [CrossRef]
80. Rossi, M.; Feese, S.; Amft, O.; Braune, N.; Martis, S.; Tröster, G. AmbientSense: A real-time ambient sound recognition system for smartphones. In Proceedings of the 2013 IEEE International Conference on Pervasive Computing and Communications Workshops (PERCOM Workshops), San Diego, CA, USA, 18–22 March 2013; pp. 230–235.
81. Garg, S.; Lim, K.M.; Lee, H.P. An averaging method for accurately calibrating smartphone microphones for environmental noise measurement. *Appl. Acoust.* **2019**, *143*, 222–228. [CrossRef]
82. Thiel, B.; Kloch, K.; Lukowicz, P. Sound-based proximity detection with mobile phones. In Proceedings of the Third International Workshop on Sensing Applications on Mobile Phones, Toronto, ON, Canada, 6 November 2012; pp. 1–4.
83. Ward, J.A.; Lukowicz, P.; Troster, G.; Starner, T.E. Activity recognition of assembly tasks using body-worn microphones and accelerometers. *IEEE Trans. Pattern Anal. Mach. Intell.* **2006**, *28*, 1553–1567. [CrossRef]
84. Murata, S.; Yara, C.; Kaneta, K.; Ioroi, S.; Tanaka, H. Accurate indoor positioning system using near-ultrasonic sound from a smartphone. In Proceedings of the 2014 Eighth International Conference on Next Generation Mobile Apps, Services and Technologies, Oxford, UK, 10–12 September 2014; pp. 13–18.
85. Rossi, M.; Seiter, J.; Amft, O.; Buchmeier, S.; Tröster, G. RoomSense: An indoor positioning system for smartphones using active sound probing. In Proceedings of the 4th Augmented Human International Conference, Stuttgart, Germany, 7–8 March 2013; pp. 89–95.
86. Sathyamoorthy, A.J.; Patel, U.; Savle, Y.A.; Paul, M.; Manocha, D. COVID-robot: Monitoring social distancing constraints in crowded scenarios. *arXiv* **2020**, arXiv:2008.06585.
87. Lee, Y.H.; Medioni, G. Wearable RGBD indoor navigation system for the blind. In Proceedings of the European Conference on Computer Vision, Zurich, Switzerland, 6–12 September 2014; pp. 493–508.
88. Kim, K.; Kim, J.; Choi, J.; Kim, J.; Lee, S. Depth camera-based 3D hand gesture controls with immersive tactile feedback for natural mid-air gesture interactions. *Sensors* **2015**, *15*, 1022–1046. [CrossRef]
89. Nagarkoti, A.; Teotia, R.; Mahale, A.K.; Das, P.K. Realtime indoor workout analysis using machine learning & computer vision. In Proceedings of the 2019 41st Annual International Conference of the IEEE Engineering in Medicine and Biology Society (EMBC), Berlin, Germany, 23–27 July 2019; pp. 1440–1443.
90. Li, M.; Leung, H. Multi-view depth-based pairwise feature learning for person-person interaction recognition. *Multimed. Tools Appl.* **2019**, *78*, 5731–5749. [CrossRef]
91. Pancholi, S.; Agarwal, R. Development of low cost EMG data acquisition system for Arm Activities Recognition. In Proceedings of the 2016 International Conference on Advances in Computing, Communications and Informatics (ICACCI), Jaipur, India, 21–24 September 2016; pp. 2465–2469.
92. Bangaru, S.S.; Wang, C.; Busam, S.A.; Aghazadeh, F. ANN-based automated scaffold builder activity recognition through wearable EMG and IMU sensors. *Autom. Constr.* **2021**, *126*, 103653. [CrossRef]
93. Zhang, X.; Chen, X.; Li, Y.; Lantz, V.; Wang, K.; Yang, J. A framework for hand gesture recognition based on accelerometer and EMG sensors. *IEEE Trans. Syst. Man Cybern.-Part A Syst. Humans* **2011**, *41*, 1064–1076. [CrossRef]
94. Kim, J.; Mastnik, S.; André, E. EMG-based hand gesture recognition for realtime biosignal interfacing. In Proceedings of the 13th International Conference on Intelligent User Interfaces, Gran Canaria, Spain, 2008; pp. 30–39.
95. Benatti, S.; Farella, E.; Benini, L. Towards EMG control interface for smart garments. In Proceedings of the 2014 ACM International Symposium on Wearable Computers: Seattle, WA, USA, 13–17 September 2014; pp. 163–170.
96. Ahsan, M.R.; Ibrahimy, M.I.; Khalifa, O.O.; et al. EMG signal classification for human computer interaction: A review. *Eur. J. Sci. Res.* **2009**, *33*, 480–501.
97. Jia, R.; Liu, B. Human daily activity recognition by fusing accelerometer and multi-lead ECG data. In Proceedings of the 2013 IEEE International Conference on Signal Processing, Communication and Computing (ICSPCC 2013), KunMing, China, 5–8 August 2013; pp. 1–4.
98. Liu, J.; Chen, J.; Jiang, H.; Jia, W.; Lin, Q.; Wang, Z. Activity recognition in wearable ECG monitoring aided by accelerometer data. In Proceedings of the 2018 IEEE international symposium on circuits and systems (ISCAS), Florence, Italy, 27–30 May 2018; pp. 1–4.
99. Zhang, X.; Yao, L.; Zhang, D.; Wang, X.; Sheng, Q.Z.; Gu, T. Multi-person brain activity recognition via comprehensive EEG signal analysis. In Proceedings of the 14th EAI International Conference on Mobile and Ubiquitous Systems: Computing, Networking and Services, Melbourne, Australia, 7–10 November 2017; pp. 28–37.
100. Kaur, B.; Singh, D.; Roy, P.P. Eyes open and eyes close activity recognition using EEG signals. In Proceedings of the International Conference on Cognitive Computing and Information Processing, Bengaluru, India, 15–16 December 2017; pp. 3–9.
101. Liu, Y.; Sourina, O.; Nguyen, M.K. Real-time EEG-based human emotion recognition and visualization. In Proceedings of the 2010 International Conference on Cyberworlds, Singapore, 20–22 October 2010; pp. 262–269.
102. Ishimaru, S.; Kunze, K.; Uema, Y.; Kise, K.; Inami, M.; Tanaka, K. Smarter eyewear: Using commercial EOG glasses for activity recognition. In Proceedings of the 2014 ACM International Joint Conference on Pervasive and Ubiquitous Computing: Adjunct Publication, Seattle, WA, USA, 13–17 September 2014; pp. 239–242.
103. Lu, Y.; Zhang, C.; Zhou, B.Y.; Gao, X.P.; Lv, Z. A dual model approach to EOG-based human activity recognition. *Biomed. Signal Process. Control* **2018**, *45*, 50–57. [CrossRef]

104. Palatini, P. Blood pressure behaviour during physical activity. *Sport. Med.* **1988**, *5*, 353–374. [CrossRef] [PubMed]
105. Lu, K.; Yang, L.; Seoane, F.; Abtahi, F.; Forsman, M.; Lindecrantz, K. Fusion of heart rate, respiration and motion measurements from a wearable sensor system to enhance energy expenditure estimation. *Sensors* **2018**, *18*, 3092. [CrossRef]
106. Brouwer, A.M.; van Dam, E.; Van Erp, J.B.; Spangler, D.P.; Brooks, J.R. Improving real-life estimates of emotion based on heart rate: A perspective on taking metabolic heart rate into account. *Front. Hum. Neurosci.* **2018**, *12*, 284. [CrossRef]
107. Li, W.; Yang, X.; Dai, A.; Chen, K. Sleep and wake classification based on heart rate and respiration rate. *IOP Conf. Ser. Mater. Sci. Eng.* **2018**, *428*, 012017. [CrossRef]
108. cheol Jeong, I.; Bychkov, D.; Searson, P.C. Wearable devices for precision medicine and health state monitoring. *IEEE Trans. Biomed. Eng.* **2018**, *66*, 1242–1258. [CrossRef]
109. Tateno, S.; Guan, X.; Cao, R.; Qu, Z. Development of drowsiness detection system based on respiration changes using heart rate monitoring. In Proceedings of the 2018 57th Annual Conference of the Society of Instrument and Control Engineers of Japan (SICE), Nara, Japan, 11–14 September 2018; pp. 1664–1669.
110. Lee, M. A Lip-reading Algorithm Using Optical Flow and Properties of Articulatory Phonation. *J. Korea Multimed. Soc.* **2018**, *21*, 745–754.
111. Gomez-Vilda, P.; Palacios-Alonso, D.; Rodellar-Biarge, V.; Álvarez-Marquina, A.; Nieto-Lluis, V.; Martínez-Olalla, R. Parkinson's disease monitoring by biomechanical instability of phonation. *Neurocomputing* **2017**, *255*, 3–16. [CrossRef]
112. Benalcázar, M.E.; Motoche, C.; Zea, J.A.; Jaramillo, A.G.; Anchundia, C.E.; Zambrano, P.; Segura, M.; Palacios, F.B.; Pérez, M. Real-time hand gesture recognition using the Myo armband and muscle activity detection. In Proceedings of the 2017 IEEE Second Ecuador Technical Chapters Meeting (ETCM), Salinas, Ecuador, 16–20 October, 2017; pp. 1–6.
113. Li, X.; Hong, K.; Liu, G. Detection of physical stress using facial muscle activity. *J. Opt. Technol.* **2018**, *85*, 562–569. [CrossRef]
114. Caulcrick, C.; Russell, F.; Wilson, S.; Sawade, C.; Vaidyanathan, R. Unilateral Inertial and Muscle Activity Sensor Fusion for Gait Cycle Progress Estimation. In Proceedings of the 2018 7th IEEE International Conference on Biomedical Robotics and Biomechatronics (Biorob), Enschede, The Netherlands, 26–29 August 2018; pp. 1151–1156.
115. Fasih Haider, P.A.; Luz, S. Automatic Recognition of Low-Back Chronic Pain Level and Protective Movement Behaviour using Physical and Muscle Activity Information. In Proceedings of the 15th IEEE International Conference on Automatic Face and Gesture Recognition (FG 2020), Buenos Aires, Argentina, 16–20 November 2020; pp. 834–838,
116. Zhang, Y.; Yang, C.; Hudson, S.E.; Harrison, C.; Sample, A. Wall++ room-scale interactive and context-aware sensing. In Proceedings of the 2018 CHI Conference on Human Factors in Computing Systems, Montreal, QC, Canada, 21–26 April 2018; pp. 1–15.
117. Cheng, J.; Amft, O.; Lukowicz, P. Active capacitive sensing: Exploring a new wearable sensing modality for activity recognition. In Proceedings of the International Conference on Pervasive Computing, Helsinki, Finland, 17–20 May 2010; pp. 319–336.
118. Zhang, Y.; Laput, G.; Harrison, C. Electrick: Low-cost touch sensing using electric field tomography. In Proceedings of the 2017 CHI Conference on Human Factors in Computing Systems, Denver, CO, USA, 6–11 May 2017; pp. 1–14.
119. Valtonen, M.; Maentausta, J.; Vanhala, J. Tiletrack: Capacitive human tracking using floor tiles. In Proceedings of the 2009 IEEE International Conference on Pervasive Computing and Communications, Galveston, TX, USA, 9–13 March 2009; pp. 1–10.
120. Noble, D.J.; MacDowell, C.J.; McKinnon, M.L.; Neblett, T.I.; Goolsby, W.N.; Hochman, S. Use of electric field sensors for recording respiration, heart rate, and stereotyped motor behaviors in the rodent home cage. *J. Neurosci. Methods* **2017**, *277*, 88–100. [CrossRef] [PubMed]
121. Wong, W.; Juwono, F.H.; Khoo, B.T.T. Multi-Features Capacitive Hand Gesture Recognition Sensor: A Machine Learning Approach. *IEEE Sens. J.* **2021**, *21*, 8441–8450. [CrossRef]
122. Chen, K.Y.; Lyons, K.; White, S.; Patel, S. uTrack: 3D input using two magnetic sensors. In Proceedings of the 26th Annual ACM Symposium on User Interface Software and Technology, St. Andrews, UK, 8–11 October 2013; pp. 237–244.
123. Reyes, G.; Wu, J.; Juneja, N.; Goldshtein, M.; Edwards, W.K.; Abowd, G.D.; Starner, T. Synchrowatch: One-handed synchronous smartwatch gestures using correlation and magnetic sensing. *Proc. ACM Interact. Mob. Wearable Ubiquitous Technol.* **2018**, *1*, 1–26. [CrossRef]
124. Lyons, K. 2D input for virtual reality enclosures with magnetic field sensing. In Proceedings of the 2016 ACM International Symposium on Wearable Computers, Heidelberg, Germany, 12–16 September 2016; pp. 176–183.
125. Pirkl, G.; Lukowicz, P. Robust, low cost indoor positioning using magnetic resonant coupling. In Proceedings of the 2012 ACM Conference on Ubiquitous Computing, Pittsburgh, PA, USA, 5–8 September 2012; pp. 431–440.
126. Parizi, F.S.; Whitmire, E.; Patel, S. Auraring: Precise electromagnetic finger tracking. *Proc. ACM Interact. Mob. Wearable Ubiquitous Technol.* **2019**, *3*, 1–28. [CrossRef]
127. Huang, J.; Mori, T.; Takashima, K.; Hashi, S.; Kitamura, Y. IM6D: Magnetic tracking system with 6-DOF passive markers for dexterous 3D interaction and motion. *ACM Trans. Graph. (TOG)* **2015**, *34*, 1–10. [CrossRef]
128. Bian, S.; Zhou, B.; Lukowicz, P. Social distance monitor with a wearable magnetic field proximity sensor. *Sensors* **2020**, *20*, 5101. [CrossRef]
129. Bian, S.; Zhou, B.; Bello, H.; Lukowicz, P. A wearable magnetic field based proximity sensing system for monitoring COVID-19 social distancing. In Proceedings of the 2020 International Symposium on Wearable Computers, Virtual Event, 12–16 September 2020; pp. 22–26.

130. Amft, O.; González, L.I.L.; Lukowicz, P.; Bian, S.; Burggraf, P. Wearables to fight COVID-19: From symptom tracking to contact tracing. *IEEE Pervasive Comput.* **2020**, *19*, 53–60. [CrossRef]
131. Bian, S.; Hevesi, P.; Christensen, L.; Lukowicz, P. Induced Magnetic Field-Based Indoor Positioning System for Underwater Environments. *Sensors* **2021**, *21*, 2218. [CrossRef]
132. Kindratenko, V.V.; Sherman, W.R. Neural network-based calibration of electromagnetic tracking systems. *Virtual Real.* **2005**, *9*, 70–78. [CrossRef]
133. Shu, L.; Hua, T.; Wang, Y.; Li, Q.; Feng, D.D.; Tao, X. In-shoe plantar pressure measurement and analysis system based on fabric pressure sensing array. *IEEE Trans. Inf. Technol. Biomed.* **2010**, *14*, 767–775. [PubMed]
134. Zhou, B.; Sundholm, M.; Cheng, J.; Cruz, H.; Lukowicz, P. Measuring muscle activities during gym exercises with textile pressure mapping sensors. *Pervasive Mob. Comput.* **2017**, *38*, 331–345. [CrossRef]
135. Kaddoura, Y.; King, J.; Helal, A. Cost-precision tradeoffs in unencumbered floor-based indoor location tracking. In Proceedings of the Third International Conference On Smart Homes and Health Telematic (ICOST), Montreal, QC, Canada, 4–6 July 2005.
136. Nakane, H.; Toyama, J.; Kudo, M. Fatigue detection using a pressure sensor chair. In Proceedings of the 2011 IEEE International Conference on Granular Computing, Taiwan, China, 8–10 November 2011; pp. 490–495.
137. Goetschius, J.; Feger, M.A.; Hertel, J.; Hart, J.M. Validating center-of-pressure balance measurements using the MatScan® pressure mat. *J. Sport Rehabil.* **2018**, *27*, 1–14. [CrossRef] [PubMed]
138. Aliau Bonet, C.; Pallàs Areny, R. A fast method to estimate body capacitance to ground. In Proceedings of the Proceedings of XX IMEKO World Congress 2012, Busan, Korea, 9–14 September 2012; pp. 1–4.
139. Aliau-Bonet, C.; Pallas-Areny, R. A novel method to estimate body capacitance to ground at mid frequencies. *IEEE Trans. Instrum. Meas.* **2013**, *62*, 2519–2525. [CrossRef]
140. Buller, W.; Wilson, B. Measurement and modeling mutual capacitance of electrical wiring and humans. *IEEE Trans. Instrum. Meas.* **2006**, *55*, 1519–1522. [CrossRef]
141. Bian, S.; Lukowicz, P. A Systematic Study of the Influence of Various User Specific and Environmental Factors on Wearable Human Body Capacitance Sensing. In Proceedings of the EAI International Conference on Body Area Networks, Virtual Event, 25–26 October 2021; pp. 247–274.
142. Goad, N.; Gawkrodger, D. Ambient humidity and the skin: The impact of air humidity in healthy and diseased states. *J. Eur. Acad. Dermatol. Venereol.* **2016**, *30*, 1285–1294. [CrossRef] [PubMed]
143. Egawa, M.; Oguri, M.; Kuwahara, T.; Takahashi, M. Effect of exposure of human skin to a dry environment. *Skin Res. Technol.* **2002**, *8*, 212–218. [CrossRef] [PubMed]
144. Jonassen, N. Human body capacitance: Static or dynamic concept?[ESD]. In Proceedings of the Electrical Overstress/Electrostatic Discharge Symposium Proceedings, 1998 (Cat. No. 98TH8347), Reno, NV, USA, 6–8 October 1998; pp. 111–117.
145. Bian, S.; Yuan, S.; Rey, V.F.; Lukowicz, P. Using human body capacitance sensing to monitor leg motion dominated activities with a wrist worn device. In Proceedings of the Sensor-and Video-Based Activity and Behavior Computing: 3rd International Conference on Activity and Behavior Computing (ABC 2021), Virtual Event, 20–22 October 2021; p. 81.
146. Cohn, G.; Morris, D.; Patel, S.; Tan, D. Humantenna: Using the body as an antenna for real-time whole-body interaction. In Proceedings of the SIGCHI Conference on Human Factors in Computing Systems, Austin, TX, USA, 5–10 May 2012; pp. 1901–1910.
147. Bian, S.; Rey, V.F.; Younas, J.; Lukowicz, P. Wrist-Worn Capacitive Sensor for Activity and Physical Collaboration Recognition. In Proceedings of the 2019 IEEE International Conference on Pervasive Computing and Communications Workshops (PerCom Workshops), Kyoto, Japan, 11–15 March 2019; pp. 261–266.
148. Bian, S.; Lukowicz, P. Capacitive Sensing Based On-board Hand Gesture Recognition with TinyML. In Proceedings of the 2021 ACM International Joint Conference on Pervasive and Ubiquitous Computing and Proceedings of the 2021 ACM International Symposium on Wearable Computers, Virtual, 21–26 September 2021; pp. 4–5.
149. Cohn, G.; Gupta, S.; Lee, T.J.; Morris, D.; Smith, J.R.; Reynolds, M.S.; Tan, D.S.; Patel, S.N. An ultra-low-power human body motion sensor using static electric field sensing. In Proceedings of the 2012 ACM Conference on Ubiquitous Computing, Pittsburgh, PA, USA, 5–8 September 2012; pp. 99–102.
150. Pouryazdan, A.; Prance, R.J.; Prance, H.; Roggen, D. Wearable electric potential sensing: A new modality sensing hair touch and restless leg movement. In Proceedings of the 2016 ACM International Joint Conference on Pervasive and Ubiquitous Computing: Adjunct, Heidelberg, Germany, 12–16 September 2016; pp. 846–850.
151. von Wilmsdorff, J.; Kirchbuchner, F.; Fu, B.; Braun, A.; Kuijper, A. An exploratory study on electric field sensing. In Proceedings of the European Conference on Ambient Intelligence, Malaga, Spain, 26–28 April 2017; pp. 247–262.
152. Bian, S.; Rey, V.F.; Hevesi, P.; Lukowicz, P. Passive Capacitive based Approach for Full Body Gym Workout Recognition and Counting. In Proceedings of the 2019 IEEE International Conference on Pervasive Computing and Communications (PerCom), Kyoto, Japan, 11–15 March 2019; pp. 1–10.
153. Yang, D.; Xu, B.; Rao, K.; Sheng, W. Passive infrared (PIR)-based indoor position tracking for smart homes using accessibility maps and a-star algorithm. *Sensors* **2018**, *18*, 332. [CrossRef]
154. Yang, B.; Luo, J.; Liu, Q. A novel low-cost and small-size human tracking system with pyroelectric infrared sensor mesh network. *Infrared Phys. Technol.* **2014**, *63*, 147–156. [CrossRef]

155. Kashimoto, Y.; Hata, K.; Suwa, H.; Fujimoto, M.; Arakawa, Y.; Shigezumi, T.; Komiya, K.; Konishi, K.; Yasumoto, K. Low-cost and device-free activity recognition system with energy harvesting PIR and door sensors. In Proceedings of the Adjunct Proceedings of the 13th International Conference on Mobile and Ubiquitous Systems: Computing Networking and Services, Hiroshima, Japan, 28 November–1 December 2016; pp. 6–11.

156. Kashimoto, Y.; Fujiwara, M.; Fujimoto, M.; Suwa, H.; Arakawa, Y.; Yasumoto, K. ALPAS: Analog-PIR-sensor-based activity recognition system in smarthome. In Proceedings of the 2017 IEEE 31st International Conference on Advanced Information Networking and Applications (AINA), Taiwan, China, 27–29 March 2017; pp. 880–885.

157. Naik, K.; Pandit, T.; Naik, N.; Shah, P. Activity Recognition in Residential Spaces with Internet of Things Devices and Thermal Imaging. *Sensors* **2021**, *21*, 988. [CrossRef] [PubMed]

158. Hossen, J.; Jacobs, E.L.; Chowdhury, F.K. Activity recognition in thermal infrared video. In Proceedings of the SoutheastCon 2015, Fort Lauderdale, FL, USA, 9–12 April 2015; pp. 1–2.

159. Chudecka, M.; Lubkowska, A.; Leźnicka, K.; Krupecki, K. The use of thermal imaging in the evaluation of the symmetry of muscle activity in various types of exercises (symmetrical and asymmetrical). *J. Hum. Kinet.* **2015**, *49*, 141. [CrossRef]

160. Al-Khalidi, F.; Saatchi, R.; Elphick, H.; Burke, D. An evaluation of thermal imaging based respiration rate monitoring in children. *Am. J. Eng. Appl. Sci.* **2011**, *4*, 586–597.

161. Ruminski, J.; Kwasniewska, A. Evaluation of respiration rate using thermal imaging in mobile conditions. In *Application of Infrared to Biomedical Sciences*; Springer: Singapore, 2017; pp. 311–346.

162. Uddin, M.Z.; Torresen, J. A deep learning-based human activity recognition in darkness. In Proceedings of the 2018 Colour and Visual Computing Symposium (CVCS), Gjovik, Norway, 19–20 September 2018; pp. 1–5.

163. Baha'A, A.; Almazari, M.M.; Alazrai, R.; Daoud, M.I. A dataset for Wi-Fi-based human activity recognition in line-of-sight and non-line-of-sight indoor environments. *Data Brief* **2020**, *33*, 106534.

164. Guo, L.; Wang, L.; Lin, C.; Liu, J.; Lu, B.; Fang, J.; Liu, Z.; Shan, Z.; Yang, J.; Guo, S. Wiar: A public dataset for wifi-based activity recognition. *IEEE Access* **2019**, *7*, 154935–154945. [CrossRef]

165. Tian, J.; Yongkun, S.; Yongpeng, D.; Xikun, H.; Yongping, S.; Xiaolong, Z.; Zhifeng, Q. UWB-HA4D-1.0: An Ultra-wideband Radar Human Activity 4D Imaging Dataset. *Lei Da Xue Bao* **2022**, *11*, 27–39.

166. Delamare, M.; Duval, F.; Boutteau, R. A new dataset of people flow in an industrial site with uwb and motion capture systems. *Sensors* **2020**, *20*, 4511. [CrossRef] [PubMed]

167. Ahmed, S.; Wang, D.; Park, J.; Cho, S.H. UWB-gestures, a public dataset of dynamic hand gestures acquired using impulse radar sensors. *Sci. Data* **2021**, *8*, 1–9. [CrossRef] [PubMed]

168. Singh, A.D.; Sandha, S.S.; Garcia, L.; Srivastava, M. Radhar: Human activity recognition from point clouds generated through a millimeter-wave radar. In Proceedings of the 3rd ACM Workshop on Millimeter-wave Networks and Sensing Systems, Los Cabos, Mexico, 25 October 2019; pp. 51–56.

169. Liu, H.; Zhou, A.; Dong, Z.; Sun, Y.; Zhang, J.; Liu, L.; Ma, H.; Liu, J.; Yang, N. M-gesture: Person-independent real-time in-air gesture recognition using commodity millimeter wave radar. *IEEE Internet Things J.* **2021**, *9*, 3397–3415. [CrossRef]

170. Kay, W.; Carreira, J.; Simonyan, K.; Zhang, B.; Hillier, C.; Vijayanarasimhan, S.; Viola, F.; Green, T.; Back, T.; Natsev, P.; et al. The kinetics human action video dataset. *arXiv* **2017**, arXiv:1705.06950.

171. Soomro, K.; Zamir, A.R.; Shah, M. UCF101: A dataset of 101 human actions classes from videos in the wild. *arXiv* **2012**, arXiv:1212.0402.

172. Chaquet, J.M.; Carmona, E.J.; Fernández-Caballero, A. A survey of video datasets for human action and activity recognition. *Comput. Vis. Image Underst.* **2013**, *117*, 633–659. [CrossRef]

173. Mohino-Herranz, I.; Gil-Pita, R.; Rosa-Zurera, M.; Seoane, F. Activity recognition using wearable physiological measurements: Selection of features from a comprehensive literature study. *Sensors* **2019**, *19*, 5524. [CrossRef] [PubMed]

174. Casale, P.; Pujol, O.; Radeva, P. Personalization and user verification in wearable systems using biometric walking patterns. *Pers. Ubiquitous Comput.* **2012**, *16*, 563–580. [CrossRef]

175. Zhang, M.; Sawchuk, A.A. USC-HAD: A daily activity dataset for ubiquitous activity recognition using wearable sensors. In Proceedings of the 2012 ACM Conference on Ubiquitous Computing, Pittsburgh, PA, USA, 5–8 September 2012; pp. 1036–1043.

176. Hanley, D.; Faustino, A.B.; Zelman, S.D.; Degenhardt, D.A.; Bretl, T. MagPIE: A dataset for indoor positioning with magnetic anomalies. In Proceedings of the 2017 International Conference on Indoor Positioning and Indoor Navigation (IPIN), Sapporo, Japan, 18–21 September 2017; pp. 1–8.

177. zhaxidelebsz. Gym Workouts Data Set. 2021. Available online: https://github.com/zhaxidele/Toolkit-for-HBC-sensing (accessed on 30 April 2022).

178. Pouyan, M.B.; Birjandtalab, J.; Heydarzadeh, M.; Nourani, M.; Ostadabbas, S. A pressure map dataset for posture and subject analytics. In Proceedings of the 2017 IEEE EMBS International Conference on Biomedical & Health Informatics (BHI), Orlando, FL, USA, 16–19 February 2017; pp. 65–68.

179. Chatzaki, C.; Skaramagkas, V.; Tachos, N.; Christodoulakis, G.; Maniadi, E.; Kefalopoulou, Z.; Fotiadis, D.I.; Tsiknakis, M. The smart-insole dataset: Gait analysis using wearable sensors with a focus on elderly and Parkinson's patients. *Sensors* **2021**, *21*, 2821. [CrossRef] [PubMed]

180. Assa, A.; Janabi-Sharifi, F. A Kalman Filter-Based Framework for Enhanced Sensor Fusion. *IEEE Sens. J.* **2015**, *15*, 3281–3292. [CrossRef]

181. Han, J.; Li, M.; Li, H.; Li, C.; Ye, J.; Yang, B. Pt-poly(L-lactic acid) microelectrode-based microsensor for in situ glucose detection in sweat. *Biosens. Bioelectron.* **2020**, *170*, 112675. doi: 10.1016/j.bios.2020.112675. [CrossRef] [PubMed]
182. Cheng, S.; Gu, Z.; Zhou, L.; Hao, M.; An, H.; Song, K.; Wu, X.; Zhang, K.; Zhao, Z.; Dong, Y.; et al. Recent Progress in Intelligent Wearable Sensors for Health Monitoring and Wound Healing Based on Biofluids. *J. Front. Bioeng. Biotechnol.* **2021**, *9*, 765987. [CrossRef] [PubMed]

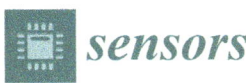

sensors

MDPI

Article

A Novel Central Camera Calibration Method Recording Point-to-Point Distortion for Vision-Based Human Activity Recognition

Ziyi Jin [1,2], Zhixue Li [3], Tianyuan Gan [1,2], Zuoming Fu [1,2], Chongan Zhang [1,2], Zhongyu He [1,2], Hong Zhang [1,2], Peng Wang [1,2], Jiquan Liu [2] and Xuesong Ye [1,2,*]

1   Biosensor National Special Laboratory, Key Laboratory of Biomedical Engineering of Ministry of Education, Zhejiang University, Hangzhou 310027, China; jinziyi@zju.edu.cn (Z.J.); gantianyuan@zju.edu.cn (T.G.); fzm21315045@zju.edu.cn (Z.F.); kevin_07@zju.edu.cn (C.Z.); jerryhe@zju.edu.cn (Z.H.); zhangh@mail.bme.zju.edu.cn (H.Z.); pengwangoptimus@zju.edu.cn (P.W.)
2   College of Biomedical Engineering and Instrument Science, Zhejiang University, Hangzhou 310027, China; liujq@zju.edu.cn
3   Independent Researcher, 181 Gaojiao Road, Yuhang District, Hangzhou 311122, China; 21106107@zju.edu.cn
*   Correspondence: yexuesong@zju.edu.cn

Abstract: The camera is the main sensor of vison-based human activity recognition, and its high-precision calibration of distortion is an important prerequisite of the task. Current studies have shown that multi-parameter model methods achieve higher accuracy than traditional methods in the process of camera calibration. However, these methods need hundreds or even thousands of images to optimize the camera model, which limits their practical use. Here, we propose a novel point-to-point camera distortion calibration method that requires only dozens of images to get a dense distortion rectification map. We have designed an objective function based on deformation between the original images and the projection of reference images, which can eliminate the effect of distortion when optimizing camera parameters. Dense features between the original images and the projection of the reference images are calculated by digital image correlation (DIC). Experiments indicate that our method obtains a comparable result with the multi-parameter model method using a large number of pictures, and contributes a 28.5% improvement to the reprojection error over the polynomial distortion model.

Keywords: camera calibration; point-to-point camera distortion calibration; vision-based human activity recognition; speckle pattern; digital image correlation

Citation: Jin, Z.; Li, Z.; Gan, T.; Fu, Z.; Zhang, C.; He, Z.; Zhang, H.; Wang, P.; Liu, J.; Ye, X. A Novel Central Camera Calibration Method Recording Point-to-Point Distortion for Vision-Based Human Activity Recognition. *Sensors* **2022**, *22*, 3524. https://doi.org/10.3390/s22093524

Academic Editor: Raffaele Gravina

Received: 23 March 2022
Accepted: 29 April 2022
Published: 5 May 2022

Publisher's Note: MDPI stays neutral with regard to jurisdictional claims in published maps and institutional affiliations.

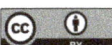
1. Introduction

In recent years, vision-based human activity recognition (HAR) has developed rapidly with many exciting achievements [1–3]. Camera calibration is the upstream task of vision-based HAR, which can establish the mapping between real space and image space. Its accuracy determines the performance of downstream tasks such as feature points recognition and 3D reconstruction, and thereby affects the final performance of vision-based HAR [4]. For instance, the fisheye camera, which has been widely used in HAR tasks in the field of monitoring and security, although it has an ultra-wide-angle field of view, the object at the edge of the fisheye image has great deformation and serious information distortion. If the distortion of the camera is not accurately calibrated, it will seriously affect the accuracy of the subsequent algorithm. So, camera calibration is of great significance to vision-based HAR, containing daily activity recognition, self-training for sports exercises, gesture recognition and person tracking [5].

Distortion calibration of the camera impacts the accuracy of other parameters' estimations. With the development of this field, distortion models' degree of freedom is increasing, thus, there is much difference compared polynomial distortion models with point-to-point distortion models. In 1992, Weng [6] summarized distortion camera models, namely, radial, decentering, and thin prism distortions, which describe the real distribution of distortion by polynomials and parameters. Polynomial distortion models are idealized models and have a gap with the actual camera imaging relationship, resulting in limited accuracy of the calibration method. For higher accuracy of distortion calibration, some general distortion models and corresponding calibration methods [7–13] are proposed.

Since radial distortion is the main distortion of the camera, some researchers [7,8] developed a general radial distortion model that does not adopt a classical two-to-six parameter radial distortion, but rather a freer form of radial distortion. Inspired by their success, more general distortion models have been developed [9–13], describing lens distortion per pixel or by some kind of interpolation. In this kind of model, as distorted points can be extracted directly, the key problem to be solved is how to determine the original position (of pixels or spaces) of distorted points. Sagawa et al. employed structured-light patterns to obtain a dense distortion sample; the camera is aligned opposite to the target to make the feature points fixed [9]. Aubrey K. et al. set a synthetic image plane and recorded distortion as bias between real camera images and images projected on the synthetic image plane [10]. Jin et al. assumed that distortion in the central area of the image plane is negligible, and calculated distortion of the surrounding area by cross-ratio invariance [13]. Based on a raxel model, Thomas S. et al.'s pipeline [11] achieved the highest accuracy, but needs a large number of images. In our method, we designed a novel objective function that treats the distortion of each pixel as a constant quantity between different images and reprojects reference images by optimization results to create "virtual photos" which can determine the original position of distorted points.

Our method is based on the central generic camera model, which assumes all lights pass through a single optical center in the imaging process. Since the rays diverge from a point in the central generic camera model, the order and spacing ratio of rays remains unchanged, and the distortion rectification map remains unchanged with distance. Accordingly, there are sufficient reasons to believe that the distortion of a pixel is consistent across images taken with the same camera, which is the basis of our objective function.

Before the iteration, using the initial estimation of parameters with Zhang's calibration method [14], we reprojected reference images to create "virtual photos" and extract dense features between "virtual photos" and original images. We designed our objective function to be a mean square error of the deformation between the "virtual photos" and original images. This objective function can remove the influence of distortion during parameter optimization, and obtain a more precise estimation of the camera parameters and target pose in each image.

To describe deformation adequately in the objective function, dense features are needed in our method. Although active phase targets can provide dense features [9,10,15,16], they are inconvenient to use. Chen et al.'s work [17] verified the accuracy and stability of feature detection methods based on digital image correlation (DIC). In Gao et al.'s work [18], the result of DIC is used to determine the accuracy of camera distortion calibration. Inspired by them, we incorporated a speckle pattern target and DIC into our camera calibration method, but unlike Chen, we did not utilize polynomial distortion models, but rather a full-pixel distortion description.

Since the polynomial distortion model is only an approximation of real distortion, the results of the camera calibration method based on the polynomial distortion model will be affected by incomplete distortion estimation. Our method can establish a point-to-point correspondence between distorted pixels and rectified pixels, which describes the camera distortion more comprehensively, and then gets a more accurate estimation of the camera parameters. Compared with methods based on the raxel model, our method needs only dozens of images, and strict experimental conditions are not required.

In our results, distortion is calculated for each point as the average value of the DIC calculation results across multiple images, which eventually formed a distortion rectification map that mapped images taken by the camera to undistorted ones. Figure 1 displays a distortion rectification map obtained by our point-to-point distortion calibration method. Figure 2 illustrates the difference between Figure 1 and the distortion rectification map obtained by Zhang's method with a polynomial distortion model using the same set of calibration images, indicating free distortion, which the polynomial distortion model cannot describe.

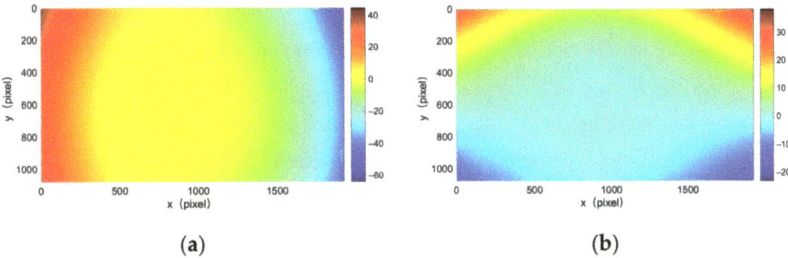

Figure 1. (**a**) Distortion rectification map of point-to-point calibration method for X directions; (**b**) Distortion rectification map of point-to-point calibration method for Y directions.

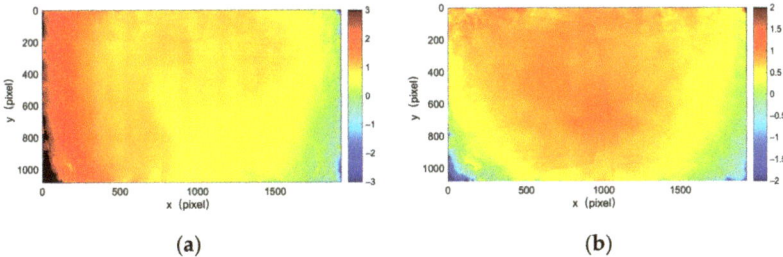

Figure 2. (**a**) Distortion rectification map of point-to-point calibration method subtracted from distortion rectification map of Zhang's calibration method for X directions; (**b**) Distortion rectification map of point-to-point calibration method subtracted from distortion rectification map of Zhang's calibration method for Y directions.

The paper is organized as follows. Section 2 illustrates relative work. Section 3 introduces the camera model and lens distortion in our method. Section 4 describes our point-to-point distortion calibration method. In Section 5, experiments are performed to verify our method's effectiveness. In Section 6, we discussed the issues not mentioned above. Finally, the conclusion is made in Section 7.

2. Related Work

2.1. Camera Model

From special to general, camera models can be classified as perspective cameras, central generic cameras, and non-central generic cameras [19]. The perspective camera is a single-view camera described by a pinhole imaging model, in which the imaging process is subjected to projective transformation, containing the finite projective camera and affine cameras [20].

The central generic camera contains the wide-angle camera, fisheye camera, and other cameras with refraction and reflection [19], which is unlikely to undergo a projective transformation and has a single focal point. In the imaging process of this camera, since the rays radiate from only one point, the order and spacing ratio of the rays remain unchanged, and the distortion rectification map remains constant with distance. That is why a distortion rectification map can describe the central generic camera's distortion. Following distortion rectification, the central generic camera is simplified to be a camera that conforms to the pinhole imaging model.

The non-central generic camera is also referred to as a general camera. It lacks a single focal point, the order and spacing ratio of the rays will vary with distance, and the distortion rectification map cannot be used for distortion correction. Michael D. Grossberg and Shree K. Nayar from Columbia University first proposed a raxel model for a general camera [21], which uses a point *p* and a direction q to describe a ray entering the camera from the outside and colliding with the sensor. Subsequent works on general camera calibration have adopted the raxel model [11,19,22–24].

2.2. Pattern Design and Feature Detection

While a chessboard or circle pattern target is usually used in camera calibration, methods for improving feature detection precision have been proposed [25–29]. Ha, and Hyowon et al. discussed a triangle pattern target [30]. The intersection of three triangles can be approximated using a series of third-order polynomials as control points. An active phase target is also used for calibration [9,10,15,16], which provides more freedom for feature setting and de-focus situations. Chen et al. utilized speckle patterns and extracted feature points using the DIC method [17]. Experiments demonstrated that calibrating with a speckle pattern produces a smaller reprojection error than calibrating with a chessboard or circle pattern.

2.3. Digital Image Correlation Method

Digital image correlation (DIC), first proposed by researchers from the University of South Carolina [31], is a method for determining material deformation. In its application there are two kinds of DIC: (1) 2D-DIC, which is used for flat materials and requires the materials to remain flat during measurement; and (2) Stereo-DIC, which is used for three-dimensional materials and deformation, and can handle more variable situations.

The core objective of DIC algorithms is to match points of interest (POI) from the speckle pattern feature on the surface of materials in images, which usually consists of two main steps: (1) obtaining an initial guess and (2) iterative optimization. In the first step, there are methods such as correlation criteria [32,33], fast Fourier transform-based cross-correlation (FFT-CC) [34], and a scale-invariant feature transform (SIFT) [35] for a path-independent initial guess. For iterative optimization, Bruck HA et al. [36] proposed the forward additive Newton–Raphson (FA-NR) algorithm, which was later improved and widely used. As calculating the gradient and the Hessian matrix in optimization progress is a noticeable burden, one feasible approach is simplifying the Hessian matrix by making some assumptions, thereby converting it to a forward additive Gauss–Newton (FA-GN) algorithm. Pan, B. et al. introduced the (IC-GN) algorithm into the DIC [37], which maintains a constant Hessian matrix and can be pre-computed.

3. Model of Camera and Lens Distortion

A camera can be regarded as a mapping between a 3D world and a 2D image. Our method was developed to address the issue of central generic camera calibration. To describe this 3D–2D mapping, we combined a pinhole camera model and a point-to-point lens distortion model.

3.1. Pinhole Camera Model

In the pinhole camera model, point **Pw** in the 3D world was transformed into a point (u, v) in an image after transformation in Equation (1) [20]. **T** (Equation (2)) is a rigid body transformation from point **Pw** in the world coordinate system to point (X, Y, Z) in the camera coordinate system, using the rotation matrix **R** and translation matrix **t**. **A** (Equation (3)) is an inner parameter matrix that transforms the point in the image coordinate system (the normalized camera coordinate system) to point (u, v) in the pixel coordinate system, where fx and fy are focal lengths in pixels, and cx and cy are pixel coordinates of the principle point. To normalize the image plane, the formula is divided by Z.

$$\begin{bmatrix} u \\ v \\ 1 \end{bmatrix} = \frac{1}{Z}\mathbf{A} \cdot d(\mathbf{T} \cdot \mathbf{P_w}) \tag{1}$$

$$\mathbf{T} = \begin{bmatrix} \mathbf{R} & \mathbf{t} \\ 0 & 1 \end{bmatrix} \tag{2}$$

$$\mathbf{A} = \begin{bmatrix} f_x & 0 & c_x \\ 0 & f_y & c_y \\ 0 & 0 & 1 \end{bmatrix} \tag{3}$$

Distortion d in Equation (1) describes the geometric deformation arising from the optical imaging system. In Zhang's method [14], distortion is employed on normalized image planes using polynomial representation [6]. However, in our method, for generality, distortion is defined as unknown mapping.

3.2. Point-to-Point Lens Distortion Model

This section will illustrate the generality of the point-to-point lens distortion model and its representation. Since $\mathbf{A}$ is a linear transformation, we can modify Equation (1) to apply distortion mapping on pixel coordinates.

$$\begin{bmatrix} u \\ v \\ 1 \end{bmatrix} = D\left(\frac{1}{Z}\mathbf{A} \cdot \mathbf{T} \cdot \mathbf{P_w}\right) \tag{4}$$

By substituting D for d, the representation and rectification progress of distortion can be simplified. The distortion calibration result obtained with this lens distortion model can be shown as a point-to-point distortion rectification map. It can describe distortion caused by any central generic camera. If we rectify a central generic camera after obtaining point-to-point distortion rectification mapping, it is simplified to be a camera that conforms to the pinhole imaging model.

Figure 3 illustrates the mechanism of rectifying a camera with point-to-point distortion rectification mapping. Point-to-point mapping contains a mapping of the X direction and a mapping of the Y direction, which is stored as two matrices. Assuming a feature point is (u_{de}, v_{de}) in a deformed image, the corresponding point with the same feature in the reference image is point (u, v). An element (u, v) in the mapping matrix of the X direction stores the displacement $d_{u,v}^x$ of feature point (u_{de}, v_{de})'s location in the deformed image relative to feature point (u, v)'s location in the reference image in the X direction. It is identical for the mapping matrix of the Y direction. Following that, the location of feature point (u_{de}, v_{de}) in the deformed image can be calculated using feature point (u, v)'s location in the reference image and element (u, v) in the mapping matrix of X and Y directions, as displayed in Equation (5).

$$\begin{aligned} u_{de} &= u + d_{u,v}^x \\ v_{de} &= v + d_{u,v}^y \end{aligned} \tag{5}$$

For every point (u, v) in the reference image, we can obtain its pixel value by copying the value of the corresponding point (u_{de}, v_{de}). If displacements $d_{u,v}^x$ and $d_{u,v}^y$ are decimals, bilinear interpolation is performed to obtain the value of the point (u_{de}, v_{de}). Going through every point (u, v) to obtain its value by Equation (5) and bilinear interpolation, a complete distortion corrected image is generated.

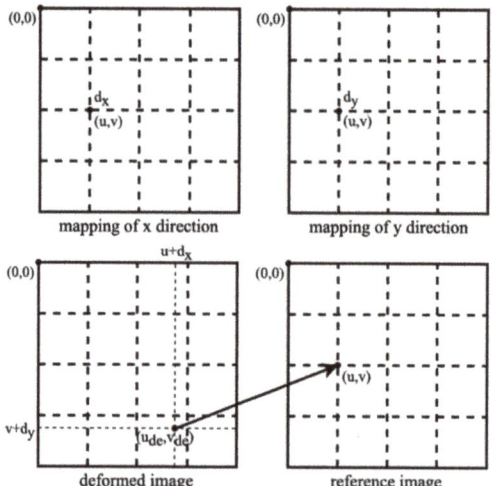

Figure 3. Mechanism of point-to-point mapping.

4. Method

Our method consists of three stages, which share the same set of calibration images. The first stage is an initial estimation. DIC method [38] is applied on images of speckle pattern calibration targets. Then, using Zhang's approach, a set of control points extracted from DIC result is used for calibration. In the second stage, all parameters and distortions are optimized using a novel object function. In the third stage, distortion rectification mapping is extracted via point-to-point calculation. We will discuss each stage in detail in the following sections.

4.1. Initial Estimation

Our calibration target is based on a speckle pattern synthesized from Equation (6) [39]. In Equation (6), n and D are the number and radius (unit in pixels) of speckle, respectively. (x_k, y_k) is the random location of the kth speckle with a random peak intensity of I_k^0. The synthesized speckle pattern image is shown in Figure 4a, which is denoted as I^r. We printed it as our calibration target. Additionally, we created a mask I^m with logical value representation, indicating the scope of the speckle pattern in image I^r, as displayed in Figure 4b.

$$I(x,y) = \sum_{k=1}^{n} I_k^0 \exp\left[-\frac{(x - x_k)^2 + (y - y_k)^2}{D^2}\right] \qquad (6)$$

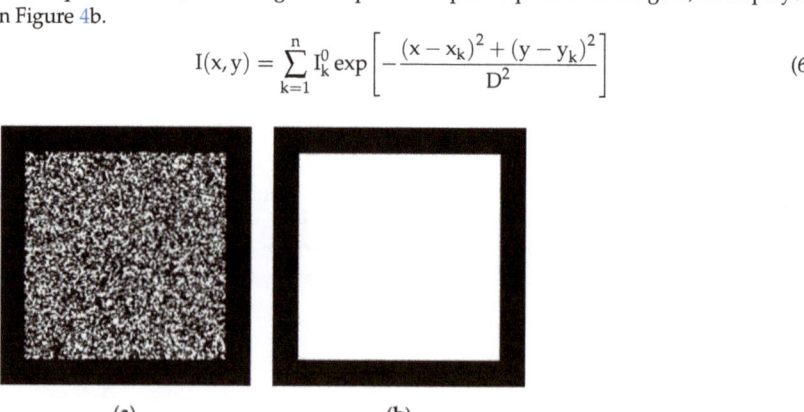

(a) (b)

Figure 4. (a) Speckle pattern image; (b) Mask of speckle pattern image.

With the camera to be calibrated, we captured 15–30 images of this camera calibration target; the ith image is denoted as I_i^d. We allowed the speckle pattern area to extend beyond the photo's edge. Figure 5 illustrates a calibration target's pose in our calibration image. A rectangle outlines the image with thick solid lines. The array of black points represents control points for initial estimation. It is a noticeable principle that the speckled area can exceed the scope of the image, as shown on the left and bottom of Figure 6, but the array of control points must remain inside the scope of the image.

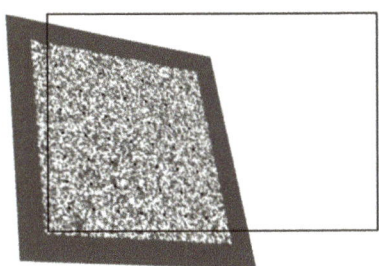

Figure 5. Taking an image of the speckle pattern calibration target.

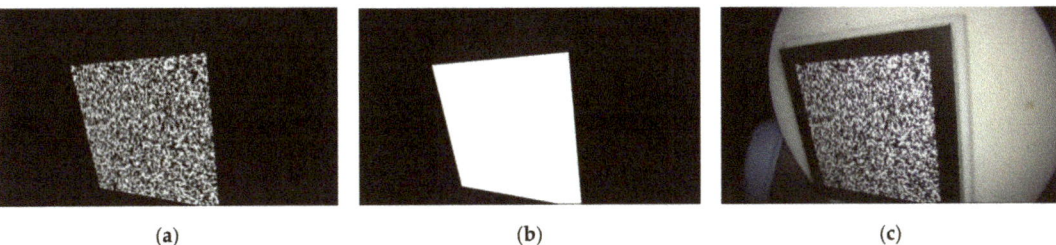

(a)   (b)   (c)

Figure 6. A group of images for DIC calculation in the second stage of our method, containing: (a) reprojection of reference image; (b) projection of mask; (c) image taken by the camera.

For initial estimation, we employ Zhang's camera calibration method. Control points are extracted from the result of the DIC calculation performed on these images. DIC calculation can determine a point-to-point correspondence between points in reference and deformed images. The result of DIC calculation is expressed as displacement of pixels in the deformed image relative to corresponding pixels in the reference image. Equation (7) represents DIC calculation, where I^r is a reference image, I^m is the mask of I^r, and I_i^d is the deformed image. The displacement of all the pixels can be denoted as two mapping matrices, M_i^x and M_i^y, corresponding to X and Y directions, respectively. If we have n deformed images, there are 2n mapping matrices.

$$M_i^x, M_i^y = \mathscr{F}_{dic}\left(I^r, I^m, I_i^d\right) \qquad (7)$$

By using the DIC approach, we can obtain the displacement of pixels in the speckle pattern area of each I_i^d relative to the corresponding point in I^r by the DIC method. We took displacement of an array of pixels in I^r and calculated their corresponding subpixel coordinates in a deformed image I_i^d using displacement and pixel coordinates in I^r, as in Equation (5). These corresponding points were saved as control points.

From initial estimation, we obtained camera parameter **A** and the pose of calibration targets $\mathbf{R}_i$ and $\mathbf{t}_i$. Radial and tangential distortion is considered to obtain a more accurate calibration result.

4.2. Optimization with a Novel Objective Function

At this stage, we performed optimization with a novel objective function, Equations (11)–(13), that is also based on DIC. $\mathbf{A}$, $\mathbf{R_i}$, and $\mathbf{t_i}$ were used as optimization variables, with initial guess calculated by Zhang's method. Then, we set radial and tangential distortion parameters to zero and reprojected reference image I^r with parameters $\mathbf{A}$, $\mathbf{R_i}$, and $\mathbf{t_i}$ to obtain "virtual photos" P_i^r, as in Equation (8). The mask I^m was also projected with the same method, as in Equation (9). Therefore, P_i^m is a mask that indicates the scope of the speckle pattern in image P_i^r.

$$P_i^r = \text{Proj}(\mathbf{A}, \mathbf{R_i}, \mathbf{t_i}, I^r) \tag{8}$$

$$P_i^m = \text{Proj}(\mathbf{A}, \mathbf{R_i}, \mathbf{t_i}, I^m) \tag{9}$$

For every pixel in the projection of reference image P_i^r, the DIC method can obtain the displacement of the corresponding point in distorted image I_i^d taken by the camera, as in Equation (10). A group of these, P_i^r, P_i^m and I_i^d, is illustrated in Figure 6. It is worth noting that P_i^r and P_i^m share the same estimation of pose corresponding to I_i^d.

$$M_i'^x, M_i'^y = \mathscr{F}_{\text{dic}}\left(P_i^r, P_i^m, I_i^d\right) \tag{10}$$

Our objective function is set as the square error of these 2n mapping matrices, as in Equations (11)–(13). $\Delta p_{u,v,i}^x$ is element (u, v) of $M_i'^x$, meaning X direction displacement of point (u, v) in image I_i^d relative to the corresponding point in image I_i^{proj}. $\overline{\Delta p_{u,v}^x}$ is average of $\Delta p_{u,v,i}^x$ for every $\Delta p_{u,v,i}^x$ that does not equal to 0, n_x is the number of $\Delta p_{u,v,i}^x$ that we took into account. $\Delta p_{u,v,i}^y$ and $\overline{\Delta p_{u,v}^y}$ are all the same for Y coordinate.

$$\min \sum_{u,v} \sum_i^n \left[\left(\Delta p_{u,v,i}^x - \overline{\Delta p_{u,v}^x} \right)^2 + \left(\Delta p_{u,v,i}^y - \overline{\Delta p_{u,v}^y} \right)^2 \right], \forall \Delta p_{u,v,i}^x \neq 0, \Delta p_{u,v,i}^y \neq 0 \tag{11}$$

$$\forall \Delta p_{u,v,i}^x \neq 0, \Delta p_{u,v,i}^y \neq 0 \tag{12}$$

$$\overline{\Delta p_{u,v}^y} = \frac{\sum_i \Delta p_{u,v,i}^y}{n_y}, \forall \Delta p_{u,v,i}^y \neq 0 \tag{13}$$

This objective function means to minimize the difference of displacements between P_i^r and I_i^d. When the optimization process was complete, we obtained new camera parameters and pose of calibration target, namely $\mathbf{A^o}$, $\mathbf{R_i^o}$, and $\mathbf{t_i^o}$.

4.3. Distortion Rectification Map Extraction

Distortion rectification maps of X and Y directions were calculated with reference image I^r, calibration images I_i^d, and parameters $\mathbf{A^o}$, $\mathbf{R_i^o}$, and $\mathbf{t_i^o}$, obtained in optimization using a novel objective function.

Using parameters $\mathbf{A^o}$, $\mathbf{R_i^o}$, and $\mathbf{t_i^o}$, we reprojected reference image I^r and its mask I^m to obtain "virtual photos" T_i^r and their mask T_i^m, as in Equations (14) and (15). DIC analysis was performed on every part of T_i^r, T_i^m, and I_i^d, as in Equation (16). $\Delta p_{u,v,i}^{o,x}$ is element (u, v) of $M_{u,v}^{o,x}$, and $\Delta p_{u,v,i}^{o,y}$ is element (u, v) of $M_{u,v}^{o,y}$. $\overline{\Delta p_{u,v}^{o,x}}$ is the average of every $\Delta p_{u,v,i}^{o,x}$ that does not equal 0, as in Equation (17). $n_{o,x}$ is the number of $\Delta p_{u,v,i}^{o,x}$ that we took into account. $\Delta p_{u,v,i}^{o,y}$ and $\overline{\Delta p_{u,v}^{o,y}}$ are all the same for Y coordinate, as in Equation (18). The result $\left(\overline{\Delta p_{u,v}^{o,y}}, \overline{\Delta p_{u,v}^{o,y}} \right)$ is displacement $\left(d_{u,v}^x, d_{u,v}^y \right)$ used in Equation (5). Therefore, point-to-point mapping of lens distortion is obtained.

$$P_i^{o,r} = \text{Proj}(\mathbf{A^o}, \mathbf{R_i^o}, \mathbf{t_i^o}, I^r) \tag{14}$$

$$P_i^{o,m} = \text{Proj}(\mathbf{A^o}, \mathbf{R_i^o}, \mathbf{t_i^o}, I^m) \tag{15}$$

$$M_i^{o,x}, M_i^{o,y} = \mathscr{F}_{\text{dic}}\left(P_i^{o,r}, T_i^{o,m}, I_i^d\right) \tag{16}$$

$$\overline{\Delta p_{u,v}^{o,x}} = \frac{\sum_{i} \Delta p_{u,v,i}^{o,x}}{n_{o,x}}, \ \forall \Delta p_{u,v,i}^{o,x} \neq 0 \tag{17}$$

$$\overline{\Delta p_{u,v}^{o,y}} = \frac{\sum_{i} \Delta p_{u,v,i}^{o,y}}{n_{o,y}}, \ \forall \Delta p_{u,v,i}^{o,y} \neq 0 \tag{18}$$

5. Experiments

We conducted experiments to ascertain our method's efficacy and priority. The convergence stability of our point-to-point distortion calibration method was proved by repeating experiments, which were repeated 10 times on 10 groups of images. Additionally, we evaluated the accuracy of the distortion rectification map calculated from the result of 7 training processes using a test set that was not used for the previous calibration. Additionally, the influence of the number of calibration images on the calibration results was investigated. We compared the performance of the distortion calibration results between our method, Zhang's method [14], and Thomas S. et al.'s method [11], using 1920 × 1080 pixels laparoscopy, demonstrating a reprojection error and RMSE of camera parameter estimation. The ablation experiment demonstrated that optimization with a novel objective function and point-to-point calculation of lens distortion contributed to the final result's improvement.

5.1. Experimental Procedures

The 2D targets employed in the experiments of Zhang's method were circular and checkerboard pattern targets. We also adopted the deltille grid target proposed by Ha et al. [30] and the speckle pattern target proposed by Chen et al. [17]. As depicted in Figure 7a, the speckle pattern was synthesized using Equation (1) with n = 1.5 × 10^4 and D = 60 pixels in a resolution of 4000 × 4000 pixels^2. It was printed on adhesive matte paper by HP Indigo 7600 and stuck on a piece of glass to serve as a calibration target of 6 × 6 cm^2. The circular pattern calibration target consisted of circulars with a 3 cm diameter and 6 cm center distance, forming a 7 × 7 array, as depicted in Figure 7b. The deltille grid pattern calibration target was composed of equilateral triangles with a side length of 6 cm and an arrangement, as demonstrated in Figure 7c. The checkerboard pattern calibration target had 6 × 6 cm^2 squares, forming an 8 × 8 array, as in Figure 7d. The circular pattern, deltille grid pattern, and checkerboard pattern calibration targets were all printed on an alumina sheet with a glass substrate. To make a comparison under the same conditions, we used 7 × 7 array features extracted from the speckle pattern as the input of the method in [11]. Calibration images of each calibration target were captured by a 1920 × 1080-pixels binocular laparoscopy. We adjusted the lighting conditions to obtain the best imaging performance for each pattern, respectively, during image recording.

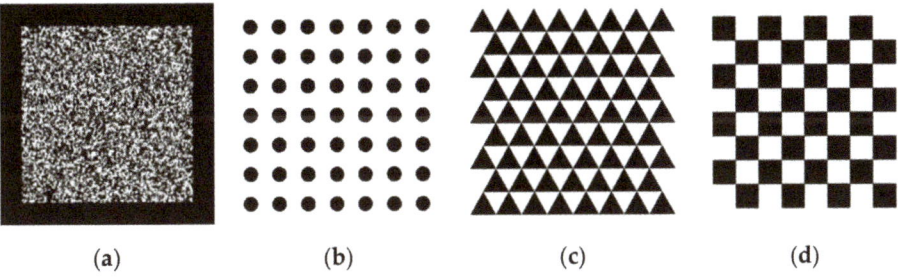

(a)   (b)   (c)   (d)

Figure 7. Two-dimensional targets used in the experiment, containing: (**a**) speckle pattern calibration target; (**b**) circular pattern calibration target; (**c**) triangle pattern calibration target; (**d**) chessboard pattern calibration target.

The experimental equipment was arranged as displayed in Figure 8. The calibration target was mounted on a mechanical arm, which was programmed to change its pose by inclination from −24° to 24° with a 6° interval. We positioned the calibration target initially in such a way that its projection covered the entire image area. The calculations were performed on a server with 256 CPUs and 512 GB of memory.

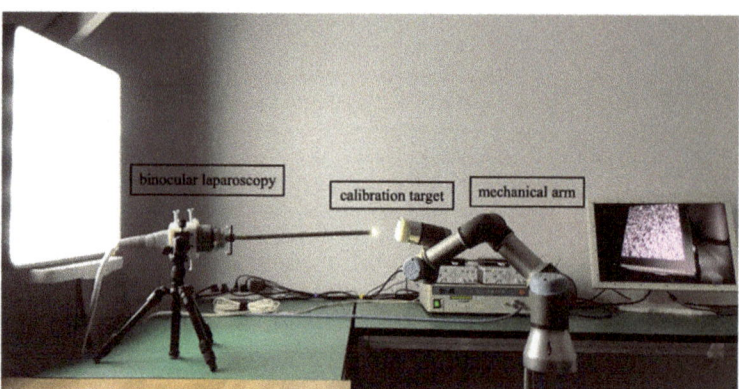

Figure 8. Experimental setup.

5.2. Validity under Different Initialization

To investigate our method's performance for each kind of calibration target, we grouped 20 images of different poses. For this, the poses of selected images had to be various, and all selected images had to cover the whole field of view. Figure 9 displays the poses of a group of selected images. We selected 10 groups of images as a training set.

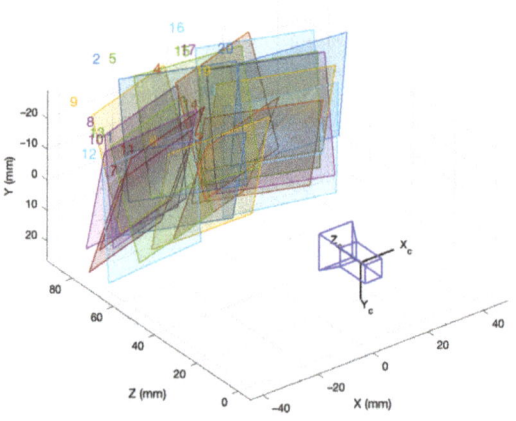

Figure 9. Poses of the target in a group of the training set.

Here, we verified the stability of our optimization's convergence under different initialization conditions by 10 training sets. The initial estimation was made by Zhang's calibration method. Then, optimization using our novel objective function was performed, and a convergence curve was recorded. Figure 10 displays the average value and range of the convergence curve in 10 training processes. The vertical axis represents the value of the objective function described in Equations (11)–(13).

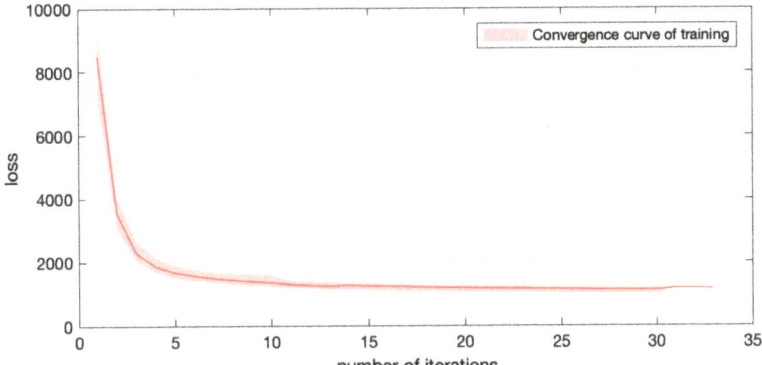

Figure 10. Average value and range of convergence curve in 10 training processes.

Additionally, we examined the distortion calibration results when different numbers of calibration images were utilized. For this purpose, the camera was calibrated 16 times, using from 10 to 40 calibration images. Then, training set images, undistorted by a distortion rectification map, were calibrated using Zhang's calibration method, assuming no distortion remains. The reprojection error was recorded, indicating the accuracy of the distortion rectification map. Figure 11 illustrates the reprojection error of calibration using different numbers of calibration images. The reprojection error calculated from training results was smaller than the initial estimation, even when only 10 images were utilized, and remained stable when more than 20 images were used.

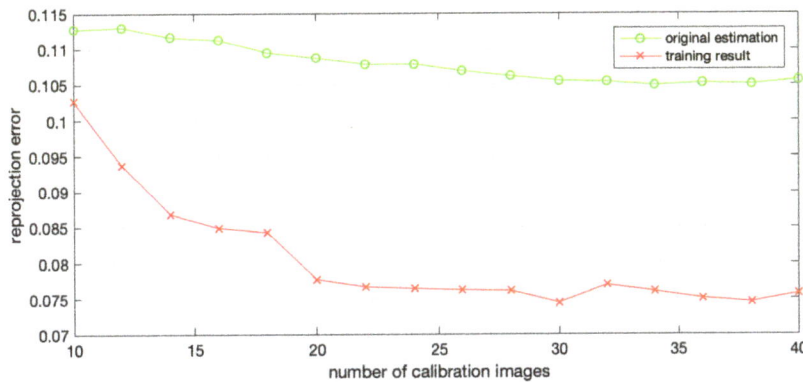

Figure 11. Reprojection error when different numbers of calibration images are used.

5.3. Ablation Study

Based on the initial estimation, we systematically added parts of our method and obtained a calibration result to demonstrate how individual parts influence the final performance. In the case of Map Extraction, the parameters obtained from the initial estimation were directly employed to calculate the point-to-point distortion rectification map, and calibration images were corrected by the point-to-point distortion rectification map. Then, assuming no distortion remained, the camera parameters were estimated using Zhang's calibration method. Each configuration of the calibration progress was repeated with 5 groups of 20 images.

As listed in Table 1, the mean reprojection error of Map Extraction was reduced by 11.48%, compared to the result of the Initial Estimation. The last configuration contained our complete calibration progress, with a mean reprojection error reduction of 30.61% compared to the initial estimation result. The reprojection errors' distribution in 5 repeated ablation experiments is showed in Figure 12. As a result, it can be inferred that in our method, both the optimizations with novel objective functions and the calculation of a point-to-point distortion rectification map are critical for improving calibration accuracy.

Table 1. The result of the ablation study.

Method	Mean Reprojection Error	Improvement (%)
Initial Estimation	0.106767	
Map Extraction	0.094512	11.48%
Map Extraction + Optimization	0.074087	30.61%

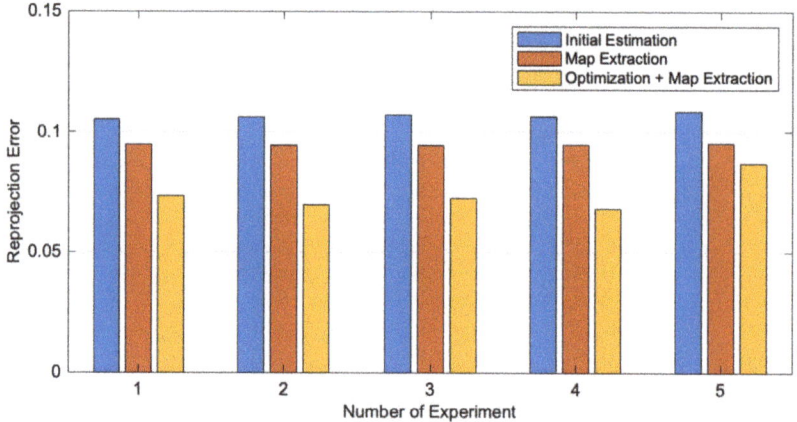

Figure 12. Reprojection errors' distribution in ablation experiments.

5.4. Benchmark Performance

This section compares the reprojection error and stability of the parameter estimation of previous methods with our novel method. Zhang's calibration method with the circle pattern target, the checkerboard pattern target, the deltille grid target, proposed by Ha et al. [30], and the speckle pattern target proposed by Chen et al. [17] are included in the comparison. For Zhang's method, using each target, we repeated the calibration progress 7 times using 7 groups of 20 pictures. A test set of 20 images was selected, excluding images in the training set. For the method of [11] and our method, we showed the reprojection error on the test set under the result of the calibration using 7 different groups of pictures. As to our method, for images in the test set, distortion was rectified using a point-to-point distortion rectification map calculated from the training result. Then, assuming no distortion remained, the camera parameters were estimated using Zhang's calibration method.

The reprojection error is shown in Table 2. The method of the top 4 lines in Table 2 is Zhang's calibration method with different calibration patterns. The reprojection errors of the chessboard, deltille grid, circle, and speckle calibration target methods were 0.34990613255, 0.115054 and 0.107224, respectively. Compared with Zhang's calibration method using different targets, the reprojection error of our novel point-to-point distortion calibration method was the smallest as it was reduced by 28.5% beyond Zhang's method using the same pattern.

The reprojection error was 0.075841 in the training result of our method, and was 0.076663 in the test result, exhibiting the performance of the distortion rectification map obtained from the training result on the new data. Although the reprojection error of the test set is slightly greater than that of the training set, it is still less than that of Zhang's calibration approach with any type of calibration target. This demonstrates that the distortion correction map calculated from our point-to-point distortion calibration method could effectively correct new images captured with the same camera and achieve the desired impact.

Table 2. Reprojection error and RMSE of internal parameters' estimation of different calibration methods, with a training set of 228 images for method of line 6, and 20 images for other methods.

Method	Mean Reprojection Error	Root Mean Squared Error			
		Fx	Fy	Cx	Cy
OpenCV (checkerboard)	0.349906	1.04336	1.070489	0.839562	0.490924
Deltille Grid [30]	0.13255	0.788706	0.841719	0.298072	0.659631
OpenCV (circle)	0.115054	0.339109	0.391043	0.334438	0.484564
Speckle [17]	0.107224	0.221421	0.186815	0.168492	0.167473
Thomas [11]	0.352319	NA	NA	NA	NA
Thomas [11] (228 pic.)	0.072295	NA	NA	NA	NA
Speckle-novel	0.076663	0.14265	0.065153	0.292851	0.164638

To compare our point-to-point distortion calibration method with the method of [11], the performance on the test set under different amounts of calibration images is shown in Table 2 and Figure 13. Assuming that 20 images were used in our method, with the same number of images, the estimation result of [11] was inferior to that of our method because of overfitting, and when 228 images were used in [11], the estimation result was superior to that of our method with 20 images.

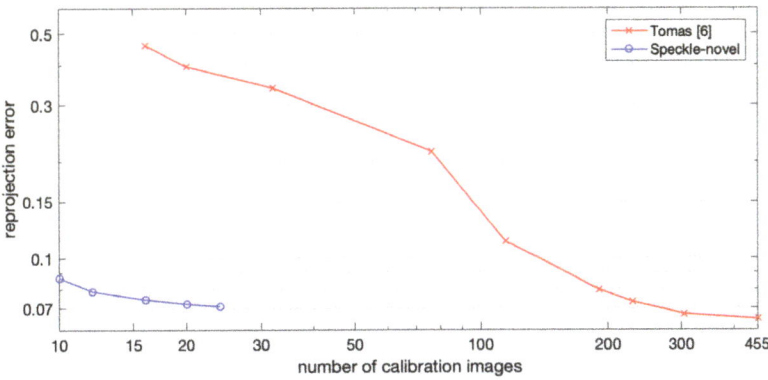

Figure 13. Reprojection error of Thomas S. et al.'s method and our point-to-point distortion calibration method on test set when different numbers of calibration images are used.

Table 2 and Figure 14 show the distributions of the internal parameters estimated using different calibration methods. The RMSE of the internal parameters' estimation is listed in Table 2. The small circle in Figure 14 represents the average value of the estimated internal parameters, and the upper and lower sides of the error bar represent the max and min value of the estimated internal parameters, respectively. It can be inferred that with the method of Chen et al. [17] and our novel method, the internal parameters' estimation in the repeated calibration is more stable than the other methods.

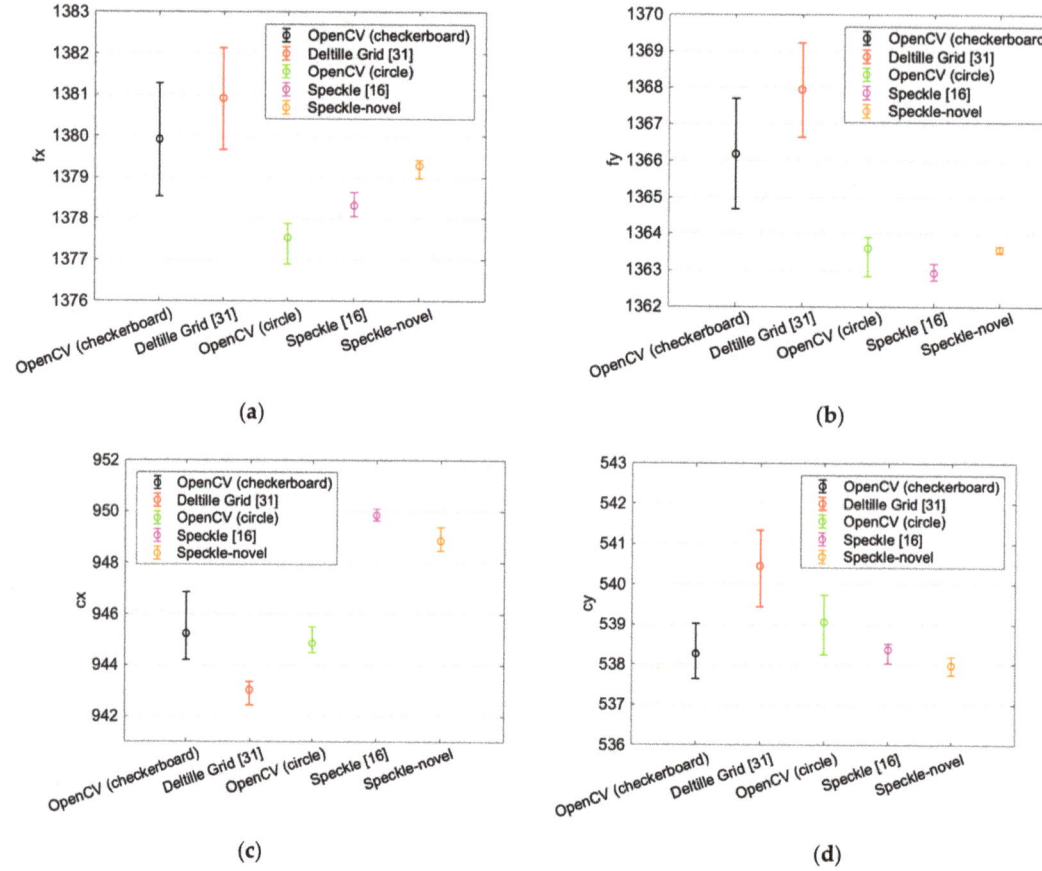

Figure 14. Distributions of internal parameters were estimated using different calibration methods. (**a–d**) are the distribution of estimated fx, fy, cx, and cy, respectively.

6. Discussion

We considered both the simulation and experimentation with a real camera when designing the experiment. In the simulation, the method employing the polynomial distortion model to simulate the camera distortion exhibits more advantages. In contrast, if we set additional distortions not limited to the polynomial distortion model, the point-to-point distortion calibration method offers more advantages. To make the experimental conditions neutral between the camera calibration method with the polynomial distortion model and point-to-point distortion calibration method, we used real cameras for our experiments.

As can be seen from the result of the validity experiment under a different initialization, the convergence curve of the optimization calculation by our method is stable, and the reprojection error is satisfactory when the number of calibration images involved in the optimization is not smaller than 20. The ablation study illustrated that the novel objective functions and the calculation of a point-to-point distortion rectification map have both resulted in a significant reduction of the reprojection error. The benchmark performance shows that the reprojection error of our method is smaller than that of methods using the polynomial distortion model. The accuracy of methods using the polynomial distortion model depends on whether the calibration pattern can achieve more accurate feature extraction and whether the features of image edges can be extracted. Our method not only uses the speckle pattern with higher feature extraction accuracy, but also adopts a full pixel distortion description and a specially designed objective function for optimization, so its reprojection error is superior to the method of the top 4 lines in Table 2.The method using the raxel model can achieve a smaller reprojection error than our method. When 228 images were used in the raxel model, the estimation result was superior to that of our method with 20 images. The following conclusion can be drawn from the findings of our experiment:

(1) For our optimization process, over 20 calibration images can completely realize the objective function convergence.

(2) Both the optimization with our new objective function and point-to-point distortion extraction significantly contributed to our method's results.

(3) The accuracy of our method is superior to methods using the polynomial distortion model. The method using the raxel model is more accurate, but with significantly more calibration images.

The setting of hyperparameters is a component in our technique that was not disclosed previously. To achieve the best performance of our method, hyperparameters were searched before calibrating different cameras in different environments. One of the hyperparameters was the subset size of the DIC calculation. The other one was the correlation coefficient threshold that determined which feature points were used in the parameter optimization.

1. Subset Size

In DIC, a larger size subset usually leads to a higher feature matching accuracy. However, an oversized subset introduces other problems, such as the complexity of deformation in the subset region. In this case, the current subset shape function cannot appropriately fit the subset deformation, resulting in decreased accuracy or failure of DIC. After a test with various subset sizes in our experiment, we used a subset with a radius of 70 pixels for DIC in the initial estimate and final verification, and a subset with a radius of 65 pixels in the parameter optimization.

2. Correlation Coefficient Cutoff

The correlation coefficient cutoff is used to determine whether the DIC results are reliable. A correlation coefficient cutoff that is set too high can introduce inaccurately matched features into the parameter optimization and reduce the accuracy of the parameter estimation. A correlation coefficient cutoff that is set too small results in large invalid regions of a calibration image that lack any features suitable for parameter optimization, which can also decrease the parameter estimation's accuracy. After testing with different cutoff values, we used 0.065 as the cutoff value of the correlation coefficient in our experiment. This implies that features matched in the DIC with a correlation coefficient of less than 0.065 will be used for parameter optimization, whereas features matched in the DIC with a correlation coefficient of more than 0.065 will be filtered out.

Our method is devoted to the accurate calibration of camera parameters and lens distortion, which paves the way for a better performance of HAR. Developing Gao et al. [18] and Chen et al.'s work [17], our method can obtain a point-to-point distortion rectification map of the camera without establishing distortion models or strictly restricting experimental conditions.

7. Conclusions

We propose a camera calibration method that requires only dozens of images to obtain point-by-point distortion calibration results and internal camera parameters. This approach extracts dense features using a speckle pattern calibration target and DIC, as well as a new objective function for parameter optimization. The distortion rectification map is calculated from the result of the parameter optimization. We can warp camera-captured images into undistorted ones using a distortion rectification map. Compared with commonly used methods, this method is not limited to the polynomial distortion model, and also allows for the pixel-level calibration of the camera distortion. We designed experiments to validate our approach's stability under various initialization conditions and compared it to the method of [11], using the same calibration target, and Zhang's calibration method, utilizing a variety of calibration targets. Our method has a lower reprojection error than that of the compared method with the same number of calibration images, as demonstrated by experiments on a test set. This proves that our method can get a more accurate estimation of the camera distortion and camera parameters, so as to better describe the mapping between real space and image space. Therefore, our method is more advantageous than calibration methods using the polynomial distortion model in downstream tasks.

Despite the advantages above, our method is limited by its single optical center assumption, and its accuracy is inferior to that of methods using the raxel model. The accuracy of the distortion rectification map of our method is also limited by the number of images. As the DIC calculation at the edge of the speckle region is not accurate enough, there are some undesirable points that cannot be ruled out in the distortion rectification map. A possible solution is not to use pixels at the edges of the speckle region during distortion rectification map extraction. Another problem is computing the resource consumption of the DIC, which increases with the size of the subset area and the number of calibration images. This can be solved with GPU-accelerated computing [40]. These topics are on which we should concentrate our future efforts.

Author Contributions: Conceptualization, X.Y., Z.J. and Z.L.; methodology, Z.J. and Z.L.; software, Z.L. and T.G.; validation, Z.J. and Z.L.; formal analysis, Z.J. and Z.L.; investigation, Z.J. and Z.L.; resources, Z.J., P.W. and J.L.; data curation, Z.L. and Z.F.; writing—original draft preparation, Z.J. and Z.L.; writing—review and editing, X.Y. and C.Z.; visualization, Z.L. and Z.H.; supervision, X.Y. and Z.J.; project administration, Z.J.; funding acquisition, H.Z. and X.Y. All authors have read and agreed to the published version of the manuscript.

Funding: This research was funded by the National Key Research and Development Project, grant number 2019YFC0117901; the National Major Scientific Research Instrument Development Project, grant number 81827804; the Robotics Institute of Zhejiang University, grant number K11806; the National Key Research and Development Project, grant number 2017YFC0110802; and the Key Research and Development Plan of the Zhejiang Province, grant number 2017C03036.

Institutional Review Board Statement: Not applicable.

Informed Consent Statement: Not applicable.

Data Availability Statement: The source code, dataset, and result files are available at https://github.com/schcat, and accessed on 22 March 2022.

Conflicts of Interest: The authors declare no conflict of interest. The funders had no role in the design of the study; in the collection, analyses, or interpretation of data; in the writing of the manuscript, or in the decision to publish the results.

References

1. Cao, Z.; Simon, T.; Wei, S.-E.; Sheikh, Y. Realtime multi-person 2d pose estimation using part affinity fields. In Proceedings of the IEEE Conference on Computer Vision and Pattern Recognition, Honolulu, HI, USA, 21–26 July 2017; pp. 7291–7299.
2. Park, S.; Ji, M.; Chun, J. 2D human pose estimation based on object detection using RGB-D information. *KSII Trans. Internet Inf. Syst. (TIIS)* **2018**, *12*, 800–816.
3. Li, J.; Liu, X.; Zhang, W.; Zhang, M.; Song, J.; Sebe, N. Spatio-temporal attention networks for action recognition and detection. *IEEE Trans. Multimed.* **2020**, *22*, 2990–3001. [CrossRef]
4. Aggarwal, J.K.; Xia, L. Human activity recognition from 3d data: A review. *Pattern Recognit. Lett.* **2014**, *48*, 70–80. [CrossRef]
5. Yadav, S.K.; Tiwari, K.; Pandey, H.M.; Akbar, S.A. A review of multimodal human activity recognition with special emphasis on classification, applications, challenges and future directions. *Knowl. Based Syst.* **2021**, *223*, 106970. [CrossRef]
6. Weng, J.; Cohen, P.; Herniou, M. Camera calibration with distortion models and accuracy evaluation. *IEEE Trans. Pattern Anal. Mach. Intell.* **1992**, *14*, 965–980. [CrossRef]
7. Claus, D.; Fitzgibbon, A.W. A rational function lens distortion model for general cameras. In Proceedings of the 2005 IEEE Computer Society Conference on Computer Vision and Pattern Recognition (CVPR'05), San Diego, CA, USA, 20–25 June 2005; pp. 213–219.

8. Hartley, R.; Kang, S.B. Parameter-free radial distortion correction with center of distortion estimation. *IEEE Trans. Pattern Anal. Mach. Intell.* **2007**, *29*, 1309–1321. [CrossRef]
9. Sagawa, R.; Takatsuji, M.; Echigo, T.; Yagi, Y. Calibration of lens distortion by structured-light scanning. In Proceedings of the 2005 IEEE/RSJ International Conference on Intelligent Robots and Systems, Edmonton, AB, Canada, 2–6 August 2005; pp. 832–837.
10. Dunne, A.K.; Mallon, J.; Whelan, P.F. Efficient generic calibration method for general cameras with single centre of projection. *Comput. Vis. Image Underst.* **2010**, *114*, 220–233. [CrossRef]
11. Schops, T.; Larsson, V.; Pollefeys, M.; Sattler, T. Why having 10,000 parameters in your camera model is better than twelve. In Proceedings of the IEEE/CVF Conference on Computer Vision and Pattern Recognition, Seattle, WA, USA, 13–19 June 2020; pp. 2535–2544.
12. Brousseau, P.-A.; Roy, S. Calibration of axial fisheye cameras through generic virtual central models. In Proceedings of the IEEE/CVF International Conference on Computer Vision, Seoul, Korea, 27–28 October 2019; pp. 4040–4048.
13. Jin, D.; Yang, Y. Using distortion correction to improve the precision of camera calibration. *Opt. Rev.* **2019**, *26*, 269–277. [CrossRef]
14. Zhang, Z. A flexible new technique for camera calibration. *IEEE Trans. Pattern Anal. Mach. Intell.* **2000**, *22*, 1330–1334. [CrossRef]
15. Huang, L.; Zhang, Q.; Asundi, A. Camera calibration with active phase target: Improvement on feature detection and optimization. *Opt. Lett.* **2013**, *38*, 1446–1448. [CrossRef]
16. Bell, T.; Xu, J.; Zhang, S. Method for out-of-focus camera calibration. *Appl. Opt.* **2016**, *55*, 2346–2352. [CrossRef] [PubMed]
17. Chen, B.; Pan, B. Camera calibration using synthetic random speckle pattern and digital image correlation. *Opt. Lasers Eng.* **2020**, *126*, 105919. [CrossRef]
18. Gao, Z.; Zhang, Q.; Su, Y.; Wu, S. Accuracy evaluation of optical distortion calibration by digital image correlation. *Opt. Lasers Eng.* **2017**, *98*, 143–152. [CrossRef]
19. Swaninathan, R.; Grossberg, M.D.; Nayar, S.K. A perspective on distortions. In Proceedings of the 2003 IEEE Computer Society Conference on Computer Vision and Pattern Recognition, Madison, WI, USA, 18–20 June 2003; pp. 594–601.
20. Andrew, A.M. Multiple view geometry in computer vision. *Kybernetes* **2001**, *30*, 1333–1341. [CrossRef]
21. Grossberg, M.D.; Nayar, S.K. A general imaging model and a method for finding its parameters. In Proceedings of the Eighth IEEE International Conference on Computer Vision, ICCV 2001, Vancouver, BC, Canada, 7–14 July 2001; pp. 108–115.
22. Ramalingam, S.; Sturm, P.; Lodha, S.K. Towards complete generic camera calibration. In Proceedings of the 2005 IEEE Computer Society Conference on Computer Vision and Pattern Recognition (CVPR'05), San Diego, CA, USA, 20–25 June 2005; pp. 1093–1098.
23. Dansereau, D.G.; Pizarro, O.; Williams, S.B. Decoding, calibration and rectification for lenslet-based plenoptic cameras. In Proceedings of the IEEE Conference on Computer Vision and Pattern Recognition, Portland, OR, USA, 23–28 June 2013; pp. 1027–1034.
24. Ramalingam, S.; Sturm, P. A unifying model for camera calibration. *IEEE Trans. Pattern Anal. Mach. Intell.* **2016**, *39*, 1309–1319. [CrossRef]
25. Förstner, W.; Gülch, E. A fast operator for detection and precise location of distinct points, corners and centres of circular features. In Proceedings of the ISPRS Intercommission Conference on Fast Processing of Photogrammetric Data, Interlaken, Switzerland, 2–4 June 1987; pp. 281–305.
26. Heikkila, J.; Silvén, O. A four-step camera calibration procedure with implicit image correction. In Proceedings of the IEEE Computer Society Conference on Computer Vision and Pattern Recognition, San Juan, PR, USA, 17–19 June 1997; pp. 1106–1112.
27. Heikkila, J. Geometric camera calibration using circular control points. *IEEE Trans. Pattern Anal. Mach. Intell.* **2000**, *22*, 1066–1077. [CrossRef]
28. Liu, Z.; Wu, Q.; Wu, S.; Pan, X. Flexible and accurate camera calibration using grid spherical images. *Opt. Express* **2017**, *25*, 15269–15285. [CrossRef]
29. Yan, F.; Liu, Z.; Pan, X.; Shen, Y. High-accuracy calibration of cameras without depth of field and target size limitations. *Opt. Express* **2020**, *28*, 27443–27458. [CrossRef]
30. Ha, H.; Perdoch, M.; Alismail, H.; So Kweon, I.; Sheikh, Y. Deltille grids for geometric camera calibration. In Proceedings of the IEEE International Conference on Computer Vision, Venice, Italy, 22–29 October 2017; pp. 5344–5352.
31. Peters, W.; Ranson, W. Digital imaging techniques in experimental stress analysis. *Opt. Eng.* **1982**, *21*, 213427. [CrossRef]
32. Tong, W. An evaluation of digital image correlation criteria for strain mapping applications. *Strain* **2005**, *41*, 167–175. [CrossRef]
33. Pan, B.; Xie, H.; Wang, Z. Equivalence of digital image correlation criteria for pattern matching. *Appl. Opt.* **2010**, *49*, 5501–5509. [CrossRef] [PubMed]
34. Jiang, Z.; Kemao, Q.; Miao, H.; Yang, J.; Tang, L. Path-independent digital image correlation with high accuracy, speed and robustness. *Opt. Lasers Eng.* **2015**, *65*, 93–102. [CrossRef]
35. Zhou, Y.; Pan, B.; Chen, Y.Q. Large deformation measurement using digital image correlation: A fully automated approach. *Appl. Opt.* **2012**, *51*, 7674–7683. [CrossRef] [PubMed]
36. Bruck, H.; McNeill, S.; Sutton, M.A.; Peters, W. Digital image correlation using Newton-Raphson method of partial differential correction. *Exp. Mech.* **1989**, *29*, 261–267. [CrossRef]
37. Pan, B.; Li, K.; Tong, W. Fast, robust and accurate digital image correlation calculation without redundant computations. *Exp. Mech.* **2013**, *53*, 1277–1289. [CrossRef]
38. Blaber, J.; Adair, B.; Antoniou, A. Ncorr: Open-source 2D digital image correlation matlab software. *Exp. Mech.* **2015**, *55*, 1105–1122. [CrossRef]

39. Bing, P.; Hui-Min, X.; Bo-Qin, X.; Fu-Long, D. Performance of sub-pixel registration algorithms in digital image correlation. *Meas. Sci. Technol.* **2006**, *17*, 1615. [CrossRef]
40. Zhang, L.; Wang, T.; Jiang, Z.; Kemao, Q.; Liu, Y.; Liu, Z.; Tang, L.; Dong, S. High accuracy digital image correlation powered by GPU-based parallel computing. *Opt. Lasers Eng.* **2015**, *69*, 7–12. [CrossRef]

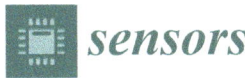

MDPI

Article

Comparing Handcrafted Features and Deep Neural Representations for Domain Generalization in Human Activity Recognition

Nuno Bento [1,*], Joana Rebelo [1], Marília Barandas [1,2], André V. Carreiro [1], Andrea Campagner [3], Federico Cabitza [3,4] and Hugo Gamboa [1,2]

1   Associação Fraunhofer Portugal Research, Rua Alfredo Allen 455/461, 4200-135 Porto, Portugal
2   Laboratório de Instrumentação, Engenharia Biomédica e Física da Radiação (LIBPhys–UNL), Departamento de Física, Faculdade de Ciências e Tecnologia (FCT), Universidade Nova de Lisboa, 2829-516 Caparica, Portugal
3   Dipartimento di Informatica, Sistemistica e Comunicazione, Università degli Studi di Milano-Bicocca, 20126 Milan, Italy
4   IRCCS Istituto Ortopedico Galeazzi, 20161 Milan, Italy
*   Correspondence: nuno.bento@fraunhofer.pt

Abstract: Human Activity Recognition (HAR) has been studied extensively, yet current approaches are not capable of generalizing across different domains (i.e., subjects, devices, or datasets) with acceptable performance. This lack of generalization hinders the applicability of these models in real-world environments. As deep neural networks are becoming increasingly popular in recent work, there is a need for an explicit comparison between handcrafted and deep representations in Out-of-Distribution (OOD) settings. This paper compares both approaches in multiple domains using homogenized public datasets. First, we compare several metrics to validate three different OOD settings. In our main experiments, we then verify that even though deep learning initially outperforms models with handcrafted features, the situation is reversed as the distance from the training distribution increases. These findings support the hypothesis that handcrafted features may generalize better across specific domains.

Keywords: human activity recognition; deep learning; domain generalization; accelerometer

Citation: Bento, N.; Rebelo, J.; Barandas, M.; Carreiro, A.V.; Campagner, A.; Cabitza, F.; Gamboa, H. Comparing Handcrafted Features and Deep Neural Representations for Domain Generalization in Human Activity Recognition. *Sensors* **2022**, *22*, 7324. https://doi.org/10.3390/s22197324

Academic Editor: Christian Haubelt

Received: 4 August 2022
Accepted: 23 September 2022
Published: 27 September 2022

Publisher's Note: MDPI stays neutral with regard to jurisdictional claims in published maps and institutional affiliations.

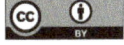
1. Introduction

Human Activity Recognition (HAR) has the objective of automatically recognizing patterns in human movement given sensor-based inputs, namely inertial measurement units (IMUs), currently available in most wearables and smartphones [1]. HAR is an important enabling technology for applications such as remote patient monitoring, locomotor rehabilitation, security, and pedestrian navigation [1].

The IMU itself may contain several sensors, such as accelerometers and gyroscopes, which possess microelectromechanical properties, allowing their capacitance to vary with movement [2]. The accelerometer measures acceleration, while the gyroscope measures angular velocity [3]. Usually, Machine Learning (ML) is applied to enable an association between the signals obtained from these sensors and specific human activities [2]. The typical HAR system comprises the following steps [4]: data acquisition, preprocessing, segmentation, feature extraction, and classification.

Similar to most ML tasks, HAR models perform well when testing on a randomly sampled subset of a carefully acquired dataset (i.e., out-of-sample validation) and struggle in Out-of-Distribution (OOD) settings (i.e., external validation). These settings occur when the source and target domains are different, such as when the models are tested across different datasets or sensor positions [5–7].

Deep learning is becoming increasingly popular in HAR applications [8]. While the typical pipeline includes a feature extraction step before training a classifier, deep neural networks automatically learn and extract features through a continuous minimization of a cost function. In principle, a neural network may have millions of learnable parameters, which translates into a large capacity to learn more complex and discriminative features [9]. These models have potential for HAR applications since sensor signals may have many inherent subtleties that may not be recognized by Handcrafted (HC) features. Although a promising approach, significant limitations have been discussed when deep learning models are deployed in real-world environments. Current methods for training deep neural networks may converge to solutions that rely on spurious correlations [10], resulting in models that lack robustness and fail in test domains that are trivial for humans [11].

On the other hand, HC features in this field are well-studied [1,12], more interpretable, and can reach high performance. In HAR, results with HC features approximate those of deep learning [13,14] even in tasks where the latter thrives, namely when the train and test sets are split by randomly shuffling the data, thus showing similar distributions [15].

Since both methods have advantages and limitations, there is a need for a more detailed comparison between them in various domains. This translates into a need for benchmarks where the similarity between train and test distributions has considerable variability.

As HAR naturally includes many kinds of possible domains, it can be considered an excellent sandbox to study the OOD generalization ability of learning algorithms (Domain Generalization), being previously used for this purpose [16].

This paper compares the performance of learning algorithms based on HC features with deep learning approaches for In-Distribution (ID) and OOD settings. For this comparison, we use five public datasets, homogenized to have the same label space and input shape, so that the models can be easily trained and tested across them. To validate whether the tasks are in fact OOD, several metrics are considered and compared with the purpose of assessing the disparity between train and test sets. To extract HC features, Time Series Feature Extraction Library (TSFEL) [12] was used. We use one-dimensional Convolutional Neural Networks (CNNs) for our deep learning baselines.

In summary, the major contributions of this work are the following:

1. A comparison between different data similarity measures and their relationship to generalization performance.
2. A validation of the hypothesis that models based on HC features can be more robust than deep learning models for several HAR tasks in OOD settings.
3. An empirical demonstration that a hybrid approach between HC features and deep representations can bridge the gap in OOD performance.

2. Related Work

Several studies compared classic ML approaches using HC features with deep learning methods. The authors from [13,14,17,18] compare CNNs with models based on support vector machines, multilayer perceptrons, and random forests. In all these studies, deep learning approaches outperformed classic methods. However, in their experiments, data splits were created by randomly shuffling the datasets, so samples from possibly different domains are represented in both the train and test sets with similar data distributions.

In regard to the use of data similarity to quantify the degree of OOD, associated with generalization, this is both an old and important question in the ML literature, as several ML methods implicitly rely on properties related to similarity (e.g., the large margin assumption in SVM learning) to guarantee good generalization performance [19]. The potential relationship between data similarity and the generalization properties of ML models was first investigated from an empirical point of view in [20], where the authors discovered that datasets found to be substantially dissimilar likely stemmed from different distributions. Based on these findings, the authors of [21] demonstrated that information about similarity can be used to understand why a model performs poorly on a validation set, while the same information can be used to understand when and how to successfully perform domain adaptation (see, for example, the recent review [22]). To that end, several metrics for measuring data similarity have been proposed in the literature. Bousquet et al. [20] developed a measure (Data Agreement Criterion, DAC) based on the Kullback–Leibler divergence, which has since become frequently used to assess the similarity of distributions [23]. More recently, Schat et al. [24] suggested a modification to the DAC measure (Data Representativeness Criterion, DRC), and investigated the link between data similarity and generalization performance. Cabitza et al. [25] proposed instead a different approach based on a multivariate statistical testing procedure to obtain a hypothesis test for OOD data, the Degree of Correspondence (DC), and also studied the correlation between DC scores and the generalization of ML models. By contrast, in the Deep Learning literature, approaches based on the use of statistical divergence measures, such as the Wasserstein distance [26] or the Maximum Mean Discrepancy (MMD) [27], have become increasingly popular to design methods for OOD detection. See also, the recent review by Shen et al. [28].

Deep learning approaches have been explored in OOD settings by testing the models on data from unseen domains [4,29–32]. Gholamiangonabadi et al. [33] verified that the accuracy went from 85.1% when validating using leave-one-subject-out (LOSO) cross-validation to 99.85% when using *k*-fold cross-validation. Bragança et al. [34] had similar results with HC features, reporting an accuracy of 85.37% for LOSO and 98% for *k*-fold. The most important features used by each model differed significantly. They concluded that LOSO would be a better validation method for generalization. Li et al. [4] and Logacjov et al. [30] compared several deep learning models with classic ML pipelines using LOSO validation. As opposed to what was verified in the previous studies involving ID settings, in the context of OOD, classic methods were mostly on par with deep learning approaches, outperforming them in some cases. Still, data acquired from different subjects of the same dataset may not be as diverse as the data encountered by HAR systems in real-world environments since datasets are usually recorded in controlled conditions with similar devices worn in the same positions. In Hoelzemann et al. [7], significant drops in performance were reported when testing on different positions and different datasets, which were then mitigated by the use of transfer learning techniques.

Transfer learning has previously been applied to HAR in cases where feature representations can be used in downstream tasks or across domains [6,35]. These methods leverage information about the target task or domain to approximate the source and target representations [5]. For example, Soleimani et al. [5] used a Generative Adversarial Network (GAN) to adapt the model to each user, outperforming other domain adaptation methods. However, the performance was poor when no transfer learning method was used (see Table 2 of [5]). The same phenomenon can be noticed in [35], where the domain adaptation methods outperformed the baseline model, which did not have access to data from the target domain. These studies illustrate the difficulty of generalizing to different domains, even when using deep learning models.

Gagnon et al. [16] included a HAR dataset in a benchmark to compare domain generalization methods applied to deep neural networks. The results indicate a 9.07% drop in accuracy from 93.35% ID to 84.28% OOD on a dataset where different devices worn in different positions characterize the possible domains. The same study showed that domain generalization techniques [11,36] did not improve results in a significant manner, and that empirical risk minimization (ERM) is still a strong baseline [37].

Boyer et al. [38] compared HC features and deep representations on an ID supervised classification task and on an OOD detection task. They concluded that, while a k-nearest neighbors (KNN) model using deep features as input outperforms the same model using HC features on the ID task, the situation partially reverts for the OOD detection task, where models based on HC features achieve the best results in two out of three datasets. However, the ID and OOD tasks are not directly comparable, since they are of different kinds and use different evaluation methods.

Trabelsi et al. [39] compared three deep learning approaches and a random forest classifier with handcrafted features as input. Similar to the experiments in our work, the datasets were homogenized by including only common activities and separated the test sets by the user. They concluded that only one of the deep learning approaches outperformed the baseline model with handcrafted features. While they formulated two different domain generalization settings (OOD-U and OOD-MD), the results for each of these settings are not directly comparable since the test sets were combined when reporting the results for the OOD-MD setting.

This paper adds to previous work by explicitly comparing the OOD robustness of HC features and deep representations in four domain generalization settings with different distances between train and test sets.

3. Methodology

3.1. Datasets

The datasets used in this study include human activity data recorded using smartphones and wearable inertial measurement units (IMUs). Table 1 contains a detailed description of these publicly available datasets.

Table 1. Description of the datasets, including activities, positions, devices, and number of subjects.

Dataset	Description	Devices	Source
PAMAP2—Physical Activity Monitoring			[40,41]
	9 subjects; 18 physical activities including sitting, lying, standing, walking, ascending stairs, descending stairs and running.	Heart rate monitor (≈9 Hz); 3 inertial measurement units each containing a triaxial accelerometer, a gyroscope and a magnetometer (100 Hz); Positions: wrist, chest and ankle.	
Sensors Activity Dataset (SAD)			[42]
	10 subjects; 7 physical activities: sitting, standing, walking, ascending stairs, descending stairs, running and biking.	5 smartphones containing an accelerometer, a gyroscope and a magnetometer (50 Hz); Positions: jeans pocket, arm, wrist and belt.	
DaLiAc—Daily Life Activities			[43]
	19 subjects; 13 physical activities including sitting, lying, standing, walking outside, ascending stairs, descending stairs and treadmill running.	4 sensors, each with a triaxial accelerometer and gyroscope (200 Hz); Positions: hip, chest and ankles.	
MHEALTH			[44,45]
	10 subjects; 12 physical activities including sitting, lying, standing, walking, climbing/descending stairs, jogging and running.	3 wearable sensors containing an accelerometer, a gyroscope and a magnetometer. One of the sensors also provides 2-lead ECG measurements (50 Hz); Positions: chest, wrist and ankle.	
RealWorld (HAR)			[46]
	15 subjects; 8 physical activities including sitting, lying, standing, walking, ascending stairs, descending stairs and running/jogging.	6 wearable sensors containing accelerometers, gyroscopes and magnetometers (50 Hz). Also includes GPS, light and sound level sensors; Positions: chest, forearm, head, shin, thigh, upper arm, and waist.	

Several criteria were followed to select the datasets for this study. Only datasets with a sampling rate close to or over 50 Hz were considered, to avoid the need for oversampling. The search was restricted to datasets that included most of the main activities seen in the literature (e.g., walk, sit, stand, run, and ascending/descending stairs). For better compatibility and to avoid large drops in performance caused by having considerably different sensor positions [7], we selected datasets that included overlapping positions with at least one of the other datasets that fulfilled the remaining criteria.

The accelerometer was the selected sensor for this work. The magnitude values were computed as the Euclidean norm of all three axes (x, y, and z), as this quantity is invariant to the orientation of the device and can give information that is more stable across domains. The magnitude signal was used along with the signal from each axis, so that all the information given by the accelerometer was retained. From those four channels, five-second windows were extracted without overlap.

All selected datasets were homogenized [47] so that a model trained on a specific dataset could be directly tested in any other. This procedure included resampling all the recordings to 50 Hz and mapping the different activity labels to a common nomenclature: walking, running, sitting, standing, and stairs. Stair-related labels were joined into a general "stairs" label, as having to distinguish between going up and down the stairs would add unnecessary complexity to the task, since it is hard to infer the direction of vertical displacement without access to a barometer [48]. The RealWorld dataset [46] generated considerably more windows than the other datasets, so one-third of these windows was randomly sampled and used in the experiments. The final distribution of windows and activities per dataset is shown in Table 2. This table contains the percentage of samples (five-second windows) of each activity in a given dataset, as well as the total number of samples and corresponding percentage of each activity and dataset. In this table, it can be seen that, while not being very well balanced, the activities have a substantial amount of samples for all the datasets. On the other hand, even with the effort of reducing samples, the RealWorld and SAD datasets have a larger influence in the experiments, which should not be an issue, since the conditions remain the same for both deep and classic approaches.

Table 2. Distribution of samples and activity labels per dataset. The # symbol represents the number of samples.

Activity	Datasets (%)					Total	
	PAMAP2	SAD	DaLiAc	MHEALTH	RealWorld	%	#
Run	10.5	16.9	20.0	33.3	19.1	18.3	7975
Sit	19.8	16.9	10.6	16.7	17.0	16.3	7102
Stairs	23.6	32.2	12.3	16.7	30.0	26.3	11,460
Stand	20.4	16.9	10.6	16.7	16.4	16.2	7047
Walk	25.7	16.9	46.5	16.7	17.5	22.8	9927
Total %	12.7	24.4	15.3	4.96	42.6	-	-
Total #	5541	10,620	6644	2160	18,546	-	43,511

3.2. Handcrafted Features

To extract HC features, TSFEL [12] was used. This library extracted features directly from the 5-second accelerometer windows generated from each public dataset. To decrease computation time, we removed the features that included individual coefficients, such as Fast Fourier Transform (FFT), empirical Cumulative Distribution Function (eCDF), and histogram values. Nonetheless, the high-level spectral features computed from the FFT were kept. We did not extract wavelet and audio-related features, such as MFCC and LPCC. The total number of features per window was 192.

After the features were computed, samples were split according to each task (see Section 4). Subsequently, features were scaled by subtracting the mean of the train set and dividing by its standard deviation (Z-score normalization). The classifiers used were Logistic Regression (LR) and a Multilayer Perceptron (MLP) with a single hidden layer of 128 neurons and Rectified Linear Unit (ReLU) activation. These classifiers were chosen to enable a fair comparison with deep learning, as they resemble the last layer(s) of a deep neural network, usually responsible for the final prediction after feature learning.

3.3. Deep Learning

Convolutional neural networks were the selected deep learning models for this study since they achieved significantly better performance and converged faster when compared with recurrent neural networks (RNN) in preliminary experiments, which was consistent with the literature [49,50]. A scheme of the baseline CNN architectures is presented in Figure 1. We chose three different architectures, which we named CNN-base, CNN-simple, and ResNet. The training process was identical for all the architectures and is explained in Section 4. CNN-simple is a simplified version of the CNN-base with only two convolutional layers and a logistic regression directly applied to the flattened feature maps. ReLU was used as the activation function for the hidden layers of both architectures. The ResNet (Figure 1c) is a residual network inspired by Ferrari et al. [18], with a few modifications. Its convolutional block is represented in Figure 2.

In an attempt to bridge the performance gap between HC features and deep representations, we built a hybrid version of each architecture. There, the HC features are concatenated with the flattened representations of each model and fed to a fusion layer before entering the final classification layer. The number of hidden units for the fusion layer was 128 on both CNN-simple and CNN-base, increasing to 256 for the ResNet. An illustration of the hybrid version of CNN-base is in Figure 3.

For all these models, the input windows were scaled by Z-score normalization, with mean and standard deviation computed across all the windows of the train set.

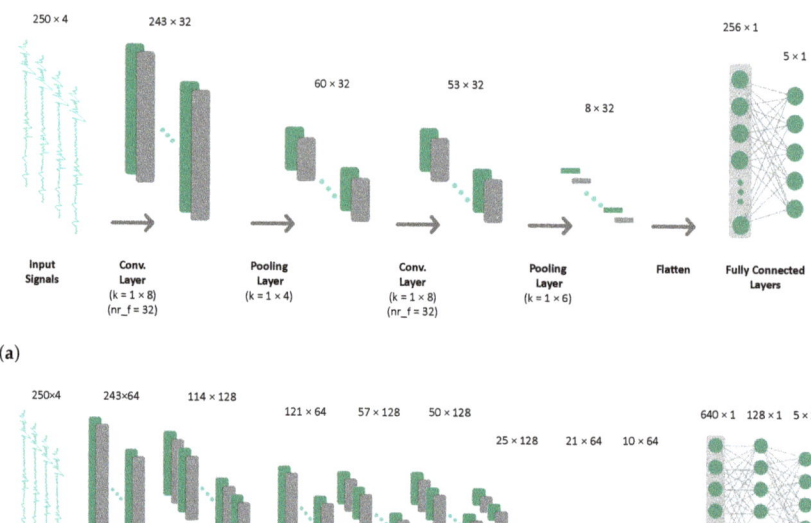

(a)

(b)

Figure 1. *Cont.*

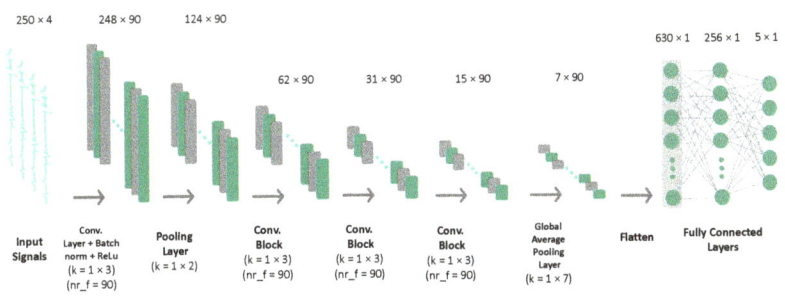

(c)

Figure 1. Convolutional neural network architectures. The values above the representation of each feature map indicate their shape (Signal length × Number of channels). Convolutional layers (1D): k = kernel size; nr_f = number of filters; stride = 1; padding = 0. Max pooling layers: k = kernel size; stride = 1; padding = 0. (**a**) CNN-simple Architecture. (**b**) CNN-base Architecture. (**c**) ResNet Architecture. The convolutional block is depicted in Figure 2.

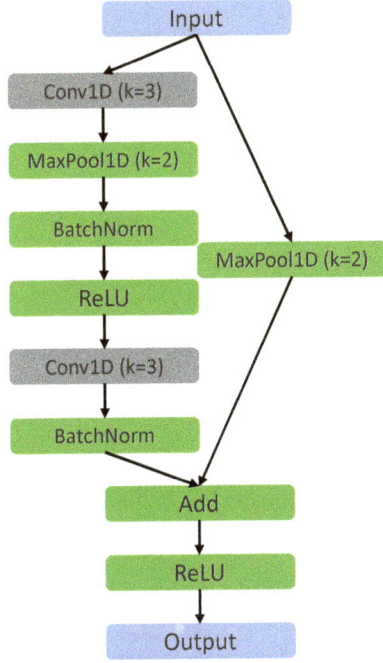

Figure 2. ResNet convolutional block. The letter k stands for "kernel size".

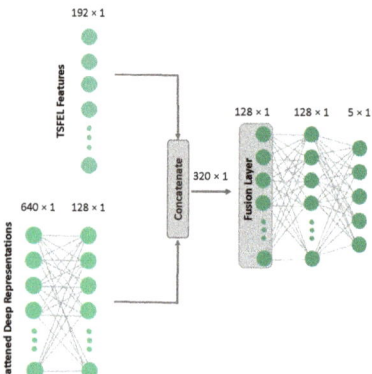

Figure 3. Simplified illustration of the hybrid version of CNN-base (excluding the CNN backbone for ease of visualization).

3.4. Evaluation

To quantify the degree to which a test domain is OOD, different metrics were applied, namely Euclidean distance, Cosine similarity, Wasserstein distance, MMD, and DC. Each metric was applied to the representations of each model before the classification stage. Regarding the Wasserstein distance [51], the Wasserstein-1 version was used and is given by:

$$W_1(X,Y) = \inf_{\pi \in \Gamma(X,Y)} \int_{\mathbb{R} \times \mathbb{R}} |x - y| \mathrm{d}\pi(x,y), \tag{1}$$

where $\Gamma(X,Y)$ is the set of distributions whose marginals are X and Y on the first and second factors, respectively. x and y are samples from each distribution $\pi(x,y)$ from the set. Intuitively, the distance is given by the optimal cost of moving a distribution until it overlaps with the other. In our experiments, x and y are the feature representations of subsets of the train and test data, thus W_1 represents the cost of mapping the distribution of x into the distribution of y (or vice versa).

Regarding the MMD , this is a kernel-based statistical procedure that aims at determining whether two given datasets come from the same distribution [52]. Given a fixed kernel function $k : X \times X \mapsto \mathbb{R}$ and two datasets X, Y with sizes $|X| = n$, $|Y| = m$, the MMD can be estimated as:

$$\mathrm{MMD}(X,Y) = \frac{1}{n(n-1)} \sum_{i \neq j} k(x_i, x_j) + \frac{1}{m(m-1)} \sum_{i \neq j} k(y_i, y_j) - \frac{2}{nm} \sum_{i,j} k(x_i, y_j) \tag{2}$$

Intuitively, the MMD measures the distance between X and Y by computing the average similarity in X and Y separately, and then subtracting the average cross-similarity between the two datasets, where the similarity between two instances is quantified by means of the selected kernel k. In this work, a simple linear kernel was selected. Furthermore, as for the Wasserstein distance, x and y represent the feature representations of subsets of the train and test data. Thus, MMD quantifies the average kernel similarity among instances in x and y, discounted by the cross-similarity between the two datasets.

The DC, by contrast, is a multivariate hypothesis testing procedure for the hypothesis that two samples of data come from the same distribution: having fixed a representative data sample, the obtained p-value, then, can be considered as a measure of how much any other data sample is OOD with respect to the representative one. In particular, scores close to 0 can be interpreted as being most likely OOD (since, assuming the null hypothesis of the two data samples coming from the same distribution, observing a p-value close to 0 has low probability). While the DC cannot be defined and computed by means of a closed-form procedure, in [25] a permutation-resampling algorithm (see Algorithm 1) was defined to compute the corresponding *p*-value, based on the selection of a base distance metric.

Algorithm 1 The algorithm procedure to compute the similarity between the two dataset *T* and *V*, using the Degree of Correspondence (DC).

---

procedure DC(*T*, *V*: datasets, *d*: distance, ∂ distance metrics)
    $d_T = \{d(t, t') : t, t' \in T\}$
    For each $v \in V$, find $t_v \in T$, nearest neighbor of v in T
    $T_{|V} = \{t \in T : \nexists v \in V s.t. t = t_v\} \cup V$
    $d_{T_{|V}} = \{d(t, t') : t, t' \in T_{|V}\}$
    $\delta = \partial(d_T, d_{T_{|V}})$
    Compute DC $= Pr(\delta' \geq \delta)$ using a permutation procedure
    return DC
end procedure

The selection of the distance metrics ∂ in Algorithm 1 is important to obtain sensible results for the DC. Intuitively, ∂ should represent the appropriate notion of distance in the instance space of interest. In [53], lacking any appropriate definition of distance in the instance space, the authors suggest the use of a general baseline, e.g., the Euclidean or cosine distance, or robust non-parametric deviation metrics, e.g., MMD or Kolmogorov–Smirnov statistics.

In previous work, model performance has been evaluated using metrics such as accuracy, sensitivity, specificity, precision, recall, and f1-score [1]. As class imbalance is common in most publicly available HAR datasets (see Table 2), f1-score is used as the main performance metric since it is more robust than accuracy in these settings [30]. To be able to compare deep learning models and classic models with HC features, the f1-scores are compared in tasks across different OOD scenarios and including five public HAR datasets.

4. Experiments and Results

The main purpose of this paper is to compare the performance of HC features and deep representations in different OOD settings for HAR. A scheme of the full pipeline used for the experiments is presented in Figure 4.

HAR is a classification task that usually involves multiple domains, easily turning into a domain generalization task if the domains are considered when splitting the data. We devise four domain generalization settings, starting with a baseline ID setting where 30% of each dataset is randomly sampled for testing, and three OOD settings: (a) splitting by user within the same dataset, where approximately 30% of the users were assigned to the test set—OOD by user (OOD-U); (b) leaving a dataset out for testing, while including all the others for training—OOD with multiple source datasets (OOD-MD); (c) training on a dataset and leaving another for testing, running all the possible combinations—OOD with a single source dataset (OOD-SD). To obtain a direct comparison, the test set of OOD-U is used as a test set for all the OOD settings. Of the three OOD settings, OOD-U is the one that is expected to be closest to the training distribution since it is drawn from the same dataset, where devices and acquisition conditions are usually similar. It is followed by OOD-MD, since joining all the datasets (except one) for training averages their distributions onto a more general space. Subsequently, as it includes only a single dataset for training, OOD-SD should capture the largest distances between train and test distributions.

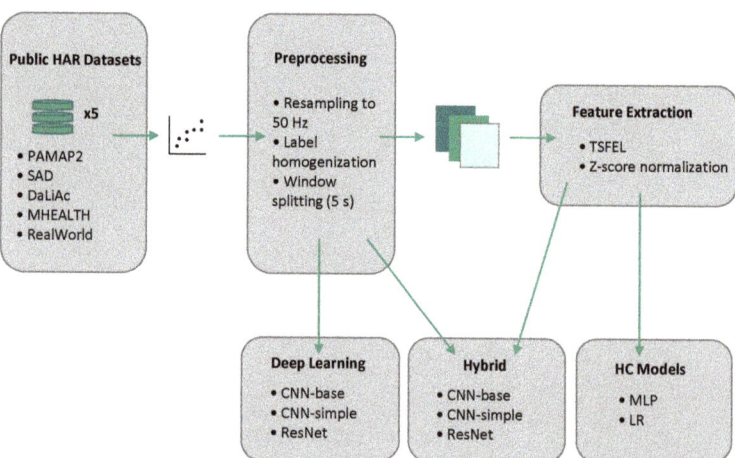

Figure 4. Scheme of the experimental pipeline.

In order to validate our hypothesis about the ordering of the distances between the train and test splits on our four settings, different metrics were applied to the feature representations. This experiment has the following objectives: (1) to validate that our three OOD settings are in fact OOD; and (2) to obtain the best metric for our main experiments, which should output values that agree with our ordering hypothesis for both HC features and deep representations. For models based on HC features, metrics were computed directly from the features. In contrast, for deep models, metrics were calculated from the hidden representations of the last layer before classification.

We note that different distance metrics have different scales, therefore, making their interpretation and comparison more difficult. For this reason, we computed distance ratios instead of raw distances, so as to make the values of the different metrics more consistent across tasks. The distance ratios were computed for each task, i.e., setting/dataset combination, using the following equation:

$$\text{Distance\_ratio} = \frac{\partial(tr_1, ts_1)}{\partial(tr_2, tr_3)},$$

(3)

where ∂ is a distance metric and tr_i and ts_i are subsets randomly sampled (with replacement) from the train and test sets, respectively. The sample size is half the minimum of the train and test set lengths. By contrast, for the DC, the raw value without any ratio-based normalization was used, since it is already normalized in the $[0, 1]$ range and is able to deal with any data representation directly.

A comparison of the considered metrics based on the TSFEL features is presented in Table 3. It is easy to observe that all the metrics agree with the OOD ordering hypothesis stated above. Indeed, the value of all metrics was higher for the OOD-U, OOD-MD, and OOD-SD (respectively, in this order) than for the ID setting. In particular, it can be seen that DC with Euclidean-based metrics saturates to values close to zero for all three OOD settings, indicating that, by the comments above on the interpretation of this score, the test sets are likely to be OOD.

Table 4 shows a comparison of the considered metrics based on the CNN-base representations. In contrast to the case of TSFEL features, the metrics showed a much lower degree of agreement with the OOD ordering hypothesis. First, it can be noted that only Wasserstein and MMD have values that clearly increase with the expected degree of OOD, being in agreement with the results of the TSFEL representations and, consequently, with our OOD ordering hypothesis. Nonetheless, it can be verified that both metrics had a large degree of variation, with the confidence intervals for the ID, OOD-U, and OOD-MD partially overlapping. In the case of DC Cosine, the score for the OOD datasets was higher than that for the ID one. This seemingly paradoxical behavior may have an intuitive geometric explanation, as it may be a consequence of the transformations that take place during training, which influence the shape of the instance space and possibly make the representations of instances that would otherwise be OOD closer to the training data manifold. In support of this hypothesis, it can be easily observed that most metrics reported a significantly different value for the OOD-SD setting than for the other OOD settings, showing that the training of the deep learning model had an important influence on the natural representation of the data manifold. In this sense, both the Wasserstein and MMD metrics seemed to be more apt at naturally adapting to this change of representation.

Table 3. Comparison of metrics over all four domain generalization settings based on the TSFEL feature representations. For each setting, values were averaged over every test set. All metrics are ratios except the ones with (*).

Metric	Setting				Avg. OOD
	ID	OOD-U	OOD-MD	OOD-SD	
Wasserstein	1.02 ± 0.04	1.42 ± 0.37	2.27 ± 1.25	3.31 ± 2.39	2.33 ± 0.91
MMD	0.95 ± 0.86	30.47 ± 56.25	800.05 ± 1513.29	1072.20 ± 2619.40	634.24 ± 1008.55
Euclidean	1.00 ± 0.01	1.08 ± 0.11	1.33 ± 0.48	1.53 ± 0.73	1.31 ± 0.29
DC Euclidean *	0.55 ± 0.10	0.05 ± 0.08	0.00 ± 0.00	0.00 ± 0.00	0.02 ± 0.03
Cosine	0.95 ± 0.33	0.85 ± 0.31	0.39 ± 0.52	0.10 ± 0.84	0.45 ± 0.35
DC Cosine *	0.60 ± 0.17	0.32 ± 0.34	0.12 ± 0.16	0.12 ± 0.21	0.19 ± 0.14

Table 4. Comparison of metrics over all four domain generalization settings based on the CNN-base representations. For each setting, values were averaged over all the datasets. All metrics are ratios except the ones with (*).

Metric	Setting				Avg. OOD
	ID	OOD-U	OOD-MD	OOD-SD	
Wasserstein	1.06 ± 0.09	1.39 ± 0.27	1.95 ± 0.45	5.71 ± 5.05	3.02 ± 1.69
MMD	1.25 ± 1.00	1.80 ± 0.92	35.23 ± 56.10	245.27 ± 402.93	94.10 ± 135.60
Euclidean	1.00 ± 0.02	1.01 ± 0.05	1.02 ± 0.15	1.12 ± 0.27	1.05 ± 0.11
DC Euclidean *	0.49 ± 0.15	0.51 ± 0.32	0.53 ± 0.45	0.10 ± 0.18	0.38 ± 0.19
Cosine	1.01 ± 0.01	0.98 ± 0.01	0.98 ± 0.03	1.03 ± 0.06	1.00 ± 0.02
DC Cosine *	0.55 ± 0.10	0.92 ± 0.10	0.65 ± 0.43	0.52 ± 0.43	0.70 ± 0.21

Thus, as a consequence of these results, we chose the Wasserstein distance ratio as our main metric to quantifiy the degree of OOD due to the fact that it agrees with our hypothesis when using both TSFEL features and deep representations as input. This metric has also been applied by Soleimani et al. [5] to compute distances between source and target distributions.

Our experiments were run on an NVIDIA (Santa Clara, CA, USA) A16-8C GPU and an AMD (Santa Clara, CA, USA) Epyc 7302 processor with python version 3.8.12 and Visual Studio Code (Microsoft, Redmond, WA, USA) as the development environment. All the learning models were implemented using the PyTorch library [54]. Adam [55] was adopted as the optimizer used for the training process. To reduce bias [16], results were averaged over nine combinations of three different batch sizes (64, 128, and 256) and three learning rates (0.0008, 0.001, and 0.003). To account for class imbalance, the percentage of instances per class in the training set was given to the cross-entropy loss function as class weights.

To make the experiments as agnostic to the training method as possible, the same procedure was used for training the classifiers based on HC features and the deep learning models. Figure 5 shows the training and validation loss over the course of training for a single task. The chosen task was the OOD-U setting on the SAD dataset, an example of a task in which there was a verified occurrence of instability in training. One of the ways to handle this instability is by ending the training process earlier—early stopping [56].

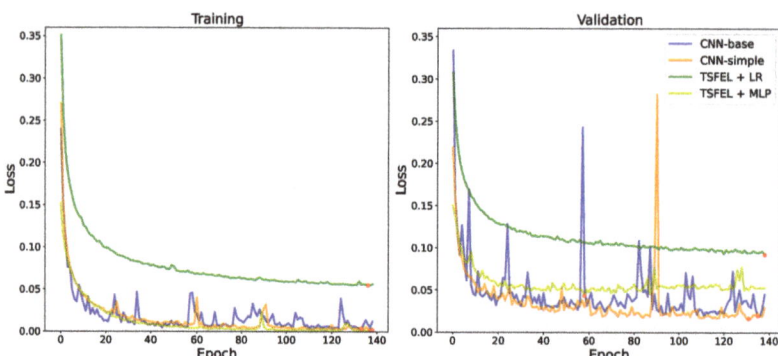

Figure 5. Evolution of loss by epoch on SAD dataset in the OOD-U setting. The red dots indicate the minimum loss of each curve.

Over all the tasks, most models reached plateaus on validation performance after 30 to 50 epochs, so the training process was limited to 140 epochs to leave a margin for models to converge, but not so much as to fully overfit the data. For validation, we randomly sampled a 10% subset of the training data without replacement. While training, a checkpoint model was saved every time the validation loss achieved its best value since the start of training. Our early stopping method consisted of stopping training if the validation loss did not improve for 30 epochs in a row, which proved helpful in cases where training was not very stable. In these cases, the validation error oscillates, increasing for a certain number of epochs before decreasing again and, on many occasions, achieving a slightly lower error rate than in any of the previous epochs, which can be seen in the loss curves for the CNN models in Figure 5. This resembles the effects of double descent [57]. In our case, one of the causes of such unstable training may be the fact that these datasets are noisy, due to the diversity in users, devices, and positions, among other factors. It may also be a consequence of overparameterization, as the phenomenon was much more pronounced when training CNNs, which have significantly more parameters than our MLP and LR models. Both these potential causes were documented by Nakkiran et al. [57].

The evolution of the f1-score over the Wasserstein distance ratio for the best performing model of each family (CNN-base and TSFEL+LR) is documented in Figure 6. For each combination of model, dataset, and setting, the average and standard deviation of the f1-score were computed over nine different runs with varying learning rates and batch sizes. The CNN-base embeddings were chosen to compute distance ratios for this figure since they contain less outliers when compared to the distance ratios computed from TSFEL representations (see Figure A2). It can be verified that, initially, the CNN model outperforms the model using HC features. However, as the distance between train and test domains increases, the situation is reverted, with the classic approach outperforming the CNN. This suggests that HC features are more robust to the shifts that occur in OOD data. The regression curves reinforce the idea of OOD stability. As expected, there is a negative correlation between f1-score and distance ratio, meaning that performance decreases as the test data becomes more distant from the distribution seen during training. In general, the distance ratios given by the Wasserstein distance appear to agree with the previously stated OOD ordering hypothesis, with OOD-SD being the most OOD of the three settings, followed by OOD-MD and OOD-U, respectively. Still, a few outliers can be seen in the figure. The higher values of standard deviation for the CNN indicate that these models are more susceptible to the choice of hyperparameters, which is reasonable due to the much larger number of trainable parameters. However, it is not always ideal to have such variability, as it indicates that the validation loss has become less correlated with the test loss. In practice, an apparently good model may perform surprisingly well in some settings while failing in situations that would otherwise be trivial to a simple model.

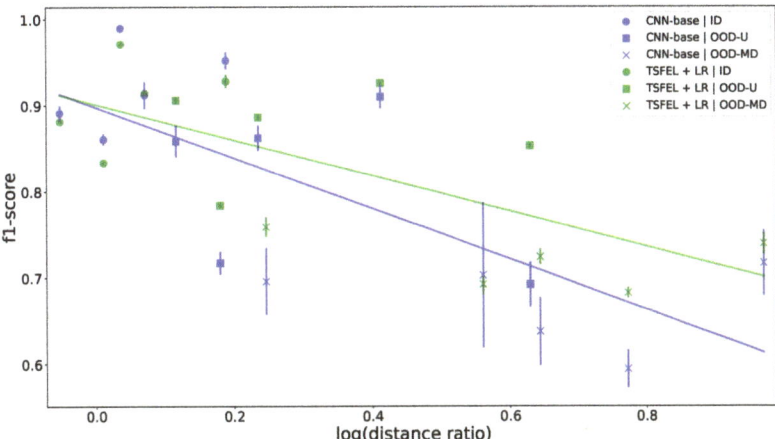

Figure 6. F1-score vs. log(distance ratio). Each marker represents a different task. Distance ratios are based on the CNN-base embeddings. Error bars represent one standard deviation away from the mean. The natural logarithm was applied to the distance ratios to make the regression curves linear.

More detailed results are presented in Table 5. For each combination of model and setting, the average and standard deviation of the f1-score were computed over all five datasets. The last column represents the average of the three OOD settings, which gives an idea of the overall generalization performance. The significant overturn from the ID to the OOD settings can be noticed in the table. TSFEL + LR, which had the worst ID f1-score (90.54%), turned out to be the best overall in the OOD regime, with an f1-score of 70% for the average of all three OOD settings. Using an MLP instead of LR slightly decreased the overall OOD performance to 69.55%, while increasing the ID performance to 92.87%, becoming closer to the deep learning results. This phenomenon may be related to an increase in the number of trainable parameters. Including HC features as an auxiliary input to deep models improved both ID and OOD results, with the hybrid version of CNN-base being the deep learning model with the strongest generalization performance (average OOD f1-score of 66.95%). However, this improvement is still insufficient to reach the OOD robustness of models solely based on HC features.

Table 5. Average f1-score in percentage over all the tasks in a given setting. Values in bold indicate the best performance for each setting.

Model	Setting				Avg. OOD
	ID	OOD-U	OOD-MD	OOD-SD	
CNN-simple	92.09 ± 5.26	79.65 ± 10.75	63.71 ± 3.54	45.21 ± 6.57	62.86 ± 4.36
CNN-base	92.10 ± 5.06	80.79 ± 9.68	66.94 ± 5.19	48.30 ± 5.41	65.34 ± 4.08
ResNet	92.46 ± 4.73	81.16 ± 9.60	67.22 ± 4.89	46.57 ± 4.84	64.98 ± 3.94
CNN-simple hybrid	93.64 ± 4.55	85.13 ± 7.69	66.60 ± 3.31	47.87 ± 2.21	66.53 ± 2.89
CNN-base hybrid	93.48 ± 4.35	85.28 ± 6.64	67.74 ± 3.37	47.84 ± 3.24	66.95 ± 2.71
ResNet hybrid	$\mathbf{93.79 \pm 4.21}$	84.71 ± 7.72	67.87 ± 3.40	47.73 ± 2.11	66.77 ± 2.90
TSFEL + MLP	92.87 ± 4.70	$\mathbf{87.09 \pm 5.35}$	70.11 ± 3.57	$\mathbf{51.45 \pm 5.31}$	69.55 ± 2.78
TSFEL + LR	90.54 ± 5.15	87.08 ± 5.55	$\mathbf{71.94 \pm 3.19}$	50.97 ± 3.29	$\mathbf{70.00 \pm 2.40}$

Despite being simpler than the ResNet, the CNN-base model achieves a slightly higher generalization performance. On the other hand, CNN-simple, the simplest deep learning model, did not perform well in OOD tasks. There appears to be an optimal number of parameters, possibly dependent on the architecture, so more studies should be conducted to understand this trade-off.

5. Discussion

This work aimed to compare the generalization performance of HC features and deep representations, focusing in particular on generalization in OOD settings.

In the first experiment, several metrics were compared to validate and quantify our OOD settings. For TSFEL representations, all the considered metrics were in agreement with our ordering hypothesis. In particular, the DC was able to clearly identify each of the OOD settings as such. In contrast, for the case of deep representations, there was some disagreement among the considered metrics. Still, the MMD and Wasserstein distance ratios remained in agreement with the adopted hypothesis. They were seen as more robust concerning the change of data representation induced by the deep learning model.

In our experiments involving HAR tasks, despite reaching lower f1-scores in the ID setting, models based on HC features were more robust in OOD settings. This difference in OOD performance supporting higher robustness for HC features may be due to their stability since they are fixed a priori based on domain knowledge, which should be valid across tasks. Conversely, deep features are automatically learned and could thus fail to identify generally helpful features, as there are known inefficiencies in the current methods for training neural networks. These are typically biased toward simple solutions [15] and rely on spurious correlations [10] rather than previous knowledge or causal relations.

In regard to the generalizability of our results to other settings, we note that even though we focused on HAR, with minor adaptations, our experiments and analyses could be replicated in a wide range of fields. For example, similar deep learning models and handcrafted features could be used and compared in fields that depend on sensor data, such as fall detection, predictive maintenance, or physiological signal processing (e.g., EEG, EMG, and ECG). Different deep learning architectures and feature extraction libraries would have to be employed for image or video processing.

Concerning practical purposes, HC features, being more robust, appear to be better suited for real-world HAR systems. However, their reimplementation in mobile or edge devices may be an arduous task. CNNs do not show this limitation, as the representations are encoded in weight matrices and can, in principle, be ported to these devices without significant effort [58]. More studies should, thus, be devoted to exploring this trade-off between increased robustness and reimplementation efforts, possibly considering the application of hybrid approaches (such as the ones also considered in this paper), as well as alternative training techniques for CNNs that attempt to improve robustness.

6. Conclusions

This paper hypothesizes that models using HC features generalize better than deep learning models across domains in HAR tasks. Three OOD settings were implemented by testing on unseen users and (single or multi-source) datasets. Five public datasets were homogenized so that they could be combined in different ways to create diverse tasks.

Several metrics were used to quantify the degree of OOD of four domain generalization settings. The DC metric was used to validate our OOD settings. In turn, the Wasserstein distance ratio was chosen as our primary metric for the study since it was able to quantify our three OOD settings in the expected order.

In our main experiments, it was verified that, although deep models have better ID performance, they are outperformed in all three OOD settings by shallow models using features that were computed based on domain knowledge. Furthermore, as the drop in f1-score in OOD settings is less accentuated for classic models, it can be inferred that HC are more robust. Hybrid models achieved intermediate results between deep and classic methods, supporting the idea that HC features can stabilize training, which helps to validate our hypothesis.

Acknowledging the limitation of current deep learning techniques in being robust with respect to OOD settings, as compared to models based on HC features, we believe our work could pave the way for further research on the development of novel training methods for making deep learning models more robust and thus bridge the generalization gap toward new, more trustworthy, gold standards in the field of HAR.

Author Contributions: Conceptualization , N.B., J.R., M.B. and A.V.C.; data curation, N.B., J.R. and M.B.; methodology, N.B., J.R., M.B., A.V.C. and A.C.; software, N.B. and J.R.; validation, N.B., J.R., M.B., A.V.C. and A.C.; formal analysis, N.B., J.R. and A.C.; writing—original draft preparation, N.B.; writing—review and editing, N.B., J.R., M.B., A.V.C., A.C., F.C. and H.G.; visualization, N.B., J.R. and M.B.; supervision, M.B., A.V.C., F.C. and H.G. All authors have read and agreed to the published version of the manuscript.

Funding: This work is financed by national funds through FCT—Fundação para a Ciência e a Tecnologia, I.P., within the scope of SAIFFER project under the Eureka Eurostars program (E!114310).

Institutional Review Board Statement: Not applicable.

Informed Consent Statement: Not applicable.

Data Availability Statement: Not applicable.

Conflicts of Interest: The authors declare no conflict of interest.

Appendix A. Supplementary Experiments

Figure A1 shows the behavior of different models over all four domain generalization settings addressed in the study in comparison to TSFEL+LR, the approach with the highest generalization performance. Similarly to the main results, an inversion tendency can be observed from the ID to the OOD regime.

Figure A1a shows a larger gap in performance for the OOD regime. This gap is mitigated in the hybrid model (Figure A1b) and becomes much smaller in Figure A1c, where handcrafted features are the only source of information.

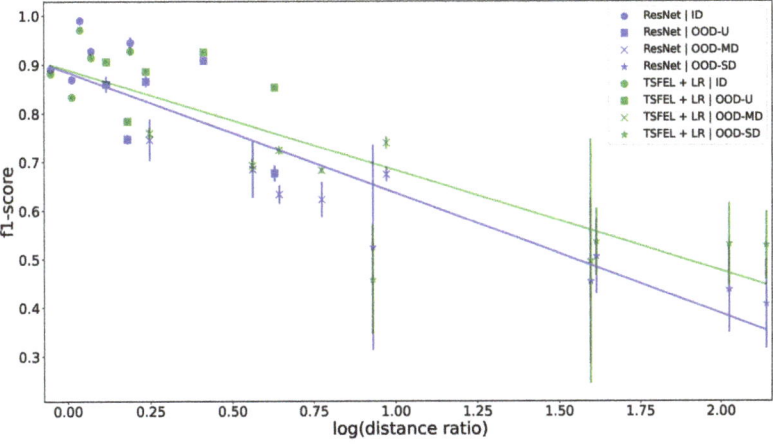

(a)

Figure A1. *Cont.*

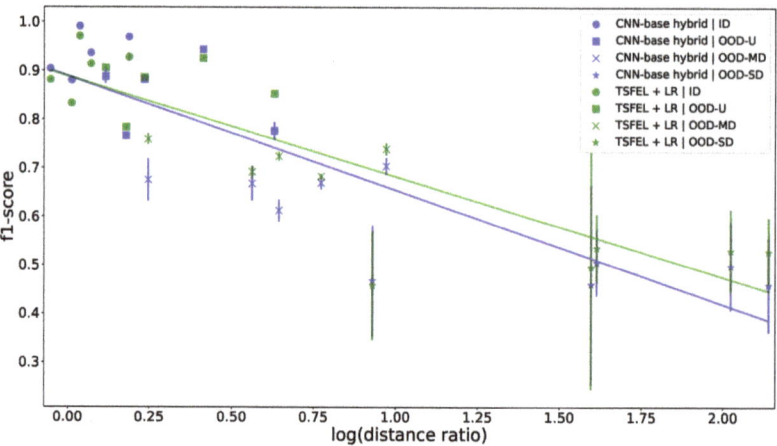

(b)

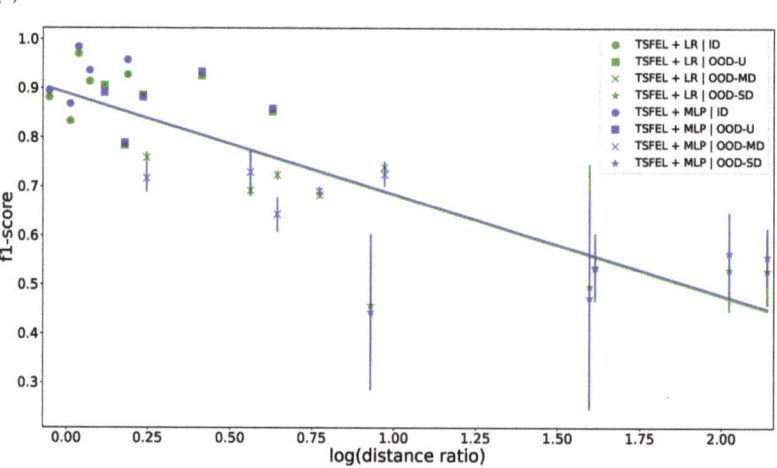

(c)

Figure A1. F1-score vs. log(distance ratio). Each marker represents a different task. Distance ratios are based on the CNN-base embeddings. Error bars represent one standard deviation away from the mean. (**a**) TSFEL + LR vs. ResNet. (**b**) TSFEL + LR vs. CNN-base hybrid. (**c**) TSFEL + LR vs. TSFEL + MLP.

By using TSFEL features to compute the distance ratios (see Figure A2), we reach the same conclusions. However, the plots in Figures 6 and A1 were based on the CNN-base embeddings, as the distance ratios presented less outliers.

Figure A3 shows the confusion matrices for the ID, OOD-U, and OOD-MD settings of the SAD dataset. It can be verified that, as expected, performance decreased in OOD settings.

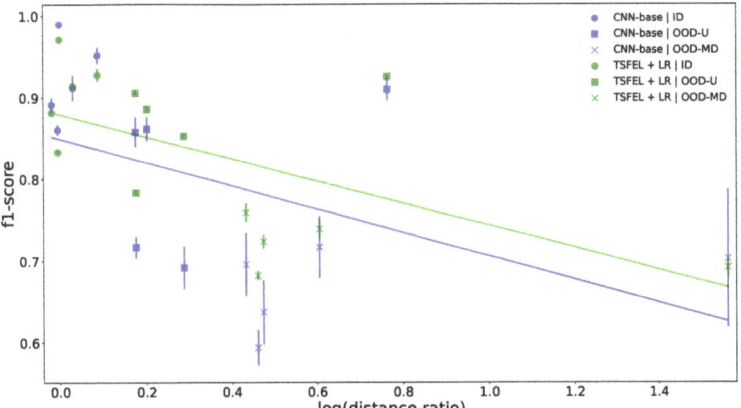

Figure A2. TSFEL + LR vs. CNN-base. Distance ratios are based on TSFEL features.

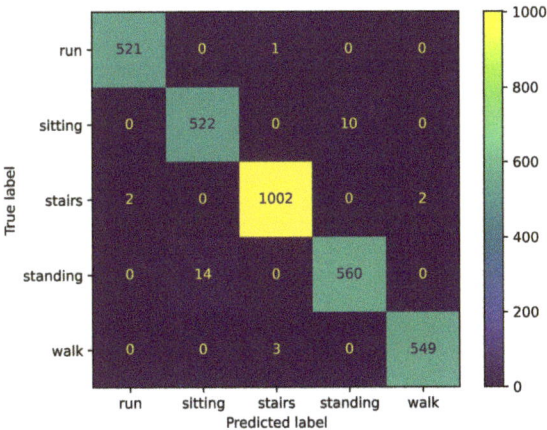

(a)

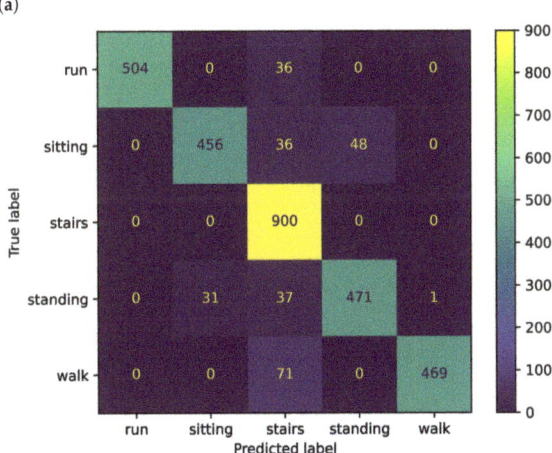

(b)

Figure A3. *Cont.*

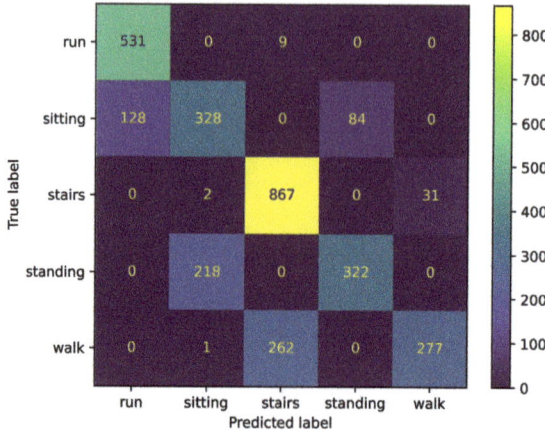

(c)

Figure A3. Confusion matrices for the SAD dataset. (**a**) In-distribution (ID). Accuracy: 99.0%, F1-score: 98.9%; (**b**) Out-of-Distribution leaving users out (OOD-U). Accuracy: 91.5%, F1-score: 91.6%; (**c**) Out-of-Distribution leaving a dataset out (OOD-MD). Accuracy: 76.0%, F1-score: 73.5%.

References

1. Sousa Lima, W.; Souto, E.; El-Khatib, K.; Jalali, R.; Gama, J. Human activity recognition using inertial sensors in a smartphone: An overview. *Sensors* **2019**, *19*, 3213. [CrossRef] [PubMed]
2. Ariza-Colpas, P.P.; Vicario, E.; Oviedo-Carrascal, A.I.; Butt Aziz, S.; Piñeres-Melo, M.A.; Quintero-Linero, A.; Patara, F. Human Activity Recognition Data Analysis: History, Evolutions, and New Trends. *Sensors* **2022**, *22*, 3401. [CrossRef] [PubMed]
3. Ahmad, N.; Ghazilla, R.A.R.; Khairi, N.M.; Kasi, V. Reviews on various inertial measurement unit (IMU) sensor applications. *Int. J. Signal Process. Syst.* **2013**, *1*, 256–262. [CrossRef]
4. Li, F.; Shirahama, K.; Nisar, M.A.; Köping, L.; Grzegorzek, M. Comparison of feature learning methods for human activity recognition using wearable sensors. *Sensors* **2018**, *18*, 679. [CrossRef] [PubMed]
5. Soleimani, E.; Nazerfard, E. Cross-subject transfer learning in human activity recognition systems using generative adversarial networks. *Neurocomputing* **2021**, *426*, 26–34. [CrossRef]
6. Wang, J.; Zheng, V.W.; Chen, Y.; Huang, M. Deep transfer learning for cross-domain activity recognition. In Proceedings of the 3rd International Conference on Crowd Science and Engineering, Singapore, 28–31 July 2018; pp. 1–8.
7. Hoelzemann, A.; Van Laerhoven, K. Digging deeper: Towards a better understanding of transfer learning for human activity recognition. In Proceedings of the 2020 International Symposium on Wearable Computers, Virtual, 12–16 September 2020; pp. 50–54.
8. Wang, J.; Chen, Y.; Hao, S.; Peng, X.; Hu, L. Deep learning for sensor-based activity recognition: A survey. *Pattern Recognit. Lett.* **2019**, *119*, 3–11. [CrossRef]
9. Nafea, O.; Abdul, W.; Muhammad, G.; Alsulaiman, M. Sensor-based human activity recognition with spatio-temporal deep learning. *Sensors* **2021**, *21*, 2141. [CrossRef]
10. Sagawa, S.; Raghunathan, A.; Koh, P.W.; Liang, P. An investigation of why overparameterization exacerbates spurious correlations. In Proceedings of the 37th International Conference on Machine Learning, Virtual Conference, 13–18 July 2020; pp. 8346–8356.
11. Arjovsky, M.; Bottou, L.; Gulrajani, I.; Lopez-Paz, D. Invariant risk minimization. *arXiv* **2019**, arXiv:1907.02893.
12. Barandas, M.; Folgado, D.; Fernandes, L.; Santos, S.; Abreu, M.; Bota, P.; Liu, H.; Schultz, T.; Gamboa, H. TSFEL: Time series feature extraction library. *SoftwareX* **2020**, *11*, 100456. [CrossRef]
13. Chen, Y.; Xue, Y. A deep learning approach to human activity recognition based on single accelerometer. In Proceedings of the 2015 IEEE International Conference on Systems, Man, and Cybernetics, Hong Kong, China, 9–12 October 2015; pp. 1488–1492.
14. Zebin, T.; Scully, P.J.; Ozanyan, K.B. Human activity recognition with inertial sensors using a deep learning approach. In Proceedings of the 2016 IEEE Sensors, Orlando, FL, USA, 30 October 2016–3 November 2016; pp. 1–3.
15. Geirhos, R.; Jacobsen, J.H.; Michaelis, C.; Zemel, R.; Brendel, W.; Bethge, M.; Wichmann, F.A. Shortcut learning in deep neural networks. *Nat. Mach. Intell.* **2020**, *2*, 665–673. [CrossRef]
16. Gagnon-Audet, J.C.; Ahuja, K.; Darvishi-Bayazi, M.J.; Dumas, G.; Rish, I. WOODS: Benchmarks for Out-of-Distribution Generalization in Time Series Tasks. *arXiv* **2022**, arXiv:2203.09978.

17. Lee, S.M.; Yoon, S.M.; Cho, H. Human activity recognition from accelerometer data using Convolutional Neural Network. In Proceedings of the 2017 IEEE International Conference on Big Data and Smart Computing (Bigcomp), Jeju, Korea, 13–16 February 2017; pp. 131–134.
18. Ferrari, A.; Micucci, D.; Mobilio, M.; Napoletano, P. Hand-crafted features vs residual networks for human activities recognition using accelerometer. In Proceedings of the 2019 IEEE 23rd International Symposium on Consumer Technologies (ISCT), Ancona, Italy, 19–21 June 2019; pp. 153–156.
19. Balcan, M.F.; Blum, A.; Srebro, N. A theory of learning with similarity functions. *Mach. Learn.* **2008**, *72*, 89–112. [CrossRef]
20. Bousquet, N. Diagnostics of prior-data agreement in applied Bayesian analysis. *J. Appl. Stat.* **2008**, *35*, 1011–1029. [CrossRef]
21. Kouw, W.M.; Loog, M.; Bartels, L.W.; Mendrik, A.M. Learning an MR acquisition-invariant representation using Siamese neural networks. In Proceedings of the 2019 IEEE 16th International Symposium on Biomedical Imaging (ISBI 2019), Venice, Italy, 8–11 April 2019; pp. 364–367.
22. Redko, I.; Morvant, E.; Habrard, A.; Sebban, M.; Bennani, Y. *Advances in Domain Adaptation Theory*; Elsevier: Amsterdam, The Netherlands, 2019.
23. Veen, D.; Stoel, D.; Schalken, N.; Mulder, K.; Van de Schoot, R. Using the data agreement criterion to rank experts' beliefs. *Entropy* **2018**, *20*, 592. [CrossRef] [PubMed]
24. Schat, E.; van de Schoot, R.; Kouw, W.M.; Veen, D.; Mendrik, A.M. The data representativeness criterion: Predicting the performance of supervised classification based on data set similarity. *PLoS ONE* **2020**, *15*, e0237009. [CrossRef]
25. Cabitza, F.; Campagner, A.; Soares, F.; de Guadiana-Romualdo, L.G.; Challa, F.; Sulejmani, A.; Seghezzi, M.; Carobene, A. The importance of being external. methodological insights for the external validation of machine learning models in medicine. *Comput. Methods Programs Biomed.* **2021**, *208*, 106288. [CrossRef]
26. Tzeng, E.; Hoffman, J.; Zhang, N.; Saenko, K.; Darrell, T. Deep domain confusion: Maximizing for domain invariance. *arXiv* **2014**, arXiv:1412.3474.
27. Zhou, F.; Jiang, Z.; Shui, C.; Wang, B.; Chaib-draa, B. Domain generalization with optimal transport and metric learning. *arXiv* **2020**, arXiv:2007.10573.
28. Shen, Z.; Liu, J.; He, Y.; Zhang, X.; Xu, R.; Yu, H.; Cui, P. Towards out-of-distribution generalization: A survey. *arXiv* **2021**, arXiv:2108.13624.
29. Ronao, C.A.; Cho, S.B. Human activity recognition with smartphone sensors using deep learning neural networks. *Expert Syst. Appl.* **2016**, *59*, 235–244. [CrossRef]
30. Logacjov, A.; Bach, K.; Kongsvold, A.; Bårdstu, H.B.; Mork, P.J. HARTH: A Human Activity Recognition Dataset for Machine Learning. *Sensors* **2021**, *21*, 7853. [CrossRef] [PubMed]
31. Xu, C.; Chai, D.; He, J.; Zhang, X.; Duan, S. InnoHAR: A deep neural network for complex human activity recognition. *IEEE Access* **2019**, *7*, 9893–9902. [CrossRef]
32. Moreira, D.; Barandas, M.; Rocha, T.; Alves, P.; Santos, R.; Leonardo, R.; Vieira, P.; Gamboa, H. Human Activity Recognition for Indoor Localization Using Smartphone Inertial Sensors. *Sensors* **2021**, *21*, 6316. [CrossRef] [PubMed]
33. Gholamiangonabadi, D.; Kiselov, N.; Grolinger, K. Deep neural networks for human activity recognition with wearable sensors: Leave-one-subject-out cross-validation for model selection. *IEEE Access* **2020**, *8*, 133982–133994. [CrossRef]
34. Bragança, H.; Colonna, J.G.; Oliveira, H.A.B.F.; Souto, E. How Validation Methodology Influences Human Activity Recognition Mobile Systems. *Sensors* **2022**, *22*, 2360. [CrossRef]
35. Ding, R.; Li, X.; Nie, L.; Li, J.; Si, X.; Chu, D.; Liu, G.; Zhan, D. Empirical study and improvement on deep transfer learning for human activity recognition. *Sensors* **2019**, *19*, 57. [CrossRef] [PubMed]
36. Ahuja, K.; Caballero, E.; Zhang, D.; Gagnon-Audet, J.C.; Bengio, Y.; Mitliagkas, I.; Rish, I. Invariance principle meets information bottleneck for out-of-distribution generalization. *Adv. Neural Inf. Process. Syst.* **2021**, *34*, 3438–3450.
37. Rosenfeld, E.; Ravikumar, P.; Risteski, A. The risks of invariant risk minimization. *arXiv* **2020**, arXiv:2010.05761.
38. Boyer, P.; Burns, D.; Whyne, C. Out-of-distribution detection of human activity recognition with smartwatch inertial sensors. *Sensors* **2021**, *21*, 1669. [CrossRef]
39. Trabelsi, I.; Françoise, J.; Bellik, Y. Sensor-based Activity Recognition using Deep Learning: A Comparative Study. In Proceedings of the 8th International Conference on Movement and Computing, Chicago, IL, USA, 22–24 June 2022; pp. 1–8.
40. Reiss, A.; Stricker, D. Introducing a New Benchmarked Dataset for Activity Monitoring. In Proceedings of the 2012 16th Annual International Symposium on Wearable Computers (ISWC), Newcastle, UK, 18–22 June 2012; IEEE Computer Society: Washington, DC, USA, 2012; pp. 108–109. [CrossRef]
41. Reiss, A.; Stricker, D. Creating and Benchmarking a New Dataset for Physical Activity Monitoring. In *Proceedings of the 5th International Conference on PErvasive Technologies Related to Assistive Environments, Heraklion, Greece, 6–8 July 2012*; Association for Computing Machinery: New York, NY, USA, 2012. [CrossRef]
42. Shoaib, M.; Bosch, S.; Incel, O.D.; Scholten, H.; Havinga, P.J. Fusion of smartphone motion sensors for physical activity recognition. *Sensors* **2014**, *14*, 10146–10176. [CrossRef]
43. Leutheuser, H.; Schuldhaus, D.; Eskofier, B.M. Hierarchical, Multi-Sensor Based Classification of Daily Life Activities: Comparison with State-of-the-Art Algorithms Using a Benchmark Dataset. *PLoS ONE* **2013**, *8*. [CrossRef] [PubMed]

44. Banos, O.; Garcia, R.; Holgado-Terriza, J.A.; Damas, M.; Pomares, H.; Rojas, I.; Saez, A.; Villalonga, C. mHealthDroid: A Novel Framework for Agile Development of Mobile Health Applications. In *Ambient Assisted Living and Daily Activities*; Pecchia, L., Chen, L.L., Nugent, C., Bravo, J., Eds.; Springer International Publishing: Cham, Switzerland, 2014; pp. 91–98. [CrossRef]
45. Banos, O.; Villalonga, C.; Garcia, R.; Saez, A.; Damas, M.; Holgado-Terriza, J.A.; Lee, S.; Pomares, H.; Rojas, I. Design, implementation and validation of a novel open framework for agile development of mobile health applications. *BioMed. Eng. Online* **2015**, *14*. [CrossRef] [PubMed]
46. Sztyler, T.; Stuckenschmidt, H. On-body Localization of Wearable Devices: An Investigation of Position-Aware Activity Recognition. In Proceedings of the 2016 IEEE International Conference on Pervasive Computing and Communications (PerCom), Sydney, NSW, Australia, 14–19 March 2016; pp. 1–9. [CrossRef]
47. Ferrari, A.; Mobilio, M.; Micucci, D.; Napoletano, P. On the homogenization of heterogeneous inertial-based databases for human activity recognition. In Proceedings of the 2019 IEEE World Congress on Services (SERVICES), Milan, Italy, 8–13 July 2019; Volume 2642, pp. 295–300.
48. Figueira, C.; Matias, R.; Gamboa, H. Body Location Independent Activity Monitoring. In Proceedings of the 9th International Conference on Bio-inspired Systems and Signal Processing, Rome, Italy, 21–23 February 2016.
49. Shakya, S.R.; Zhang, C.; Zhou, Z. Comparative study of machine learning and deep learning architecture for human activity recognition using accelerometer data. *Int. J. Mach. Learn. Comput.* **2018**, *8*, 577–582.
50. Shiranthika, C.; Premakumara, N.; Chiu, H.L.; Samani, H.; Shyalika, C.; Yang, C.Y. Human Activity Recognition Using CNN & LSTM. In Proceedings of the 2020 5th International Conference on Information Technology Research (ICITR), Online, 2–4 December 2020; pp. 1–6.
51. Arjovsky, M.; Chintala, S.; Bottou, L. Wasserstein generative adversarial networks. In Proceedings of the 34th International Conference on Machine Learning, Sydney, Australia, 6–11 August 2017; pp. 214–223.
52. Gretton, A.; Borgwardt, K.M.; Rasch, M.J.; Schölkopf, B.; Smola, A. A kernel two-sample test. *J. Mach. Learn. Res.* **2012**, *13*, 723–773.
53. Cabitza, F.; Campagner, A.; Sconfienza, L.M. As if sand were stone. New concepts and metrics to probe the ground on which to build trustable AI. *BMC Med. Inform. Decis. Mak.* **2020**, *20*, 1–21. [CrossRef] [PubMed]
54. Paszke, A.; Gross, S.; Massa, F.; Lerer, A.; Bradbury, J.; Chanan, G.; Killeen, T.; Lin, Z.; Gimelshein, N.; Antiga, L.; et al. Pytorch: An imperative style, high-performance deep learning library. In Proceedings of the 33rd Conference on Neural Information Processing Systems (NeurIPS 2019), Vancouver, BC, Canada, 8–14 December 2019.
55. Kingma, D.P.; Ba, J. Adam: A method for stochastic optimization. *arXiv* **2014**, arXiv:1412.6980.
56. Heckel, R.; Yilmaz, F.F. Early stopping in deep networks: Double descent and how to eliminate it. *arXiv* **2020**, arXiv:2007.10099.
57. Nakkiran, P.; Kaplun, G.; Bansal, Y.; Yang, T.; Barak, B.; Sutskever, I. Deep double descent: Where bigger models and more data hurt. *J. Stat. Mech. Theory Exp.* **2021**, *2021*, 124003. [CrossRef]
58. Bai, J.; Lu, F.; Zhang, K. ONNX: Open Neural Network Exchange. Available online: https://github.com/onnx/onnx (accessed on 26 September 2022).

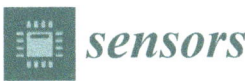

MDPI

Article

Semi-Supervised Adversarial Learning Using LSTM for Human Activity Recognition

Sung-Hyun Yang, Dong-Gwon Baek and Keshav Thapa *

Department of Electronic Engineering, Kwangwoon University, Seoul 01897, Korea; shyang@kw.ac.kr (S.-H.Y.); whitedk@kw.ac.kr (D.-G.B.)
* Correspondence: kshavthapa@kw.ac.kr

Abstract: The training of Human Activity Recognition (HAR) models requires a substantial amount of labeled data. Unfortunately, despite being trained on enormous datasets, most current models have poor performance rates when evaluated against anonymous data from new users. Furthermore, due to the limits and problems of working with human users, capturing adequate data for each new user is not feasible. This paper presents semi-supervised adversarial learning using the LSTM (Long-short term memory) approach for human activity recognition. This proposed method trains annotated and unannotated data (anonymous data) by adapting the semi-supervised learning paradigms on which adversarial learning capitalizes to improve the learning capabilities in dealing with errors that appear in the process. Moreover, it adapts to the change in human activity routine and new activities, i.e., it does not require prior understanding and historical information. Simultaneously, this method is designed as a temporal interactive model instantiation and shows the capacity to estimate heteroscedastic uncertainty owing to inherent data ambiguity. Our methodology also benefits from multiple parallel input sequential data predicting an output exploiting the synchronized LSTM. The proposed method proved to be the best state-of-the-art method with more than 98% accuracy in implementation utilizing the publicly available datasets collected from the smart home environment facilitated with heterogeneous sensors. This technique is a novel approach for high-level human activity recognition and is likely to be a broad application prospect for HAR.

Keywords: HAR; semi-supervised learning; adversarial learning; syn-LSTM; smart home

Citation: Yang, S.-H.; Baek, D.-G.; Thapa, K. Semi-Supervised Adversarial Learning Using LSTM for Human Activity Recognition. *Sensors* **2022**, *22*, 4755. https://doi.org/10.3390/s22134755

Academic Editors: Christian Haubelt, Hugo Gamboa, Tanja Schultz and Hui Liu

Received: 13 May 2022
Accepted: 20 June 2022
Published: 23 June 2022

Publisher's Note: MDPI stays neutral with regard to jurisdictional claims in published maps and institutional affiliations.

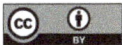

1. Introduction

Human activity recognition has been a concern in Artificial intelligence (AI) research for decades. However, the many proposed approaches face challenges in recognizing human activity accurately and precisely. The HAR system has gained popularity in recent years because of the progress of ubiquitous sensing devices and their capacity to solve specified problems like privacy [1]. HAR systems deployments to the real world in applications such as ambient assisted living (AAL), personal health [2], elderly care [3], defences [4], astronauts [5], and smart homes [6] are potentially increasing. However, there are challenges in the existing techniques to recognize activities substantially since they are now required to account for all unanticipated changes in the real-time scenario.

For example, in this pandemic situation, a COVID-19 patient needs isolation and can be monitored and treated without hospitalization to reduce the burden on isolation centres and hospitals. Sometimes users might modify their schedule of activities without prior knowledge. However, we could anticipate that the system could swiftly understand such new changes; in real-world situations, all these changes are inevitable [7].

Current efforts at HAR focus primarily on detecting changes—finding new activities [8,9] and learning actively—acquiring user annotations about new activities [10]. When a new activity class is added, they must reconstruct and retrain the model from scratch. Some researchers have investigated how an activity model with different activities might develop automatically [11]. This capacity, however, offers the advantage of keeping the knowledge in the business model that has been built through time while lowering training costs, manual configuration and manual feature engineering. Various supervised [12] and semi-supervised [13] methods for activity recognition have been presented. These models provide good accuracy with sufficient data on training. However, their performance from new, undiscovered distributions drops drastically. Therefore, detecting a new user's activity remains challenging for the model. Most machine learning [14] and deep learning [15] are not conceptually aware of all activities, but they can efficiently recognize human activity with the proper learning and models. The deep neural network is the underlying model for many artificial intelligence models and state-of-art methods. However, deep learning demands a significant amount of data to be a label for learning. Nonetheless, due to practical constraints, some fields of inquiry have data collecting and labeling limitations. As a result, providing enough labeled data in many circumstances is not viable. In the AAL domain, particularly the sensor-based Human Activity Recognition (HAR) problem, data acquisition and labeling tasks necessitate the involvement of human annotators and the use of pervasive and intrusive sensors. Furthermore, the expense of manual annotation, especially for massive datasets, is prohibitively high.

There are two needs for recognizing human activity: improving accuracy, developing trustworthy algorithms to tackle new users, and changing regular activity schedule issues. Therefore, our strategy ensures that the activity identification is addressed mainly through improved performance over previous approaches. This work emphasizes recognition activity by accompanying semi-supervised and adversarial learning on a synchronized LSTM model. To need a system to have the relevant data and ensure that no labels based on the previously learned data can be fully anticipated. Furthermore, this technique could improve performance by utilizing fewer labeling classes. Our method's highlights are as follows:

- We present semi-supervised and adversarial learning using a synchronized LSTM model to recognize human activity with competitive accuracy.
- The model understands new changes and learns accordingly with reduced error rates; in real-world situations, all these changes are inevitable.
- LSTM is the unsupervised model, but we train it in a semi-supervised feature with a synchronized parallel manner. Therefore, the proposed approach is also an adapted version of LSTM.
- The proposed joint model can structure and learn Spatio-temporal features directly and automatically from the raw sensor data without manual feature extraction. As a result, the model can train unannotated data more easily and conveniently.
- This framework can likely be applied to various recognition domains, platforms, and applications such as natural language processing (NLP), PQRS-detection, fault detection, facial recognition, etc.
- This method could be the best-suited state-of-the-art method for human activity recognition because of its high-level activity recognition ability with reduced errors and increased accuracy.

The proposed method can be used as the external sensor deployment method for a mix of several sensor deployment methods like wearable, external, camera, or all For the user's convenience. But we evaluated and compared using fully-added real-world data sets collected from external sensors deployed in various corners of the house and apartment from Kasteren and Adaptive System Advanced Studies Center (CASAS). The remaining documents are arranged accordingly. Section 2 describes related work. Section 3 shows our recommended technique. Section 4 provides the experiment set-up, analysis and assessment. Finally, the paper ends in Section 5.

2. Related Work

The activity was identified via heterogeneous sensors, wearable sensors, and cameras for ambient assistive living and monitoring [16]. An innovative HAR method uses body-worn sensors that partition the activity into sequences of shared, meaningful and distinguishing states known as Motion Units [17], i.e., a generalized sequence modeling method. However, the external sensor is on researchers' choice because of body and personal issues [18]. Many approaches that use techniques like deep learning, transfer learning, and adversarial learning are proposed in the state-of-art strategies for HAR. In [19], active learning methodologies for scaling activity recognition apply dynamic k-means clustering. Active learning reduces the labeling effort in the data collecting and classification pipeline. On the other hand, feature extraction is considered a classification problem. [20] evaluates human activities based on unique combinations of interpretable categorical high-level features with applications to classification, learning, cross comparison, combination and analysis of dataset and sensor. Despite all of the improvements made in the suggested model, such as the computational cost reduction, the approaches are still prone to underfitting due to their poor generalization capacity [21].

A machine learning Naive Bayes classifier recognizes the most prolonged sensor data sequences [22]. A progressive learning technique dubbed the dynamic Bayesian network has been explored by re-establishing previously learned models to identify activity variation [23]. To extract task-independent feature representations from early generative models, deep learning approaches have been employed on Boltzman machines [24]. More sophisticated models like CNN [25,26] were effectively utilized in complex HAR tasks. Likewise, some suitable methods are employed to categorize certain sorts of activity, such as multilayer perceptrons [27], vector support machine [28], Random forest [29], decision-making tree [30], and an updated HMM [31]. This research aimed to record sensor changes or changes in discrimination models to recognize human activities. Valuable data means data, especially for lesser amounts, which may be employed to generate high performance. These ultimately save on labelling. For this purpose, several techniques are used in the study. Cameras were also used as external HAR sensors. Indeed, significant research has identified activities and actions in video sequences [32,33]. The mentioned work is particularly suited for safety applications and interactive applications. However, video sequences have particular problems with HAR, privacy and pervasiveness.

Adversarial machine learning has gained increasing interest with the advent of Generative Adversarial Networks (GANs) [34], and it now achieves excellent performance in a wide range of fields, including medicine [35,36], text and image processing [37,38], and architecture [39,40]. GANs work by pitting generator and discriminator algorithms against one another in order to distinguish between produced and real-world data. Deep learning is used to create discriminators that continually learn the best set of features, making it difficult for the generator to pass the discriminator test [41]. The difficulty of providing synthetic data was addressed in the first attempts to use adversarial machine learning for HAR. However, improving categorization algorithms remains the most pressing issue in this sector.

It is challenging to obtain labelled data from users for practical applications. However, unlabeled data can be collected. Since semi-supervised learning uses both the labelled and unlabeled data for model training, the respective models can capture the characteristics of unlabeled data left-out users and further enhance validation performance. Furthermore, adversarial semi-supervised learning models compete with a state-of-the-art method for many areas, such as the classification of images [42] and material recognition [43]. Therefore, the adversarial semi-supervised [44] model is a viable solution. However, unlike other semi-supervised learning techniques, adversarial semi-supervised learning methods are generally applied to circumstances in which unlabeled data is available [45,46].

3. Proposed Method

Human activity recognition systems consist of data acquisition, pre-processing, feature extraction and training/testing phases. Our approach also contains the same process, but the driving factor is new in HAR. The workflow of our proposed method is shown in Figure 1. Heterogeneous sensors were deployed in the apartment's different locations. The data from the sensors are pre-processed by doing segmentation and filtrations. As we use the deep learning model, the feature is extracted automatically. Then, we train and classify the activity and recognize it. If data is unannotated, we reprocessed it and classified it. Finally, we add some perpetuation to develop the self-immune system to the network as an adversarial learning mechanism. We can benefit from training the unlabeled data and labeled data. Similarly, it minimized the error by adversarial learning techniques that can boost the accuracy of the HAR. Hence, we present the Semi-supervised adversarial learning mechanism to detect the human activity facilitated by the synchronized LSTM model that is novel in HAR to this date.

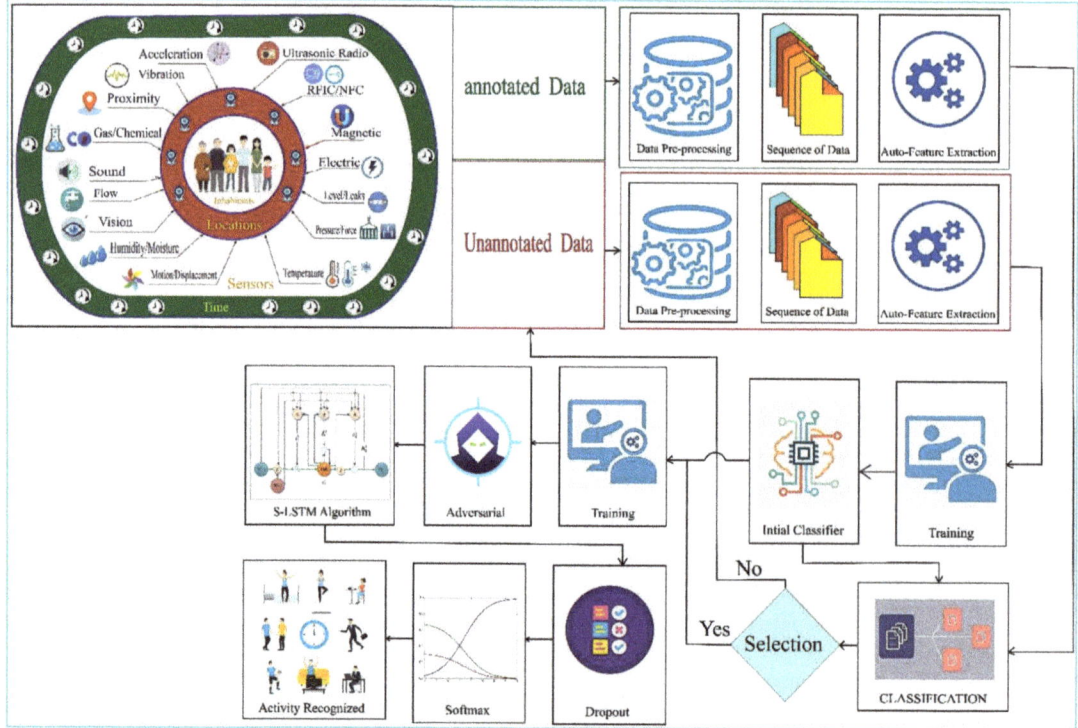

Figure 1. System workflow of our proposed method for HAR.

3.1. Semi-Supervised Learning

Supervised learning [47] is a strategy employed by learning data and labels in many domains or environments. Supervised learning knows and uses labelled data and is helpful for large-scale issues. Various machine learning and deep learning approaches have been used as the supervised learning mechanism. However, hundreds to millions of learning data can be provided to train, and labelling each data is vital. Therefore, supervised learning cannot be used without sufficient learning data because of these issues. Semi-supervised learning is a mechanism to address these deficiencies [48]. It is a technique used to recognize unlisted data with essential criteria like thresholds and re-learn models using available learning data to increase performance based on the projected values of the learned sequences. The semi-supervised method reduces manual annotation and helps develop a self-learning model, which gains robust knowledge and eventually increases the recognition efficiency or accuracy of the recognition model. The feedback properties of LSTM are used to send the unannotated. Then the unannotated data is trained and annotated.

3.2. Sync LSTM

Sync LSTM is the adapted LSTM based on artificial recurrent networks (RNN). The insight of the LSTM and unfolded sync-LSTM network is shown in Figure 2a,b, respectively. It can handle multiple data streams at a time [49]. A conventional LSTM neuron takes a lengthy time to process a signal with significant time steps. As a result, we simultaneously deployed numerous LSTM units to process different data streams. The input streams of data are vectored as $x \in \mathbb{R}(I \times F \times S \times V \times P)$ in which I and F are the initial and final end times. Similarly, S denotes the sensor ID, V is the sensor's data value, and P represents the sensor location. $x_t^m = \left(x_t^1, x_t^2, x_t^3 \ldots x_t^N\right)$ is Sync-LSTM sample inputs where each data is a individual set $m = 1, 2, 3, \ldots N$ sampled at time $t = 1, 2, 3, \ldots N-1$. The input data vector $bx_t^1, x_t^2 \ldots x_t^N \in \mathbb{R}$ $[(S_1 \times E_1 \times I_1 \times V_1 \times L_1), (E_2 \times I_2 \times V_2 \times L_2), \ldots (S_N \times E_N \times I_N \times V_N \times L_N)]$. $Y_t^1, Y_t^2, Y_t^3 \ldots Y_t^N$ resembles the output through the hidden states $h_t^1, h_t^2, h_t^3 \ldots \ldots h_t^N$ at the time t.

$$i_t^m = \sigma\left(w_{xi} \times x_t^m + w_{hi} \times h_{t-1}^m + w_{ci} \times c_{t-1}^m + b_i\right) \tag{1}$$

$$f_t^m = \sigma\left(w_{xf} \times x_t^m + w_{hf} \times h_{t-1}^m + w_{cf} \times c_{t-1}^m + b_f\right) \tag{2}$$

$$o_t^m = \sigma\left(w_{xo} \times x_t^m + w_{ho} \times h_{t-1}^m + w_{co} \times c_{t-1}^m + b_o\right) \tag{3}$$

$$c_t^m = f_t^m \times c_{t-1}^m + i_t^m \times tanh \times \left(w_{xc} x_t^m + w_{hc} h_{t-1}^m + b_c\right) \tag{4}$$

$$h_t^m = o_t^m \times tanh \times c_t^m \tag{5}$$

$$h_t^m = \mathrm{H}\left(w_{x^m h^m} \times x_t^m + w_{h^m h^m} \times h_{t-1}^m + b_h^m\right) \tag{6}$$

$$Y_t^m = \left(w_{y^m h^m} \times h_{t-1}^m + b_y^m\right) \tag{7}$$

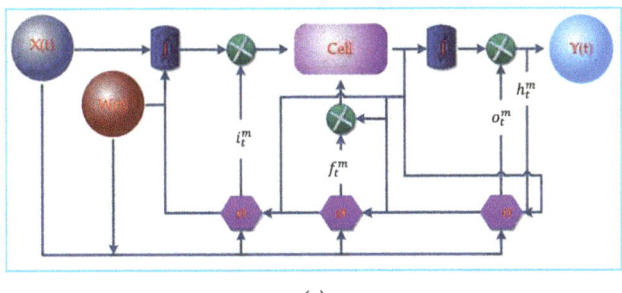

(a)

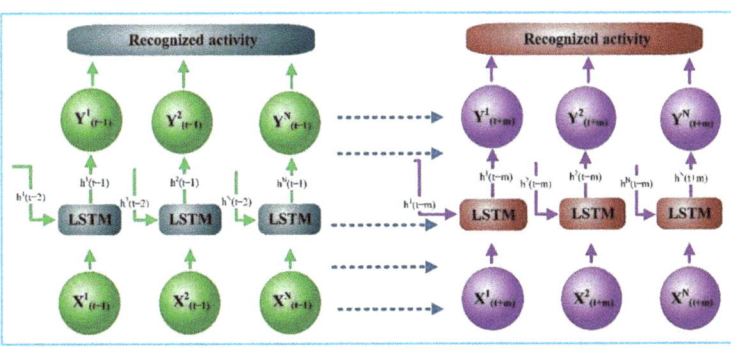

(b)

Figure 2. (**a**) Internal Architecture of sync-LSTM; (**b**) Unfold of sync-LSTM.

H is the composite function, where the i_t^m; input gate, f_t^m; the forget gate, o_t^m; the output gate and the c_t^m; cell memory with W(t); weight matrix. Every given gate has its activation functions σ; sigmoid and ∫; hyperbolic tangent.

It comprises an input layer, the LSTM parallel layers, and the outputs wholly linked. In the last stage, the result is summed up as n × h, where h is the number of neurons buried in each LSTM unit. After each step, the LSTM layers update their inner state. Finally, the weight, bais, and hidden layers are allocated to 128. The number of classes determines the final number of parameters.

3.3. Adversarial Training

Adversarial learning is a technique to regularize neural networks that improve the prediction performance of the neural network or approaches to deep learning by adding tiny disturbances or noises with training data that increases the loss of a more profound learning model. The schematic diagram of the adversarial learning is shown in Figure 3. However, it proposed that small perturbations to deep learning input may result in incorrect decisions with high confidence [50]. If x and θ are the input and different parameters for a predictive model, adversarial learning adds the following terms to its cost function in the training phase to classify the correct class.

$$\log p \ (Y_t^m | X_t^m + r_t^m ; \theta) = where \ r_t^m = argmin \log p \ (Y_t^m | X_t^m + r_t^m ; \hat{\theta}) \qquad (8)$$

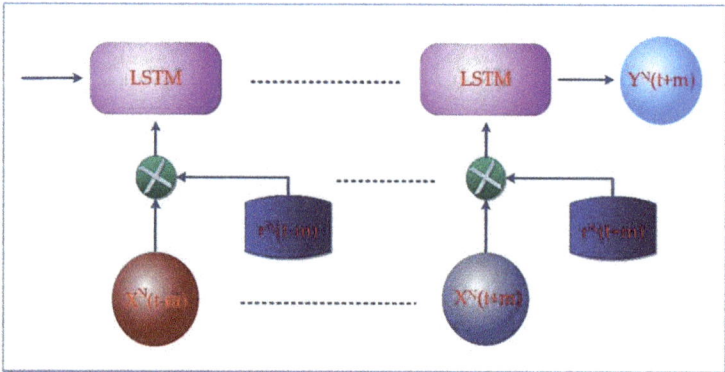

Figure 3. Adding of Adversarial Function.

From Equation (8), r is adversarial in the input data. $\hat{\theta}$, is a set of the constant parameter of the recognition model. At each training, the proposed algorithm identifies the worst-case perturbations r_t^m Against the currently trained model to θ. Contrary to other techniques of regularization, such as dropout, that add random noise, adversarial training creates disturbances or random noise that may readily be misclassified in the learning model by changing input instances.

Algorithm 1 represents the detailed steps of the recognition system, adding the adversarial function. The adversarial function is a small perturbation that maximizes the loss function. As a result, the predictive accuracy or predictive model is eventually improved by reducing the cumulative loss function of the predictive models.

Algorithm 1 Sync-LSTM Model with Adversarial Training

Step 1. initialize network
Step 2. reset: inputs = 0, activations = 0
Step 3. initialize the inputs
Step 4. Create forward and backward sync-LSTM
    Calculate the gate values:
    input gates: i_t^m
    forget gates: f_t^m
    loop over the cells in the block
    output gates: o_t^m
    update the cell: c_t^m
    final hidden state/ $h_t^m = \mathrm{H}\left(w_{x^m h^m} x_t^m + w_{h^m h^m} h_{t-1}^m + b_h^m\right)$
    final output: $Y_t^m = \left(w_{y^m h^m} h_{t-1}^m + b_y^m\right)$
Step 5. Predict and calculate the loss function
    Calculate seq2seq loss
    Calculate class loss using cross-entropy
Step 6. Add random perturbations,
    $\log p\left(Y_t^m \middle| X_t^m + r_t^m; \theta\right) = where\ r_t^m = arg\min \log p\left(Y_t^m \middle| X_t^m + r_t^m; \hat{\theta}\right)$
Step 7. Calculate loss function by adding adversarial loss
Step 8. Optimize the model based on AdamOptimizer

Algorithm 2 presents a semi-supervised learning framework that guides how unannotated from multiple inputs can be incorporated into a sync-LSTM recognition model.

Algorithm 2 Semi-Supervised Sync-LSTM Model

Step 1. Recognize unlabeled data based on Algorithm 1
Step 2. Add recognized dataset to original training dataset
Step 3. Retrain the model using Algorithm 2

---

4. Experimental Configurations and Parameters

The detailed results in both the training and recognition are presented in this section. First, several design hypotheses are assigned and processed. Then, the proposed model is trained with the labelled and unlabeled data, and the results are compared with the existing model outputs. Finally, Milan, Aruba, and the House-C datasets are considered for the experimental analysis of the proposed approach from the CASAS dataset and Kasteren house.

4.1. Datasets

The Kasteren dataset [51] and CASAS dataset [52] from WSU have been used to evaluate our proposed method. Table 1 shows an overview of the datasets. The data was collected in an apartment with more than five rooms. In Milan, 33 sensors are installed, whereas in house-C, 21 sensors are installed, and in Aruba, 34 sensors are installed. For the Milan dataset, motion, door, and temperature sensors are the primary sources of sensor events. A woman and a dog were the primary annotated resident in the Milan dataset. The woman's children occasionally visited the house as an unlabeled resident. The seventy-two days were spent collecting the data from the Milan house. A total of fifteen activities are recorded as the annotated data. One resident in the House-C dataset performed sixteen different activities for twenty days. The sensors show the change of state according to the occupant's action. The data for the Kasteren House-C is recorded using radiofrequency identification, a wireless sensor network, mercury contacts, a passive infrared-PIR, float sensors, a pressure sensor, a reed switch, and temperature sensors. CASAS Aruba dataset is another trademark dataset that collected eleven annotated activities for two hundred and twenty-two days. The schematic layout of the sensor deployment is shown in Figure 4.

Table 1. Outlines of Datasets.

Description	Milan	House-C	Aruba
Setting	Apartment	House	Apartment
Rooms	6	6	5
Senors	33	21	34
Activities	15	16	11
Residents	1	1	1
period	72 days	20 days	220 days
Activities Performed	Bed-to-Toilet, Chores, Dining_Rm_Activity, Eve_meds, Guest_Bathroom, Kitchen_Activity, Leave_Home, Master_Bathroom, Meditate, Watch_TV, Sleep, Read, Morning_Meds, Master_Bedroom_Activity	Brushing teeth, Drinking, Dressing, Eating, Leaving House, Medication, Others, Preparing Breakfast, Preparing Lunch, Preparing Dinner, Relax, Sleeping, Showering, Snack, Shaving, Toileting	Meal_Preparation, Relax, Eating, Work, Sleeping, Wash_Dishes, Bed_to_Toilet, Enter Home, Leave Home, Housekeeping, Resperate

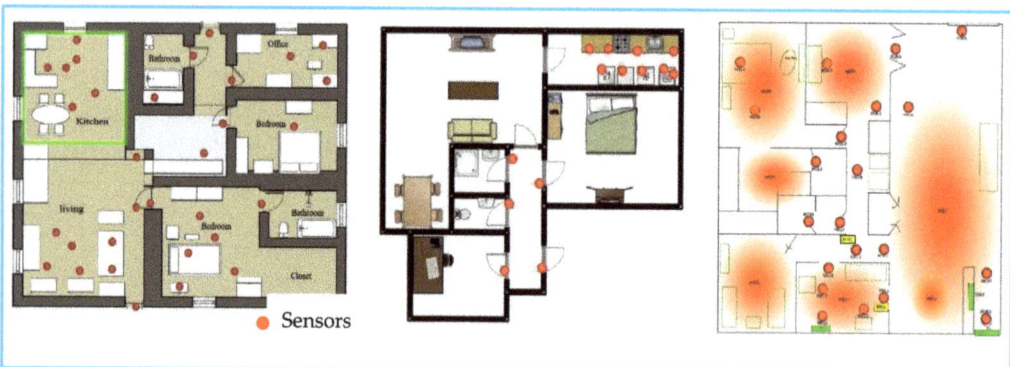

Figure 4. Floor Plan and Sensor Deployment.

4.2. Parameter Setting and Training

The proposed method is trained and tested using the TensorFlow_GPU1.13.1 library and scikit-learn. The obtained data is pre-processed and sampled in overlapping sliding windows with a fixed width of 200 ms with a window length ranging from 0.25 s to 7 s. Our algorithm is examined using an i7 CPU topped with 16 GB RAM and GTX Titan GPU processed on CUDA 9.0 using the cuDDN 7.0 library. The CPU and GPU are employed to minimize the amount of memory used. The dataset is divided into three sections: a training set, validation, and testing. 70% of data is used for training, 10% for validation, and the rest for testing. The data is validated using the k-fold CV (cross-validation). We used 10-fold cross-validation (K = 10) to confirm our findings. The outcome of the accuracy test is averaged, and the error is determined as follows.

$$CV = \frac{1}{p} \sum_{p=1}^{10} E \ (error) \tag{9}$$

The dropout rate is adjusted to 0.5 during training to eliminate unnecessary neurons from each hidden layer to alleviate overfitting. Random initialization and training parameter optimization can also help to reduce training loss. To avoid overfitting and make the model stable, cross-entropy and L2 normalization are incorporated.

$$L = -\frac{1}{k} \sum_{k=1}^{n} y_t^m . log y_t^{m'} + \Gamma.||W||, \tag{10}$$

In Equation (10), k is the number of samples per batch and w denotes the weighting parameter. y_t^m is the recognized output, and $y_t^{m'}$; the label. L2 normalization reduces the size of weighting parameters, preventing overfitting. Adversarial learning is a technique for regularizing neural networks. It also improves the neural network's prediction performance. It perhaps approaches deep learning by adding tiny disturbances or noises to the network with training data that increases the loss of a more profound learning model for regularization, improving recognition ability as adversarial training. If r_t^m is the adversarial input, then is θ the perturbations, which is written as

$$= argmin \log p \ (Y_t^m | X_t^m + r_t^m; \hat{\theta})$$

We strive to tune the optimum hyperparameters, as indicated in Table 2, so that the learning rate and L2 weight decrease and the difference decreases, resulting in the most significant possible performance. For the Milan, House-C, and Aruba datasets, we employ a learning rate of 0.005, 0.004, and 0.006 and a batch value of 100 for each epoch to train the model. For all sets, learning begins at 0.001. The training lasts roughly 12,000 epochs and ends when the outputs are steady. The Adam optimizer is an adaptive moment estimator that generates parameter-independent adaptive learning rates. The input dimension is set to 128, and the output dimension is set to 256. The gradient crossover threshold is reduced by adjusting gradient clipping to 5, 4, and 5.

Table 2. Hyperparameter Configurations.

Hyperparameters	Values		
	Milan	**House-C**	**Aruba**
Time Steps of input	128	128	128
Initial Learning Rate	0.001	0.001	0.001
Learning Rates	0.005	0.004	0.006
Momentum	0.5	0.5	0.5
Optimizer (Bi-LSTM)	Adam	Adam	Adam
Batch Size	100	100	100
Dropout Rate	0.5	0.5	0.5
Batch Size	100	100	100
Epochs	12,000	12,000	12,000

4.3. Evaluation Parameters

Accuracy, F1-score, and training time evaluate the model's performance. These can be calculated using the confusion matrix, where the row represents the predicted class, and the column represents the actual class. Human activity recognition is evaluated according to their computational recognition accuracy, resulting from the Precision and Recall parameters. Precision is the proportion of correctly recognized instances from perceived activity occurrences. A recall is the proportion of correctly identified instances out of the total events. The f-score is the weighted average of Precision and Recall between 0 and 1. The better performance indicated if closer to 1

$$Precision = \frac{tp}{tp + fp} \times 100 \tag{11}$$

$$Recall = \frac{tp}{tp + fn} \times 100 \tag{12}$$

$$Accuracy = \frac{tp + tn}{tp + tn + fp + fn} \times 100 \tag{13}$$

$$f - score = \frac{2 \times Precision \times Recall}{Precision + Recall} \tag{14}$$

where tp; true-positive, tn; true-negative, fp; false-positive, and fn; false-negative. The tp is the number of true activities detected in positive instances, while an fp indicates the false activities detected in negative instances. The fn score indicates the exact number of false activities detected in positive instances, whereas the tn score reflects the correct non-detection of activities in negative instances.

5. Results and Evaluations

5.1. Recognition Analysis

The activity is recognized according to the proposed smart home development method. The method shows a tremendous recognition result. Table 3 shows the confusion matrix of Milan, showing the correctly recognized instances out of the perceived activity occurrences and correctly recognized instances out of the total occurrences. Thus, all the activities have more than 95% of recognition accuracy to the given instances. According to the confusion matrix, the *Bed-to-Toilet* activity was correctly detected with 95% accuracy but still has an activity error of 5%. The *Bed-to-Toilet* may create confusion with *Sleep* activity and *Morning_Meds* these activities are very closely related. Fortunately, *Eve_Meds* has a 100% confusion accuracy. The activities *Chores, Desk_Activity, Dining_RM_Activity, Guest_Bathroom, Kitchen_Activity, Leave_Home, Master_Bathroom, Mediate, Watch_TV, Sleep, Read,* and *Master_Bedroom_Activity* recognition accuracies of 98%, 98%, 99%, 97%, 97%, 96%, 99%, 98%, 99%, 97%, 96%, 95% and 95%, respectively. Although the obtained result is good enough, we still struggle to get the 100%, letting some errors. The errors arise because of confusion between similar activities, activities performed in the same room, and the different activities performed simultaneously with the same instances. Sometimes we performed the same activities with different people, which was unannotated.

Table 3. Confusion matrix for Milan dataset.

	Activity	1	2	3	4	5	6	7	8	9	10	11	12	13	14	15	Recall
1	Bed-to-Toilet	95	0	0	0	0	0.3	0	0	0	0	0	0	0	1	0.3	98.344
2	Chores	0	98	0	0	0	0	1	0.2	0.05	0	0	0	0	0	0	98.741
3	Desk_Activity	0	0	98	0	0	0	0	0	0	0	2	0.3	0	0	0	97.707
4	Dining_Rm_Activity	0	0.8	0	99	0	2	0	0.1	0	0	0	0	0	0	0	97.154
5	Eve_Meds	0	0	0	0	100	0	0	0	0	0	0	0	0	0	0	100.000
6	Guest_Bathroom	0	0	0	0.3	0.2	97	0	1.2	1	0	0	0	0	0	0	97.292
7	Kitchen_Activity	0	1.2	0	1.2	0	0	97	0	0.3	0	0	0	0.6	0	0	96.710
8	Leave_Home	0	0	0	2	0	0	1.2	96	0.9	0	0	0	1	0	0	94.955
9	Master_Bathroom	0	1.1	0	0	0	0	1	0.4	99	0	0	0	0.2	0	0	97.345
10	Meditate	0	0	0	0	0.3	0	0	0	0	98	0.6	0	0	0	0	99.090
11	Watch_TV	0	0	0	0	0	0	0	0	0	0	99	0	0	0	0	100.000
12	Sleep	2	0	0	0	0	0	0	0	0	0	0	97	0	1	0.5	96.517
13	Read	0	0	0	1	0	1	0	0	0	0	0	0	96	0	0.9	97.068
14	Morning_Meds	1	0	0.5	0	0	0	0.8	0	0	0	0	0	0	95	0.033	97.603
15	Master_Bedroom_Activity	0	0	0	0	0	0	0	0	0	0	0	0	0	0.2	95	99.790
	Precision	96.939	96.934	99.492	95.652	99.502	96.710	96.040	98.059	97.778	100.000	97.441	99.692	98.160	97.737	98.208	

In this dataset, the house owner's daughter often visited her house, performed the same task, and was recognized more accurately. The confusion matrix for House-C is shown in Table 4. The number of activity instances is relatively few, so errors are relatively low, and recognizing the activity with true positive value results in 98.01% accuracy.

House-C has achieved 98.11% precision, 98.109% recall, and 0.98 f1-score. Activities such as *brushing teeth* (95% accurate), *Showering* (97%), *Shaving* (95%) *toileting* (93%) create confusion and errors because all the activities happen in one location. However, the errors that occur are comparatively low, so that they can be neglected. Furthermore, *Preparing Breakfast* (97%), *Preparing Lunch* (96%), *Preparing Dinner* (98%), *Snacks* (97%) and *Eating* (99%) have good recognition accuracy but still have some errors because of confusion among these activities as they share some sensor values. House-C's dataset is insufficient to establish the experimental concept fully and has 100% recognition accuracy. Although the accuracy is good, more data and training could be needed to find actual recognition.

Table 4. Confusion matrix for House-C.

	Activity	1	2	3	4	5	6	7	8	9	10	11	12	13	14	15	16	Recall
1	Brushing Teeth	95	0	0	0	0	0.3	0	0	0	0	0	0	0	0.3	0.3	0.5	98.548
2	Drinking	0	98	0	0	0	0	1	0.2	0.05	0	0	0	0	0	0	0.2	98.542
3	Dressing	0	0	98	0	0	0	0	0	0	0	0.5	0.3	0	0	0	0.1	99.090
4	Eating	0	0.3	0	99	0	2	0	0.1	0	0	0	0	0	0	0	0.05	97.585
5	Leaving House	0	0	0	0	100	0	0	0	0	0	0	0	0	0	0	0.1	99.900
6	Medication	0	0	0	0.3	0.2	97	0	0.2	1	0	0	0	0	0	0	0.4	97.881
7	Preparing Breakfast	0	0.2	0	0.2	0	0	97	0	0.3	0	0	0	0.3	0	0	0.5	98.477
8	Preparing Lunch	0	0	0	2	0	0	1.2	96	0.9	0	0	0	0.5	0	0	0.1	95.333
9	Preparing Dinner	0	0.1	0	0	0	0	1	0.4	99	0	0	0	0.2	0	0	0.3	98.020
10	Relax	0	0	0	0	0.3	0	0	0	0	98	0.6	0	0	0	0	0.5	98.592
11	Sleeping	0	0	0	0	0	0	0	0	0	0	99	0	0	0	0	0.43	99.568
12	Showering	1	0	0	0	0	0	0	0	0	0	0	97	0	1	0.5	0.2	97.292
13	Snacks	0	0	0	1	0	1	0	0	0	0	0	0	96	0	0.4	0.1	97.462
14	Shaving	1	0	0.5	0	0	0	0.8	0	0	0	0	0	0	95	0.033	0.4	97.204
15	Toileting	0	0	0	0	0	0	0	0	0	0	0	0	0	0.2	93	0.11	99.668
16	Others	0.2	0	0.1	0.2	0.3	0.2	0.3	0.11	0.2	0.1	0	0.58	0.3	0.5	0.2	93	96.583
	Presicion	97.737	99.391	99.391	96.397	99.206	96.517	95.755	98.959	97.585	99.898	98.901	99.101	98.664	97.938	98.483	95.886	

Nevertheless, we confirm that our proposed approach for human activity recognition is feasible. In Aruba, the number of instances per activity type varies considerably as shown in the Table 5. The proposed system allows most activities to be recognized with an overall accuracy of 98.34% and an F1-score of 0.98. However, some activities have 100% accuracy and some have less recognition accuracy, such as Enter Home of 95%. The *Enter_House* and *Leave_House* activities involve the same main door and sensors, taking their occurrences into account. Likewise, *Wash_Dishes* gets mistaken with *Meal_Preparation* since both are done in the kitchen, sharing the same occurrences. The *Wash_Dishes* action may also be performed during *Meal_Preparation* and can therefore be regarded as concurrent.

Table 5. Confusion matrix for Aruba.

	Activities	1	2	3	4	5	6	7	8	9	10	11	Recall
1	Meal_Preparation	98	1.3	0.7	0	0	1.1	0	0	0	0	0	96.934
2	Relax	0	98	0	1	1	0	0.3	0	0	0	0.1	97.610
3	Eating	0	0	97	0	0	1	0	0	0.5	0.1	0	98.377
4	Work	0.6	1.2	0.2	95	0.1	0.6	0.4	1	0.3	0	0	95.573
5	Sleeping	0	0	0	0	97	0	0	1	0	0	0	98.980
6	Wash_Dishes	0	0	0	0.3	0.2	99	0	0	0	0	0	99.497
7	Bed_to_Toilet	0	0	0	0	0	0	98	1	0	0	0	98.990
8	Enter_Home	0	0.4	0	0	2	0	1.54	98	0	0	0	96.135
9	Leave_Home	0	0	0	0	0	0	0	0	100	0	0	100.000
10	Housekeeping	0.2	0	0	0	0	0	0	0	0	98	0	99.796
11	Resperate	0	0	0	0	0	0	0	0	0	0	97	100.000
	Precision	99.190	97.126	99.081	98.650	96.710	97.345	97.765	97.030	99.206	99.898	99.897	

5.2. Recognition Comparison

The accuracy and loss curves of Milan, House-C, and Aruba are shown in Figures 5–7. The gap between the training and testing accuracy in the graphs is comparatively tiny, indicating the model's effectiveness. Furthermore, the gap between training and test loss is very narrow, explaining that dropout techniques, adversarial training, and semi-supervised learning are beneficial.

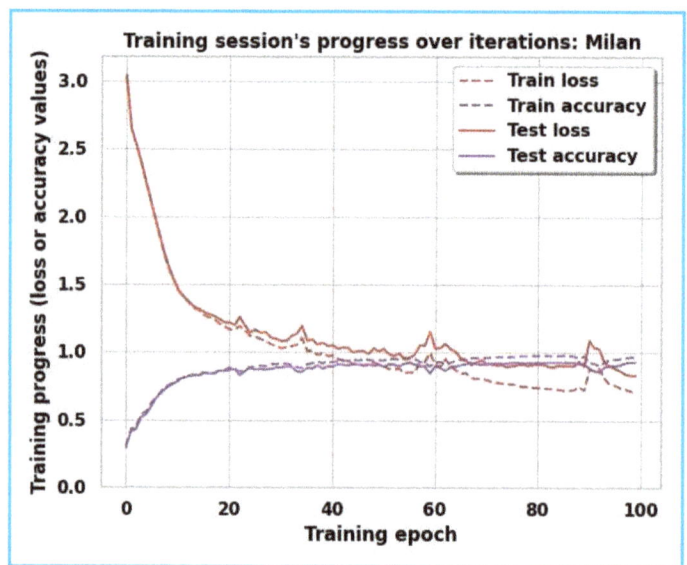

Figure 5. Training/Test Accuracy/Loss for Milan.

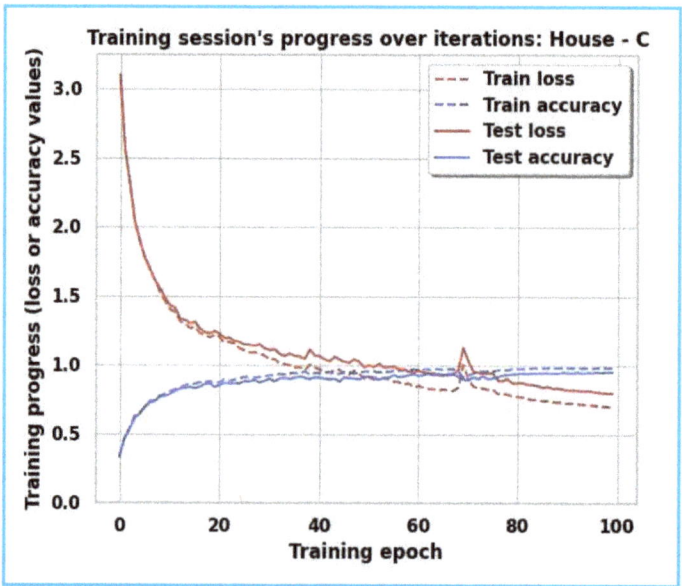

Figure 6. Training/Test Accuracy/Loss for House-C.

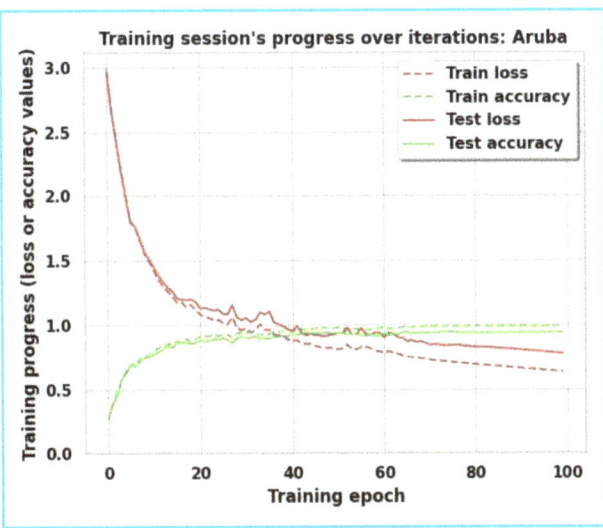

Figure 7. Training/Test Accuracy/Loss for Aruba.

The average accuracy was 98.154%, and the average error was 0.1571. The performance result of the proposed approach with the existing framework, such as HMM, LSTM, and sync-LSTM methods (algorithms), is based on average precision, recall, and accuracy, as shown in Figure 8a and f-score in Figure 8b. The accuracy of our work is more than 98%, and the f1-score is more than 0.98. The sync-LSTM also has competitive accuracy with our method but cannot deal with new or unannotated data. The analysis reveals that the presentation method can be more accurate than the current approaches.

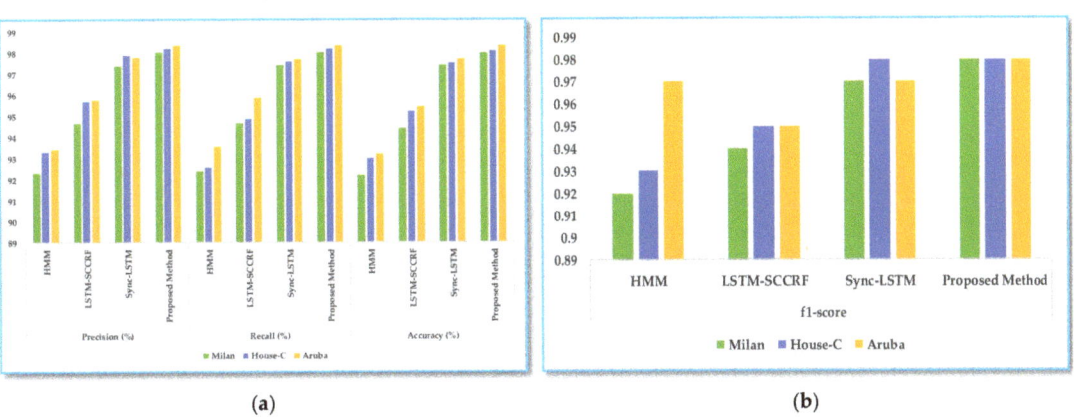

Figure 8. (**a**) the average precision, recall, and accuracy and (**b**) the f1-score comparison with different models.

6. Conclusions

The presented work in this paper shows that semi-supervised adversarial sync-LSTM can produce a feasible solution for detecting human activities in the intelligent home scenario—a comprehensive comparison with recently introduced activity recognition techniques, such as HMM, LSTM, and sync-LSTM. LSTM can work with single data sequences, and sync-LSTM can accept multiple inputs and generate synchronized and parallel outputs. Still, these techniques fail to address the new and unknown data in the sequence. Many approaches have been researched on annotated and regular activity detection. However, few of them have tried to detect complex and unannotated activity. The proposed method used the improvised LSTM and its semi-supervised learning ability to recognize complex and unannotated human activity from the data collected from the sensors in the smart home. The adversarial learning technique increases learning ability by adding tiny disturbances or noises to the network. Accuracy, processing complexity, complex activity and unannotated activity recognition are still challenging issues in human activity recognition. However, the precision and recall are also excellent, resulting in an f1 score of more than 0.98 and 98% accuracy.

Nevertheless, the accuracy is not equal or tends to be one hundred percent due to shared location, sensor timing, noise interference, and limited data. The existing best-performing model faces several real-time challenges while dealing with different datasets. The number of activities performed, sensor types, sensor deployment, number of inhabitants, and periods are vital parameters affecting model performance. In addition, the window size also plays a crucial role in model performance because small windows may not contain all the information, and large windows may lead to overfitting and overload. Recognizing the unannotated data and processing it in parallel is beneficial for highly imbalanced datasets.

The computational complexity is $O(W)$, where W is the weight and relies on the number of weights. The weight is determined by the number of output units, cell storage units, memory capacity, and hidden unit count. The amount of units connected with forwarding neurons, memory cells, gate units, and hidden units also impacts. The length of the input sequence has no bearing on the computational complexity. Using an LSTM framework for the labelled and unlabeled data adds time complexity, yet our method has a reasonable calculation time of 9 s.

Besides detecting unannotated activity, the proposed method can automatically extract Spatio-temporal information by consuming less pre-processing time and manual feature extraction. In addition, external sensors were used instead of body-worn and video sensors to protect the user's privacy and avoid body hurdles. Furthermore, more complex, multi-user, and multi- variants activities can be recognized by enhancing and upgrading the proposed method in the future. Moreover, we can take advantage of cloud computing, edge computing and IoT services to process a large amount of data for better performance. Finally, our approach can be used in other domains and environments like sign language detection, cognitive abilities, etc. Hence, our suggested approach is a better state-of-art method for HAR.

Author Contributions: Conceptualization, K.T. and S.-H.Y.; methodology, K.T.; software, D.-G.B.; validation, K.T., S.-H.Y. and D.-G.B.; formal analysis, K.T.; investigation, S.-H.Y.; resources, D.-G.B.; data curation, D.-G.B.; writing—original draft preparation, K.T.; writing—review and editing, S.-H.Y. and K.T.; visualization, K.T.; supervision, S.-H.Y.; project administration, D.-G.B.; funding acquisition, S.-H.Y. All authors have read and agreed to the published version of the manuscript.

Funding: This research was supported by the Ministry of Trade, Industry & Energy of the Republic of Korea as an AI Home Platform Development Project (20009496).

Acknowledgments: This is work is conducted under a research grant from Kwangwoon University in 2022. The work reported in this paper was conducted during the sabbatical year of Kwangwoon University in 2020.

Conflicts of Interest: The authors declare no conflict of interest.

References

1. Wan, S.; Qi, L.; Xu, X.; Tong, C.; Gu, Z. Deep Learning Models for Real-Time Human Activity Recognition with Smartphones. *Mob. Netw. Appl.* **2019**, *25*, 743–755. [CrossRef]
2. Ordóñez, F.J.; Roggen, D. Deep convolutional and LSTM recurrent neural networks for multimodal wearable activity recognition. *Sensors* **2016**, *16*, 115. [CrossRef] [PubMed]

3. Van Kasteren, T.L.M.; Englebienne, G.; Kröse, B.J.A. An activity monitoring system for elderly care using generative and discriminative models. *Pers. Ubiquitous Comput.* **2010**, *14*, 489–498. [CrossRef]

4. Shi, X.; Li, Y.; Zhou, F.; Liu, L. Human activity recognition based on deep learning method. In Proceedings of the 2018 International Conference on Radar (RADAR), Brisbane, Australia, 27–31 August 2018.

5. Das, A.; Jens, K.; Kjærgaard, M.B. Space utilization and activity recognition using 3D stereo vision camera inside an educational building. In *Adjunct Proceedings of the 2020 ACM International Joint Conference on Pervasive and Ubiquitous Computing and Proceedings of the 2020 ACM International Symposium on Wearable Computers, 12–17 September 2020*; ACM: New York, NY, USA, 2020.

6. Thapa, K.; Al, Z.M.A.; Lamichhane, B.; Yang, S.H. A deep machine learning method for concurrent and interleaved human activity recognition. *Sensors* **2020**, *20*, 5770. [CrossRef]

7. Abdallah, Z.S.; Gaber, M.M.; Srinivasan, B.; Krishnaswamy, S. AnyNovel: Detection of novel concepts in evolving data streams: An application for activity recognition. *Evol. Syst.* **2016**, *7*, 73–93. [CrossRef]

8. Fang, L.; Ye, J.; Dobson, S. Discovery and recognition of emerging human activities using a hierarchical mixture of directional statistical models. *IEEE Trans. Knowl. Data Eng.* **2020**, *32*, 1304–1316. [CrossRef]

9. French, R.M. Catastrophic forgetting in connectionist networks. *Trends Cogn. Sci.* **1999**, *3*, 128–135. [CrossRef]

10. Hossain, H.M.S.; Roy, N.; Al Hafiz Khan, M.A. Active learning enabled activity recognition. In Proceedings of the 2016 IEEE International Conference on Pervasive Computing and Communications (PerCom), Sydney, Australia, 14–19 March 2016.

11. Ye, J.; Dobson, S.; Zambonelli, F. Lifelong learning in sensor-based human activity recognition. *IEEE Pervasive Comput.* **2019**, *18*, 49–58. [CrossRef]

12. Kabir, M.H.; Hoque, M.R.; Thapa, K.; Yang, S.H. Two-layer hidden Markov model for human activity recognition in home environments. *Int. J. Distrib. Sens. Netw.* **2016**, *12*, 4560365. [CrossRef]

13. Oh, S.; Ashiquzzaman, A.; Lee, D.; Kim, Y.; Kim, J. Study on human activity recognition using semi-supervised active transfer learning. *Sensors* **2021**, *21*, 2760. [CrossRef]

14. Zhang, L.; Wu, X.; Luo, D. Human activity recognition with HMM-DNN model. In Proceedings of the 2015 IEEE 14th International Conference on Cognitive Informatics & Cognitive Computing (ICCI*CC), Beijing, China, 6–8 July 2015.

15. Nair, R.; Ragab, M.; Mujallid, O.A.; Mohammad, K.A.; Mansour, R.F.; Viju, G.K. Impact of wireless sensor data mining with hybrid deep learning for human activity recognition. *Wirel. Commun. Mob. Comput.* **2022**, *2022*, 1–8. [CrossRef]

16. Vrigkas, M.; Nikou, C.; Kakadiaris, I.A. A review of human activity recognition methods. *Front. Robot. AI* **2015**, *2*. [CrossRef]

17. Hartmann, Y.; Liu, H.; Lahrberg, S.; Schultz, T. Interpretable High-level Features for Human Activity Recognition. In Proceedings of the 15th International Joint Conference on Biomedical Engineering Systems and Technologies, Online, 8–10 February 2022; pp. 40–49. [CrossRef]

18. Lara, O.D.; Labrador, M.A. A survey on human activity recognition using wearable sensors. *IEEE Commun. Surv. Tutor.* **2013**, *15*, 1192–1209. [CrossRef]

19. Wang, X.; Lv, T.; Gan, Z.; He, M.; Jin, L. Fusion of skeleton and inertial data for human action recognition based on skeleton motion maps and dilated convolution. *IEEE Sens. J.* **2021**, *21*, 24653–24664. [CrossRef]

20. Liu, H.; Hartmann, Y.; Schultz, T. Motion units: Generalized sequence modeling of human activities for sensor-based activity recognition. In Proceedings of the 2021 29th European Signal Processing Conference (EUSIPCO), Dublin, Ireland, 23–27 August 2021. [CrossRef]

21. Wang, J.; Zheng, V.W.; Chen, Y.; Huang, M. Deep transfer learning for cross-domain Activity Recognition. *arXiv* **2018**, arXiv:1807.07963. [CrossRef]

22. Gao, L.; Bourke, A.K.; Nelson, J. Evaluation of accelerometer based multi-sensor versus single-sensor activity recognition systems. *Med. Eng. Phys.* **2014**, *36*, 779–785. [CrossRef]

23. Hammerla, N.Y.; Halloran, S.; Ploetz, T. Deep, convolutional, and recurrent models for human activity recognition using wearables. *arXiv* **2016**, arXiv:1604.08880. [CrossRef]

24. Ignatov, A. Real-time human activity recognition from accelerometer data using Convolutional Neural Networks. *Appl. Soft Comput.* **2018**, *62*, 915–922. [CrossRef]

25. Raziani, S.; Azimbagirad, M. Deep CNN hyperparameter optimization algorithms for sensor-based human activity recognition. *Neurosci. Inform.* **2022**, 100078. [CrossRef]

26. Prasad, A.; Tyagi, A.K.; Althobaiti, M.M.; Almulihi, A.; Mansour, R.F.; Mahmoud, A.M. Human Activity Recognition using cell phone-based accelerometer and Convolutional Neural Network. *Appl. Sci* **2021**, *11*, 12099. [CrossRef]

27. Talukdar, J.; Mehta, B. Human action recognition system using good features and multilayer perceptron network. In Proceedings of the 2017 International Conference on Communication and Signal Processing (ICCSP), Chennai, India, 6–8 April 2017.

28. Schuldt, C.; Laptev, I.; Caputo, B. Recognizing human actions: A local SVM approach. In Proceedings of the 17th International Conference on Pattern Recognition, ICPR 2004, Cambridge, UK, 26 August 2004.

29. Fan, L.; Wang, Z.; Wang, H. Human activity recognition model based on decision tree. In Proceedings of the 2013 International Conference on Advanced Cloud and Big Data, Nanjing, China, 13–15 December 2013.

30. Kabir, M.; Thapa, K.; Yang, J.Y.; Yang, S.H. State-space based linear modeling for human activity recognition in smart space. *Intell. Autom. Soft Comput.* **2018**, *25*, 1–9. [CrossRef]

31. Candamo, J.; Shreve, M.; Goldgof, D.B.; Sapper, D.B.; Kasturi, R. Understanding transit scenes: A survey on human behavior-recognition algorithms. *IEEE Trans. Intell. Transp. Syst.* **2010**, *11*, 206–224. [CrossRef]

32. Ahad, M.A.R.; Tan, J.K.; Kim, H.S.; Ishikawa, S. Human activity recognition: Various paradigms. In Proceedings of the 2008 International Conference on Control, Automation and Systems, Seoul, Korea, 14–17 October 2008.

33. Goodfellow, I.J.; Pouget-Abadie, J.; Mirza, M. Generative Adversarial Networks. *arXiv* **2014**, arXiv:1406.2661. [CrossRef]

34. Kumar, A.; Sattigeri, P.; Fletcher, P.T. Semi-supervised learning with GANs: Manifold invariance with improved inference. *arXiv* **2017**, arXiv:1705.08850. [CrossRef]

35. Erickson, Z.; Chernova, S.; Kemp, C.C. Semi-supervised haptic material recognition for robots using generative adversarial networks. *arXiv* **2017**, arXiv:1707.02796. [CrossRef]

36. Kingma, D.P.; Rezende, D.J.; Mohamed, S.; Welling, M. Semi-supervised learning with deep generative models. *arXiv* **2014**, arXiv:1406.5298.

37. Qi, G.J.; Zhang, L.; Hu, H.; Edraki, M.; Wang, J.; Hua, X.S. Global versus localized generative adversarial nets. *arXiv* **2017**, arXiv:1711.06020. [CrossRef]

38. Nouretdinov, I.; Costafreda, S.G.; Gammerman, A. Machine learning classification with confidence: Application of transductive conformal predictors to MRI-based diagnostic and prognostic markers in depression. *Neuroimage* **2011**, *56*, 809–813. [CrossRef]

39. Scudder, H. Probability of error of some adaptive pattern-recognition machines. *IEEE Trans. Inf. Theory* **1965**, *11*, 363–371. [CrossRef]

40. Alzantot, M.; Chakraborty, S.; Srivastava, M.B. SenseGen: A deep learning architecture for synthetic sensor data generation. *arXiv* **2017**, arXiv:1701.08886. [CrossRef]

41. Sung-Hyun, Y.; Thapa, K.; Kabir, M.H.; Hee-Chan, L. Log-Viterbi algorithm applied on second-order hidden Markov model for human activity recognition. *Int. J. Distrib. Sens. Netw.* **2018**, *14*, 155014771877254. [CrossRef]

42. Bidgoli, A.; Veloso, P. DeepCloud. The application of a data-driven, generative model in design. *arXiv* **2019**, arXiv:1904.01083. [CrossRef]

43. Soleimani, E.; Khodabandelou, G.; Chibani, A.; Amirat, Y. Generic semi-supervised adversarial subject translation for sensor-based Human Activity Recognition. *arXiv* **2020**, arXiv:2012.03682. [CrossRef]

44. Sudhanshu, M. Semi-Supervised Learning for Real-World Object Recognition Using Adversarial Autoencoders. Master's Thesis, Royal Institute of Technology (KTH), Stockholm, Sweden, 23 May 2018.

45. Balabka, D. Semi-supervised learning for human activity recognition using adversarial autoencoders. In Proceedings of the 2019 ACM International Joint Conference on Pervasive and Ubiquitous Computing and Proceedings of the 2019 ACM International Symposium on Wearable Computers, UbiComp/ISWC'19, London, UK, 9–13 September 2019.

46. van Engelen, J.E.; Hoos, H.H. A survey on semi-supervised learning. *Mach. Learn.* **2020**, *109*, 373–440. [CrossRef]

47. Nafea, O.; Abdul, W.; Muhammad, G.; Alsulaiman, M. Sensor-based human activity recognition with spatio-temporal deep learning. *Sensors* **2021**, *21*, 2141. [CrossRef]

48. Zhu, X.; Goldberg, A.B. Overview of semi-supervised learning. In *Introduction to Semi-Supervised Learning*; Springer: Cham, Switzerland, 2009; pp. 9–19.

49. Thapa, K.; AI, Z.M.A.; Sung-Hyun, Y. Adapted long short-term memory (LSTM) for concurrent\\human activity recognition. *Comput. Mater. Contin.* **2021**, *69*, 1653–1670. [CrossRef]

50. Pauling, C.; Gimson, M.; Qaid, M.; Kida, A.; Halak, B. A tutorial on adversarial learning attacks and countermeasures. *arXiv* **2022**, arXiv:2202.10377. [CrossRef]

51. van Kasteren, T.L.M.; Englebienne, G.; Kröse, B.J.A. Human activity recognition from wireless sensor network data: Benchmark and software. In *Activity Recognition in Pervasive Intelligent Environments*; Atlantis Press: Paris, France, 2011; pp. 165–186.

52. Cook, D.J.; Schmitter-Edgecombe, M. Assessing the quality of activities in a smart environment. *Methods Inf. Med.* **2009**, *48*, 480–485. [CrossRef]

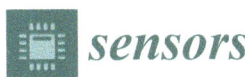

MDPI

Article

Device-Free Multi-Location Human Activity Recognition Using Deep Complex Network

Xue Ding [1], Chunlei Hu [1], Weiliang Xie [1], Yi Zhong [2,*], Jianfei Yang [3] and Ting Jiang [4]

1   Mobile and Terminal Technology Research Department, China Telecom Research Institute, Beijing 102209, China
2   School of Information and Electronics, Beijing Institute of Technology, Beijing 100081, China
3   School of Electrical and Electronics Engineering, Nanyang Technological University, Singapore 639798, Singapore
4   School of Information and Communication Engineering, Beijing University of Posts and Telecommunications, Beijing 100876, China
*   Correspondence: yi.zhong@bit.edu.cn

Abstract: Wi-Fi-based human activity recognition has attracted broad attention for its advantages, which include being device-free, privacy-protected, unaffected by light, etc. Owing to the development of artificial intelligence techniques, existing methods have made great improvements in sensing accuracy. However, the performance of multi-location recognition is still a challenging issue. According to the principle of wireless sensing, wireless signals that characterize activity are also seriously affected by location variations. Existing solutions depend on adequate data samples at different locations, which are labor-intensive. To solve the above concerns, we present an amplitude- and phase-enhanced deep complex network (AP-DCN)-based multi-location human activity recognition method, which can fully utilize the amplitude and phase information simultaneously so as to mine more abundant information from limited data samples. Furthermore, considering the unbalanced sample number at different locations, we propose a perception method based on the deep complex network-transfer learning (DCN-TL) structure, which effectively realizes knowledge sharing among various locations. To fully evaluate the performance of the proposed method, comprehensive experiments have been carried out with a dataset collected in an office environment with 24 locations and five activities. The experimental results illustrate that the approaches can achieve 96.85% and 94.02% recognition accuracy, respectively.

Keywords: human activity recognition; Wi-Fi sensing; multi-location; deep complex network

Citation: Ding, X.; Hu, C.; Xie, W.; Zhong, Y.; Yang, J.; Jiang, T. Device-Free Multi-Location Human Activity Recognition Using Deep Complex Network. *Sensors* **2022**, *22*, 6178. https://doi.org/10.3390/s22166178

Academic Editors: Hugo Gamboa, Tanja Schultz and Hui Liu

Received: 19 July 2022
Accepted: 13 August 2022
Published: 18 August 2022

Publisher's Note: MDPI stays neutral with regard to jurisdictional claims in published maps and institutional affiliations.

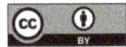
1. Introduction

Human Activity Recognition (HAR) has been considered as an indispensable technology in many Human-Computer Interaction (HCI) applications, such as smart homes, health-care services, security surveillance, entertainment, etc [1,2]. Both the device-based and device-free sensing approaches attract widespread attention [3–6]. Owing to their superiority involving sensing accuracy and robustness, sensor-based [7,8] and camera-based [9,10] HAR methods have been widely used in various fields. However, these techniques experience varied limitations in some applications. Specifically, sensor-based methods require the users to equip themselves with additional devices, which is inconvenient. Although the camera-based technique is successfully applied to various scenarios, it is restricted to well-lit conditions and fails to work in a non-line-of-sight (NLOS) scene. More critically, it raises privacy concerns.

Recently, device-free sensing technology based on wireless signals has been widely studied owing to its capacity to overcome the above defects effectively [11,12]. Since only radio frequency (RF) signals are utilized, it naturally has the strengths of working in darkness and NLOS circumstances and protecting users' privacy in the meantime.

Compared with the other wireless signals, such as Frequency Modulated Continuous Wave (FMCW) [13,14], millimeter-wave (MMW) [15,16], and Ultra-Wide Band (UWB) [17,18], Wi-Fi has an overwhelming advantage due to its ubiquity in daily life. Leveraging commercial off-the-shelf (COTS) devices, Wi-Fi-based human activity recognition obviates the need for additional specialized hardware. Consequently, study of the Wi-Fi-based HAR technique has proliferated rapidly over the past decade [19–22].

Although Wi-Fi-based HAR approaches have made significant achievements at a fixed location, it is still challenging in multi-location sensing. When it comes to intelligent control in smart homes, it will be seriously inconvenient for users if they can only control the smart devices at a specified location in a room. Moreover, a target that can be detected at one position but fails to be identified at other positions is not desired. Therefore, multi-location sensing is one of the most essential capabilities for the HAR system. According to the principle of RF signal propagation, when encountering an obstacle, the signal will be reflected, refracted, and scattered, leading to the superposition of multipath [23,24]. Therefore, both the activity and its location affect signal transmission to a certain extent. Consequently, even for the same human activity, different locations would result in signals having different patterns, which will lead to a serious decline in multi-location sensing accuracy. Furthermore, owing to the rapid development of the deep learning technique, the performance of human activity recognition has been effectively improved [25]. However, these methods usually rely on abundant labeled or unlabeled samples, which have never been easily accessible for labor-intensive and time-consuming. In addition, it is quite difficult to obtain large amounts of data for all locations. Therefore, a multi-location human activity recognition method using small-scale data needs to be explored.

Literature [26] is the state-of-the-art multi-location human activity recognition method. An activity decomposition network (ActNet) is proposed to decompose the training samples into activity features and location features. In addition, data from different locations are assembled for training to mitigate the data limitation issue. The performance is evaluated at 24 sampling locations in the perceptual range. Using only 10 training samples for each position can achieve promising recognition accuracy.

Existing Wi-Fi-based sensing approaches for human activity recognition are mostly dependent on the amplitude of Channel State Information (CSI) because phase information contains certain errors caused by the hardware and software of the transceiver, including Sampling Time Offsets (STO) and Carrier Frequency Offsets (CFO) [27,28]. The proposed phase offsets removal method and phase difference make it possible to utilize phase information in Wi-Fi-based sensing [29,30]. However, it inevitably loses some useful information. Despite both amplitude and phase providing a wealth of activity-related information, only very few studies have used them simultaneously. In multi-location HAR, although the same activity conducted in different locations will lead to different signal delays at the receiver, the time delay generated by the same action may change with a certain rule, which is unrelated to the locations and will be reflected in the phase information. Therefore, leveraging the amplitude and phase information of CSI effectively at the same time can extract the feature representation that is more related to the activity. Furthermore, since more abundant features can be obtained, the sample size can be reduced to some extent. Although deep learning-based HAR methods emerge due to the key merit of automatically learning representative features, the amplitude and phase information are usually applied as the input of the neural network separately.

In this paper, inspired by the Deep Complex Network (DCN) [31,32] which is designed to extract meaningful information from the real and imaginary parts of complex numbers, we propose a multi-location human activity recognition system based on the Deep Complex Network. Firstly, we propose a multi-location human activity identification method based on Amplitude and Phase enhanced Deep Complex Network (AP-DCN), which can make efficient use of amplitude and phase information. Specifically, complex Convolutional Neural Network (CNN), complex Batch Normalization (BN), and the complex ReLU activation function are used for feature extraction. Softmax is used for activity classification.

Under the condition of limited data samples, high accuracy multi-location human activity recognition is realized. Moreover, considering the imbalanced number of samples in different positions and the more restricted number of training samples in some positions, the transfer learning method is used to realize the sharing of human activity characteristics in distinct locations. A novel human activity sensing method based on Deep Complex Network-Transfer Learning (DCN-TL) is proposed. The model is trained with sufficient activity samples from source domain locations to learn the common features of the source domain and target domain, as well as the specific characteristics of the source domain. Then, the model is fine-tuned with a small number of samples from target domain locations to learn the specific characteristics of the target domain. Thereby, in the case of unbalanced samples at different locations, multi-location human activity recognition can be achieved.

The main contributions of this paper can be summarized as follows:

- First, the effects of amplitude and phase information on Wi-Fi-based human activity recognition are analyzed. In order to make full use of the information in CSI, the AP-DCN-based recognition method is designed to improve the recognition accuracy of multi-location sensing.
- Second, in order to alleviate the problem of unbalanced samples at different locations, the DCN-TL-based human activity recognition method is proposed to reduce the dependence of the perception method on the number of activity samples at a specific location.
- Third, comprehensive experiments are conducted to evaluate the performance of the proposed AP-DCN-based and DCN-TL-based multi-location sensing methods. Experimental results demonstrate that the proposed approach can achieve satisfactory multi-location human activity recognition accuracy with very few samples.

The remainder of this article is organized as follows. In Section 2, the preliminaries of Wi-Fi sensing are introduced. In Section 3 provides an overview of the proposed system and a detailed description of the AP-DCN-based and DCN-TL-based multi-location human activity recognition methods. In Section 4, the experiment setup and performance evaluation are elaborated. Our conclusions are presented in Section 5.

2. Preliminaries

In this section, the measured signal is analyzed to verify the multi-location issue mentioned above. Firstly, the signal metric leveraged in Wi-Fi-based HAR is introduced. Then, the influence of location variations on Wi-Fi signals is investigated to reveal the encountered challenges. More importantly, both amplitude and phase information are presented.

2.1. Channel State Information

Wi-Fi-based HAR leverages the impact of human movements on the propagation of the wireless signal for sensing. In a Multiple Input Multiple Output (MIMO) and Orthogonal Frequency Division Multiplexing (OFDM) wireless communication system, this process can be described by the fine-grained CSI, which represents the state of the communication link between the transmitter (TX) and the receiver (RX).

Letting y and x denote the received signal and transmitted signal, the relation between them can be modeled as:

$$y = Hx + n \tag{1}$$

where n is the noise vector and H is the CSI channel matrix which is made up of complex numbers, namely $H = H_R + iH_I$. For the s-th subcarrier between the i-th transmitting antenna and the j-th receiving antenna, it is given by

$$H_{ij}^s = \left\| H_{ij}^s \right\| e^{j\angle H_{ij}^s}, s \in [1, N_s], i \in [1, N_t], j \in [1, N_r] \tag{2}$$

where $\left\|H_{ij}^{s}\right\|$ and $\angle H_{ij}^{s}$ denote amplitude and phase, respectively. N_t and N_r stand for the number of antennas at the TX and RX. And i and j are the indices of TX and RX antennas. N_s is the number of subcarriers for each pair of transceiver antenna.

2.2. Problem Analysis

To demonstrate the challenge of multi-location HAR using Wi-Fi signals, the CSI amplitudes of the activities at the same and distinct locations are analyzed and presented in Figures 1 and 2. The horizontal axis represents the frame length, and the ordinate indicates the amplitude of CSI. The dataset will be presented in more detail in Section 4. As demonstrated in Figure 1, each subgraph depicts a kind of activity. The two curves in each subgraph represent two samples of the same activity. The measured signals for the same action at a fixed location seem to have similar waveforms. In the left figures of Figure 1, the variation trends of the two samples are different to some extent, which is because there are slight differences in the amplitude, speed, and starting position of each movement performed by the volunteers, resulting in differences among different samples of the same activity. Therefore, in the process of activity recognition, it is necessary to extract similar feature patterns between different samples of the same action that represent the changing trend of the activity itself as much as possible. Furthermore, it can be observed that diverse human activities will generate different characteristic patterns in the received signals at the same location. These are the foundation of wireless sensing. However, the measured signals for the same activity possess varying CSI amplitudes at different locations. As illustrated in Figure 2, five curves correspond to the same activity at five different locations. As can be seen, although it is relatively easy to identify the types of human activities by interpreting the CSI patterns at a single location, it may not be possible to ensure good classification accuracy for multi-location sensing.

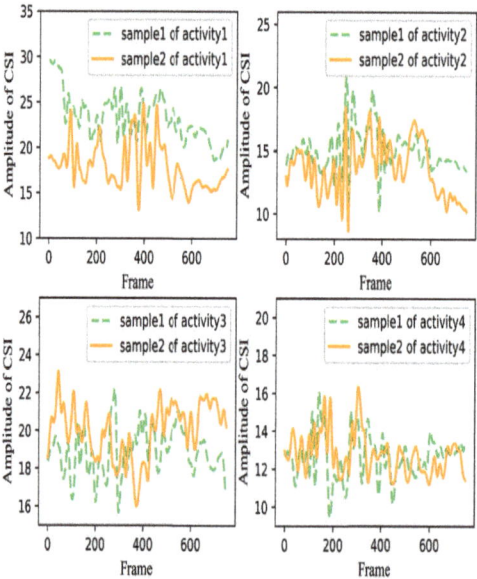

Figure 1. CSI amplitude of four different activities at the same location.

In addition to the amplitude of CSI, the phase of the activity is also analyzed and shown in Figure 3. As can be seen, the phase can also reflect the characteristics of the activity. Therefore, both amplitude and phase should be utilized effectively. According to the above observation, just in terms of amplitude and phase, apart from the types of activities, the location variations can also obviously affect signal transmission. Therefore, both kinds of information should be strongly integrated, which can provide more accurate representative features so as to achieve multi-location sensing with limited data.

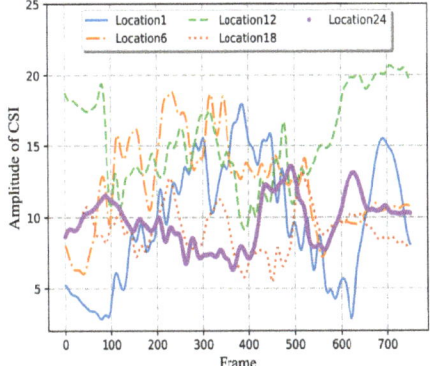

Figure 2. CSI amplitude of the same activity at five different locations.

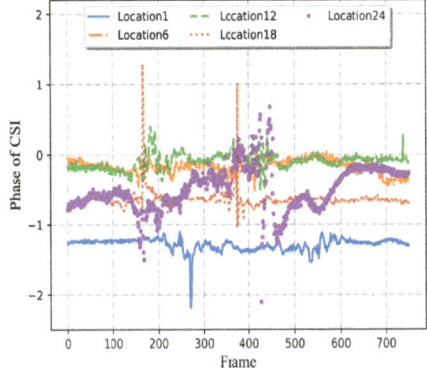

Figure 3. CSI phase of the same activity at five different locations.

3. System Model

3.1. Overview

In this part, the framework of the multi-location human activity recognition system is introduced, as shown in Figure 4. First of all, the Wi-Fi communication system is set up to collect CSI data in the Wi-Fi environment. The details will be described in Section 4. Then, feature extraction is carried out on CSI samples that are affected by human activities, and activity categories are distinguished according to the differences in features to realize human activity recognition.

To meet the requirement of high accuracy multi-location human activity recognition, a sensing method based on AP-DCN was proposed. High-accuracy multi-location sensing depends on adequate activity data from various positions. When data samples are restricted, sufficient activity information should be mined from the limited data. According to the above analysis, both the amplitude and phase of the Wi-Fi signal carry information related to human activities. Compared with the real-valued deep learning method based on the single amplitude or phase, the deep complex network simulates complex space computation through real-number space computation and can extract richer feature information. AP-DCN is designed to fully mine human activity information in amplitude and phase of CSI by using the complex convolution operation.

In some application scenarios, besides the lack of data samples, there is also the problem of unbalanced sample numbers provided at different positions. Therefore, a multi-location human activity perception method based on transfer learning named DCN-TL is proposed to transfer the common features of human activities learned from some locations with sufficient activity data to other locations with insufficient data so as to alleviate the impact of unbalanced data samples and limited sample number.

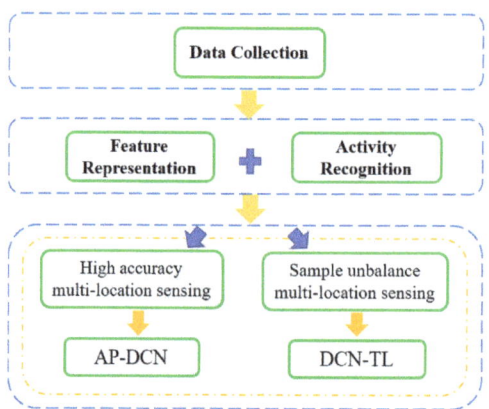

Figure 4. The framework of multi-location human activity recognition system.

3.2. Ap-Dcn

3.2.1. Network Architecture of AP-DCN

In this section, AP-DCN, which makes full use of the amplitude and phase information of CSI for multi-location human activity recognition, is designed. The architecture of the proposed AP-DCN is shown in Figure 5. With CSI as the input, in order to efficiently guide the network to learn meaning information, the calculated amplitude and phase are input to the backbone network as the real and imaginary parts of the new complex matrix, respectively.

The network consists of two complex convolution blocks, each of which contains a two-dimensional complex convolution layer, a complex batch normalization layer, and a complex activation function layer. When it comes to the number of network layers, theoretically, the more layers, the more effectively features can be extracted. However, in our scenario, the data samples are limited, and too many layers will easily lead to overfitting of the model. In addition, considering the complexity of the network in general, we designed the network using two complex convolutional blocks. Specifically, the two complex convolutional layers use 32 and 16 complex convolutional kernels, respectively. The kernel size is 3 × 3. Batch normalization layers correspond to 32 and 16 channels, respectively. Rectified Linear Unit (ReLU) is used as the activation function of the network. In order to reduce the number of model parameters and alleviate the over-fitting problem to some extent, the adaptive average pooling is applied to the real part and the imaginary part, and the size of the output feature map is 1 × 1. Subsequently, a complex linear layer follows, which is equivalent to the full connection layer of a real-valued neural network. The input size of the linear layer is 16, and the output size is 5, corresponding to five activity categories. Finally, since human activity recognition is defined as a classification problem, a softmax layer is connected to the end of the network to predict the category of the activity. The details are presented in the following.

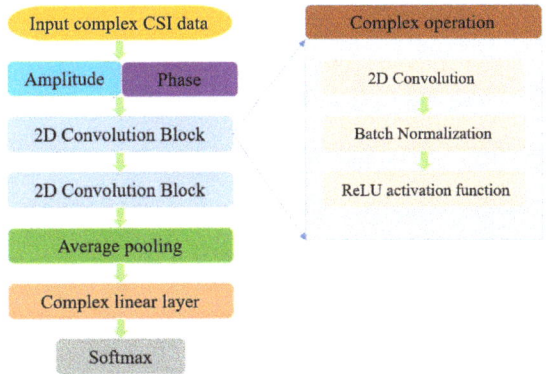

Figure 5. The architecture of the AP-DCN.

3.2.2. Network Layer of AP-DCN

For the CSI channel matrix $H = H_R + iH_I$, $H_R \in R$, $H_I \in R$, where each element is a complex number. The amplitude and the phase can be expressed as:

$$A = \|H\| = \sqrt{H_R^2 + H_I^2} \tag{3}$$

$$P = \angle H = \arctan(H_I/H_R) \tag{4}$$

As described in the literature [31], to perform the two-dimensional convolution operations in the complex domain, complex filter matrix (complex convolution kernel) $W = W_R + iW_I$, where W_R and W_I are real matrices, is to be convolved by a complex matrix $C = A + iP$. The calculation process of complex convolution can be expressed as:

$$
\begin{aligned}
W * C &= (W_R + iW_I) * (A + iP) \\
&= (W_R * A - W_I * P) + i(W_I * A + W_R * P)
\end{aligned}
\tag{5}
$$

where $*$ represents the convolution operation. The real and imaginary parts of the convolution operation can be expressed in matrix notation as follows:

$$
\begin{bmatrix} \Re(W * C) \\ \Im(W * C) \end{bmatrix} = \begin{bmatrix} W_R & -W_I \\ W_I & W_R \end{bmatrix} * \begin{bmatrix} A \\ P \end{bmatrix}
\tag{6}
$$

where $\Re$ and $\Im$ denote taking the real and imaginary parts of a complex number, respectively. The complex convolution operation is demonstrated in Figure 6.

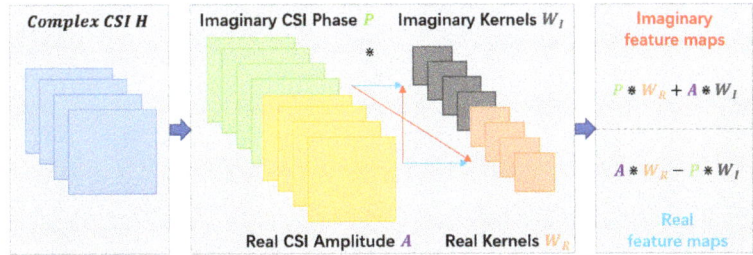

Figure 6. Complex convolution operation.

To ensure the same distribution of the neural network input of each layer in the training process, and to effectively avoid the issue of the training gradient disappearing, complex batch normalization is used for transforming the input value of each layer to standard normal distribution with an average of 0 and variance of 1, so as to accelerate convergence speed of the deep model. Taking the input $x = \{x_1, x_2, \ldots, x_m\}$ as an example, the output of the complex batch normalization layer can be obtained via the following process:

$$\tilde{x} = (V)^{-\frac{1}{2}}(x - \mathbb{E}[x]) \tag{7}$$

where the expectation $\mathbb{E}$ is calculated as follows:

$$\mathbb{E}(x) = \begin{bmatrix} \mathbb{E}(\Re(x)) \\ \mathbb{E}(\Im(x)) \end{bmatrix} = \begin{bmatrix} \frac{1}{m}\sum_{i=1}^{m}\Re(x_i) \\ \frac{1}{m}\sum_{i=1}^{m}\Im(x_i) \end{bmatrix} \tag{8}$$

The covariance matrix V is

$$V = \begin{pmatrix} V_{rr} & V_{ri} \\ V_{ir} & V_{ii} \end{pmatrix}$$
$$= \begin{pmatrix} Cov(\Re\{x\}, \Re\{x\}) & Cov(\Re\{x\}, \Im\{x\}) \\ Cov(\Im\{x\}, \Re\{x\}) & Cov(\Im\{x\}, \Im\{x\}) \end{pmatrix} \tag{9}$$

where Cov implies the covariance calculation. Take $Cov(\Im(x), \Re(x))$ as an example

$$Cov(\Im(x), \Re(x)) = \frac{\sum_{i=1}^{m}(\Im(x_i) - \mathbb{E}(\Im(x_i)))(\Re(x_i) - \mathbb{E}(\Re(x_i)))}{m} \tag{10}$$

In order to maintain the original feature distribution, the scale transformation and translation transformation follow the calculation process in reference [31].

The complex ReLU (CReLU) activation function is applied on both the real and the imaginary part of a neuron. For a complex input z, it is given by

$$CReLU(z) = ReLU(\Re(z)) + iReLU(\Im(z)) \tag{11}$$

The complex linear layer is computed similarly to the complex convolution operation by replacing the convolution operation with the multiplication operation. Then, the module value of complex output z of the complex linear layer is calculated to obtain:

$$z' = \sqrt{(\Re(z))^2 + (\Im(z))^2} \tag{12}$$

In the training phase, cross-entropy loss is employed. Letting L denote a real-value loss function, the back-propagation (BP) can be written as:

$$\nabla_L(H) = \frac{\partial L}{\partial H} = \frac{\partial L}{\partial H_R} + i\frac{\partial L}{\partial H_I} = \frac{\partial L}{\partial \Re(H)} + i\frac{\partial L}{\partial \Im(H)}$$
$$= \Re(\nabla_L(H)) + i\Im(\nabla_L(H)) \tag{13}$$

$$\nabla_L(W) = \frac{\partial L}{\partial W} = \frac{\partial L}{\partial W_R} + i\frac{\partial L}{\partial W_I}$$
$$= \Re(\nabla_L(H))\left(\frac{\partial H_R}{\partial W_R} + \frac{\partial H_R}{\partial W_I}\right)$$
$$+ \Im(\nabla_L(H))\left(\frac{\partial H_I}{\partial W_R} + \frac{\partial H_I}{\partial W_I}\right) \tag{14}$$

The loss function is minimized with Adam [33] to optimize the network parameters. The exponential decay rate $\rho 1$ and $\rho 2$ are empirically set as 0.9 and 0.999, and the learning rate is set as 0.001. ReduceLROnPlateau learning rate policy is utilized. The learning rate will be reduced by half when there is no improvement in the training loss over eight epochs. The total epoch is set up as 50.

3.3. Dcn-Tl

3.3.1. Human Activity Recognition Method Based on DCN-TL

The process of the DCN-TL-based sensing method mainly consists of feature representation and recognition, and model fine-tuning based on transfer learning. A feature representation and classification recognition method based on a one-dimensional complex convolutional network was proposed to extract features and predict categories of human activities. The network is trained through the human activity samples with sufficient data in the source domain to obtain the pre-trained model. Then, a small number of target domain samples are used to update the pre-trained model by the transfer learning method. In practical application scenarios, the model pre-training and the model update are completed offline. After the optimal parameters are obtained, the activity prediction can be realized online without affecting the system response speed during use.

3.3.2. Feature Representation Method Based on One-Dimensional Complex Convolution

Before knowledge transfer, it is necessary to learn as much activity-related experiential knowledge as possible from the data samples in the source domain. In order to effectively mine the time-dimension information of CSI data, a human activity feature representation method based on a one-dimensional complex convolutional network is proposed. The activity features contained in the amplitude and phase of CSI data are extracted by one-dimensional convolution which is suitable for sequence information extraction. Table 1 shows the structure of the feature extraction network model. The 750×30 complex CSI matrix is used as the input, and its amplitude and phase are calculated to input the backbone network. The network consists of two one-dimensional complex convolutional layers, two complex batch normalization layers, an adaptive averaging pooling layer, and two complex linear layers. In Table 1, ($\times 4$) represents the convolution operation or linear multiplication operation between the real/imaginary parts and the two corresponding network weights four times. ($\times 2$) represents two corresponding operations on the real and imaginary parts. Complex convolution operations and complex linear operations are computed in the same way as AP-DCN. The softmax classifier is still used for classification and recognition. Specific network parameters are set as follows: the number of convolution kernels corresponding to the two convolution layers is 128; the kernel size is 3; for one-dimensional convolution, that is, three times the number of input channels. For example, the size of the convolution kernel at the first layer is 3×30, and the size of the convolution kernel at the second layer is 3×128. The step size and the padding are set to 1.

Table 1. The model structure of feature extraction network.

Layer	Output Size
Input layer	$(-1, 30, 750)$
Complex convolution layer 1 ($\times 4$)	$(-1, 128, 750)$
Complex batch normalization layer 1 ($\times 2$)	$(-1, 128, 750)$
Complex convolution layer 2 ($\times 4$)	$(-1, 128, 750)$
Complex batch normalization layer 2 ($\times 2$)	$(-1, 128, 750)$
Adaptive average pooling layer ($\times 2$)	$(-1, 128)$
Complex linear layer 1 ($\times 4$)	$(-1, 64)$
Complex linear layer 2 ($\times 4$)	$(-1, 5)$

Figure 7 shows the specific one-dimensional convolution operation process for the real or imaginary part of the complex input matrix. Taking the amplitude or phase of CSI data with an input size of $T \times s$ as an example, it is composed of T time slices, and each time slice corresponds to s subcarrier information, which can be regarded as the feature vector with the dimension of s.

The convolution kernel is used to conduct a one-dimensional convolution operation with input data. Different from the two-dimensional convolution operation, the convolution kernel of the one-dimensional convolution operation moves only along the time axis. The convolution kernel is a feature detector, which is equivalent to a sliding time window in the time dimension. We define the number of convolution kernels as N and the size of the convolution kernels as k. The number of convolution kernels determines the dimension of the output vector, which is the number of features obtained. The size of the convolution kernel determines the time length of the activity involved in each convolution operation. The length of the input data and the size of the convolution kernel determine the number of output neurons. Taking step size 1 and padding size 0 as an example, after a layer of convolution operation, the output matrix with size $N \times (T - k + 1)$ is obtained. For the network mentioned above, the same loss function calculation method, model optimization method, and parameter setting are still used to train the model and obtain the pre-training model for the next stage of knowledge transfer.

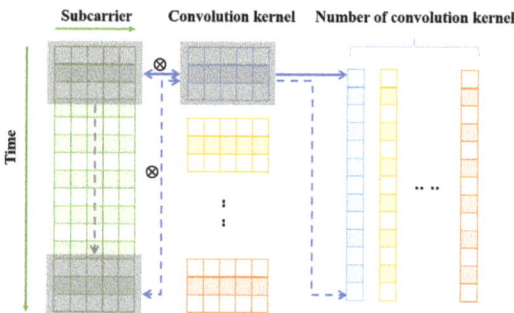

Figure 7. One-dimensional convolution operation.

3.3.3. Recognition Method Based on Transfer Learning

The above feature representation and learning methods can be used to train the basic model with strong discriminant ability from relatively sufficient source domain data. At this point, the learned knowledge contains the basic characteristics of CSI data and the general characteristics of activities at different source domain locations. When data samples from different locations are unbalanced, to adapt the model to the target domain location where the data sample is further constrained, the model needs to have the ability to transfer knowledge learned from the source domain locations to the target domain locations. Therefore, a multi-location activity recognition scheme based on transfer learning is proposed. The model fine-tuning of transfer learning can realize knowledge sharing with very few target domain samples. The low-level parameters of the network are obtained from sufficient source domain data, and the high-level parameters are learned from the target domain data with limited samples.

The transfer learning scheme is based on the pre-training model. Figure 8 shows the architecture of the transfer learning network. The specific process is as follows: Firstly, the network model is pre-trained using the source domain training data set composed of several positions to obtain the optimal model parameters. These parameters are then used to initialize the network and freeze the network layer before the linear layer. Finally, the two linear layers are trained with very few data samples from the target domain locations. Based on the pre-training model, the activity feature representation of source domain learning is transferred to the target domain, which greatly reduces the need for training samples in the target domain and effectively alleviates the problem of sample imbalance. The forward and back-propagation of traditional network training involve all layers of the whole network, while the transfer learning process only involves the last two layers, which can effectively reduce training parameters and shorten training time.

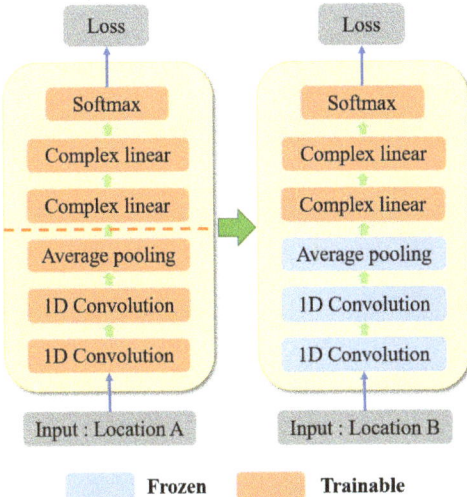

Figure 8. Architecture of transfer learning network.

4. Experiment and Evaluation

In order to validate the performance of our proposed AP-DCN-based and DCN-TL-based multi-location HAR method, a series of experiments have been conducted. The experiment setup and the experiment results are reported in this section.

4.1. Experiment Setup

To fully evaluate the performance of the proposed method, a dataset has been collected in a cluttered office. The experimental scene is shown in Figure 9. Halperin et al. develop Linux 802.11n CSI Tool [34] based on Intel 5300 Network Interface Card (NIC) which is leveraged to acquire the fine-grained CSI data. The transmitter (TX) and the receiver (RX) work in 802.11n, and operate on a 5 GHz frequency band, with a bandwidth of 20 MHz. They are both equipped with three antennas. CSI with 30 groups of subcarriers from each TX-RX pair can be obtained. It is worth noting that the CSI data from only one of the antenna pairs, namely 30 subcarriers, can be alternatively used.

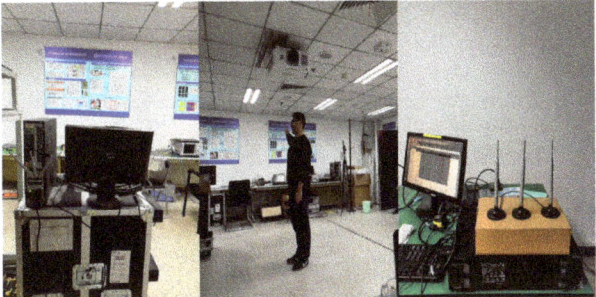

Figure 9. Data collection experimental scene.

To explore the multi-location HAR method, data samples at 24 different locations within a region between the transceivers are collected. The specified location is depicted in Figure 10. The distance between adjacent sampling locations is approximately 0.6 m. The room size is approximately 6 m × 8 m. The distance between TX and RX is 4 m. We predefined five activities, including drawing a circle (O), drawing across (X), lifting up and laying down two arms (UP), pushing and opening with two arms (PO), and sitting down (ST). Five volunteers (one female and four males ranging from 23–30 years old) conducted 50 samples for each activity at each location. There are 24 × 50 = 1200 samples for each activity of each person. Since the initial sampling rate is 200 frames per second, and the actual duration of the actions is 3.5∼4 s, namely 700∼800 frames, 750 frames is cut as a sample.

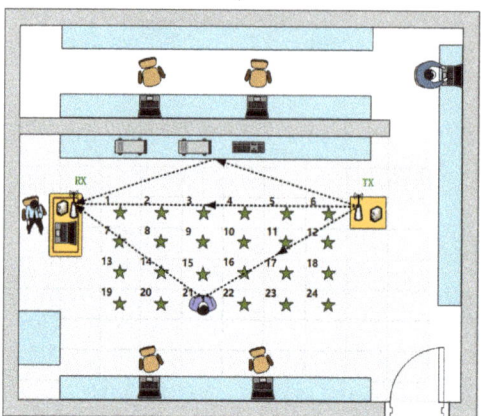

Figure 10. The layout of data collection locations.

4.2. Experiment Results of Ap-Dcn

The evaluation contains the following three parts. Firstly, the feasibility and effectiveness of the approach are explored. Then, the reliability is discussed. Finally, the proposed method is compared with other approaches to prove the superiority of our system.

Overall performance. To verify the feasibility of the multi-location sensing method, 50 samples for each activity at 24 locations of one person are randomly divided into three parts, the training set, the validation set, and the testing set, which accounts for 20%, 20%, and 60%, respectively. It is worth noting that, to reduce the computational burden, only 30 subcarriers from one TX-RX antenna and five training samples from each location are used. The size of the sample is 750 × 30, each is a complex number with its real and imaginary parts. The average accuracy of the proposed method for the five activities of one person is 96.53%. The confusion matrix is demonstrated in Figure 11. It can be seen that all the activities can obtain an acceptable recognition accuracy. In particular, the activity ST achieved 99.86% recognition accuracy. Since X and O are both movements in front of the body after raising the right arm, they are easier to be confused than other activities. In summary, our proposed method performs well in multi-location human activity sensing.

The enhancement effect of amplitude and phase information on multi-location recognition is analyzed. The comparison of recognition accuracy of different methods is demonstrated in Table 2. CNN represents the real-valued convolutional neural network corresponding to AP-DCN network structure. DCN represents complex convolutional networks with the same network structure that are not enhanced by amplitude and phase calculation. Through the comparison between CNN and DCN, it can be seen that complex convolution calculation plays a certain role in extracting richer activity information. The comparison between DCN and AP-DCN shows that manual calculation of amplitude and phase can effectively guide the network to learn more accurate information, so as to achieve higher accuracy of human activity perception.

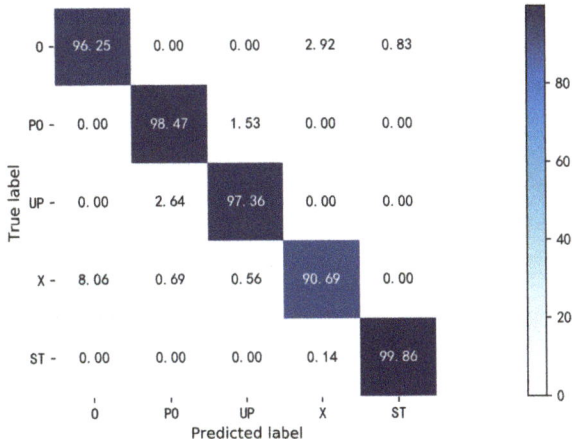

Figure 11. The confusion matrix of AP-DCN recognition accuracy.

Table 2. Comparison of recognition accuracy of different methods.

Sensing Method	Accuracy (%)
CNN	92.23
DCN	94.92
AP-DCN	96.53

Performance of multi-location HAR in terms of different location areas. According to the principle of wireless sensing, when the target is farther away from the transmitter and the receiver, the delay of the reflected signal generated by the target may be larger. After multi-path superposition, the influence on the received signal is relatively small. Therefore, when the target and the perceptual location area are far from the transceiver, the sensing effect will decrease. To evaluate the reliability of the proposed method in different location areas, four perceptual regions from near and far relative to the transceiver are selected. Table 3 shows the recognition accuracy of different perception areas. Loc1-Loc6 indicates the training and testing samples are selected from location 1–6 in Figure 10. As can be seen, as the location region expands, although the perceptual effect slightly declines, high recognition accuracy can be obtained in each perception area. Although the perception effect is slightly decreased, high recognition accuracy can be obtained in each perception area. For 24 sampling positions covering almost the whole space, the recognition accuracy is still satisfied.

Table 3. The AP-DCN recognition accuracy of different sensing areas.

Sensing Area	Accuracy (%)
Loc 1~Loc 6	98.44
Loc 1~Loc 12	98.27
Loc 1~Loc 18	97.99
Loc 1~Loc 24	96.53

Performance of multi-location HAR for different number of training samples. Intuitively, the more samples involved in training, the richer the activity features can be provided. The number of training samples involving 4, 6, 8, and 10 for each activity at each location are investigated. The recognition accuracy with different numbers of training samples is shown in Table 4. As can be seen, the proposed method can provide satisfied recognition accuracy of 95.81% with four training samples. When the number of training samples increases from four to ten, the recognition accuracy is further improved.

Table 4. The recognition accuracy for different number of training samples.

Number of Training Samples	4	6	8	10
Accuracy (%)	95.81	96.85	97.39	98.11

Performance of multi-location HAR for different number of subcarriers with different sampling rates. This paper, in addition to implementing human activity recognition for multi-location, also aims to reduce the computational burden, which is more suitable for real-time applications. Therefore, a small sample size is desired. CSI measurements are collected at the initial transmission rate of 200 packets per second, and the 750 CSI series are down-sampled to 375, 250, 150, and 75. Furthermore, the number of subcarriers of 10, 20, and 30 are investigated. It is worth noting that only five training samples for each activity at each location are utilized. The recognition accuracy with different numbers of subcarriers and sampling rates are shown in Figure 12. As can be seen, the proposed method can provide satisfied recognition accuracy with very few subcarriers and low sampling rates. As far as the sampling rate is concerned, when the sampling rate decreases to 20 frames/s, the method can still obtain 88.61% with only 10 subcarriers.

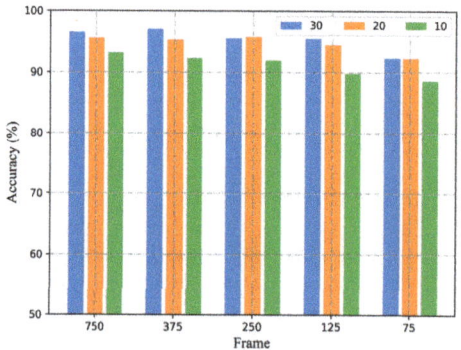

Figure 12. The recognition accuracy with different number of subcarriers and sampling rates.

Performance of multi-location HAR for different persons. To verify the reliability of the system for different users, we collected the data samples involving five subjects marked as User1–User5. Their heights range from 160–180 cm, while the age is from 23–30 years old. The recognition results of the five users for five activities at 24 locations are shown in Table 5. As illustrated, the average recognition accuracy is 96.85%. Consequently, our method can work well for different users.

Table 5. The AP-DCN recognition accuracy for different users.

Users	User1	User2	User3	User4	User5	Average
Accuracy (%)	96.53	98.00	96.28	95.00	98.42	96.85

Comparison with different recognition methods. In this part, to evaluate the superiority, four typical approaches are compared with our system. ActNet [26] is the state-of-the-art multi-location HAR method, which decomposes the input samples into the location-irrelevant activity features and activity-irrelevant location features. It jointly learns different activities from multi-locations to mitigate the issue of insufficient data. SqueezeNet [35] and Alexnet [36] are two classical deep learning methods. WiHand [37] utilizes the low rank and sparse decomposition (LRSD) algorithm to separate activity signal from background information, thus making it adapt to location variation. It is worth noting that, in order to keep the settings as similar as possible to the original literature, all five methods use 10 training samples. In addition, the first three use 270 subcarriers, while the last two use 30 subcarriers. As can be seen in Table 6, our system outperforms these three methods in multi-location HAR, even using fewer subcarriers.

Table 6. Comparison with different recognition methods.

Methods	Accuracy (%)
ActNet [26]	94.60
SqueezeNet [35]	90.07
Alexnet [36]	89.00
WiHand [37]	88.22
AP-DCN	98.11

4.3. Experiment Results of Dcn-Tl

This section still uses the data set composed of five human activities collected at 24 positions in Section 4.1 to evaluate the performance of the multi-location human activity recognition method based on DCN-TL. 50 samples of each activity collected by volunteers at each location are divided into three parts: model training, knowledge transfer, and performance test, accounting for 60%, 20%, and 20%, respectively. For any volunteer, a maximum of 30 training samples, 10 transfer samples, and 10 test samples are available for an activity at each location. This section still uses 750 frame length and 30 subcarriers as input. The parameters of the pre-training network are the same as in the previous section.

Overall performance. In order to verify the perceptual performance of the method when the number of training samples at different locations is unbalanced and the number of samples at some locations is further limited, for the 24 sampling locations in the data set, we take the example of sufficient samples at six locations and insufficient samples at other locations to evaluate the feasibility of the method. The six training positions are selected starting from the first position in Figure 10 at equal intervals, taking one for every four positions from location 1 to 24. Three samples were randomly selected from 10 transfer samples for model transfer learning. The testing set consists of testing samples involving five activities at 24 positions, with a total of $24 \times 5 \times 10 = 1200$ samples. Experimental results show that the average recognition accuracy of DCN-TL is 93.00%. The confusion matrix is shown in Figure 13. Among them, ST can obtain 100% recognition accuracy. Other activities can also obtain satisfactory recognition accuracy. Therefore, DCN-TL performs well in the multi-location human activity sensing when the number of training samples at different positions is unbalanced and the number of samples at some positions is further limited.

Performance of multi-location HAR in terms of different location areas. We discuss the performance of human activity recognition based on the DCN-TL recognition method when the perception area gradually expands. At the 24 sampling positions shown in Figure 10, location 1–6 in the first row parallel to the transceiver is defined as perception area 1, and the experiment number is marked as N1. Training positions 2 and 5 are symmetrically selected. One row is added at a time to gradually expand the perception area, forming evaluation experiments numbered N2, N3, and N4. The training position of the latter perception area is increased based on the training position of the former perception area. For example, "N1+8/11" represents that the training positions 8 and 11 are added on the basis of N1, namely, the four positions participating in the model pre-training are 2/5/8/11. Table 7 shows the recognition accuracy of different perception areas. It can be seen that, with the expansion of the perception area, the recognition accuracy gradually improves. This is because the model can learn more knowledge in the pre-training stage due to the gradual increase of training positions.

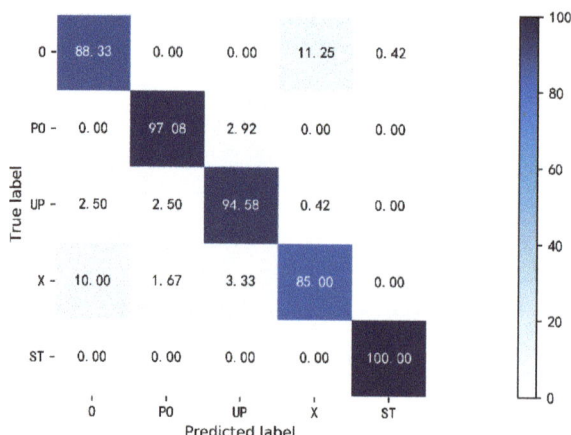

Figure 13. The confusion matrix of DCN-TL recognition accuracy.

Table 7. The DCN-TL recognition accuracy of different sensing areas.

Number	Training Locations	Testing Locations	Accuracy (%)
N1	2/5	Loc 1~Loc 6	88.33
N2	N1+8/11	Loc 1~Loc 12	90.83
N3	N2+14/17	Loc 1~Loc 18	91.78
N4	N3+20/23	Loc 1~Loc 24	93.42

Performance of multi-location HAR in terms of different number of training locations. The number of positions involved in pre-training is a critical factor affecting perceptual performance. The influence of the number of locations involved in pre-training on recognition accuracy is discussed in this part. A total of 12, 8, 6, and 4 pre-training positions are sampled at equal intervals from 24 positions. As shown in Table 8, when only four positions participate in training, and three samples are provided for each transfer location, the recognition accuracy can still be 90.42%. When there are 12 training positions, the recognition accuracy is 94.64%. With the increase of the number of training positions, the recognition accuracy increases gradually.

Table 8. The recognition accuracy of different numbers of pre-trained locations.

Number of Training Locations	24	12	8	6	4
Accuracy (%)	98.58	94.64	93.33	93.00	90.42

Performance of multi-location HAR in terms of different number of transfer samples. The influence of the number of samples involved in knowledge transfer on recognition accuracy is discussed. This part takes six pre-training positions as examples and tests the method at 24 positions. A total of 1–5 transfer samples are randomly selected from the transfer sample set. The recognition accuracy is shown in Table 9. When only one transfer sample is provided, the recognition accuracy is 90.55%. Using five transfer samples, the recognition accuracy can reach 97.44%. With the increase in the number of transfer samples, the model can learn more activity characteristics of the target domain location based on the experiential knowledge of source domain location learning, so as to improve the recognition accuracy.

Table 9. The recognition accuracy of different numbers of transfer samples.

Number of Transfer Samples	1	2	3	4	5
Accuracy (%)	90.55	93.17	94.75	96.33	97.44

Performance of multi-location HAR for different users. To verify the reliability of the proposed method for different users, the performance of human activity data involving five volunteers are evaluated. Five volunteers are marked as User 1–User 5. Six positions are used for training, 24 positions are tested, and three transfer samples are provided for each position. Table 10 shows the recognition accuracy of 5 activities at 24 positions by different volunteers. The average recognition accuracy is 94.02%. Experimental results show that this method can be well applied to different users.

Table 10. The DCN-TL recognition accuracy for different users.

Users	User1	User2	User3	User4	User5	Average
Accuracy (%)	93.50	93.00	94.75	93.67	95.17	94.02

5. Discussion

In the evaluation for this paper, 24 positions with an interval of 0.6m are sampled in a typical indoor area. When the range of sensing area is fixed, increasing the number of sampling locations will improve the perception effect. If the sensing area continues to expand, such as in a larger room, the perception effect will be decreased to some extent. When the sensing target is far away from the transmitter and receiver, the influence on signal transmission will be weakened. Theoretically speaking, the sensing performance decreases with the increase of the distance between the sensing target and the sensing device. For the number of activities, there may be more activities in practice scenarios. As for the experimental settings in most literature, five to eight activities are usually recognized in a typical smart home control scenario. If the number of activities continues to increase, the recognition accuracy will decrease to a certain extent, because some actions may have similar features and be easily confused. This is still a challenging issue for Wi-Fi-based human activity recognition, which will be further explored in future work.

6. Conclusions

In this paper, Wi-Fi-based multi-location human activity recognition technique is explored. A novel AP-DCN-based method that fully leverages the amplitude and phase information is presented. The complex convolution layer, complex batch normalization layer, and complex ReLU activation function are leveraged for feature representation. Furthermore, considering the unbalanced sample number at different locations, a perception method based on DCN-TL is proposed. To verify the performance of the method, a dataset involving five activities at 24 positions in an office is built. The experiment results indicate that the AP-DCN-based method can achieve an average accuracy of 96.85% for five people with only five training samples at each of the 24 locations. Furthermore, the proposed method is also applicable to the training samples with a low sampling rate and fewer subcarriers. In the case of unbalanced number of data samples at different locations, the recognition accuracy is 94.02%. Therefore, it is concluded that the presented method is feasible for multi-location human activity recognition with limited data samples, which promisingly promotes the generalization performance of the device-free sensing system.

Author Contributions: Conceptualization, X.D., C.H., W.X. and T.J.; methodology, X.D.; software, X.D.; validation, X.D.; formal analysis, X.D., C.H., W.X., Y.Z. and J.Y.; investigation, X.D. and Y.Z.; resources, W.X., C.H. and T.J.; data curation, X.D.; writing—original draft preparation, X.D.; writing—review and editing, X.D., C.H., W.X., Y.Z., J.Y. and T.J.; visualization, X.D.; supervision, T.J., C.H. and W.X.; project administration, C.H., W.X. and T.J.; funding acquisition, T.J., Y.Z. All authors have read and agreed to the published version of the manuscript.

Funding: This work is supported by the National Natural Sciences Foundation of China (No. 62071061), and Beijing Institute of Technology Research Fund Program for Young Scholars.

Institutional Review Board Statement: Not applicable

Informed Consent Statement: Not applicable

Data Availability Statement: Not applicable

Conflicts of Interest: The authors declare no conflict of interest.

References

1. Kumar, P. Human Activity Recognition with Deep Learning: Overview, Challenges & Possibilities. *Ccf Trans. Pervasive Comput. Interact.* **2021**, *339*, 1–29.
2. Liu, J.; Liu, H.; Chen, Y.; Wang, Y.; Wang, C. Wireless sensing for human activity: A survey. *IEEE Commun. Surv. Tutor.* **2019**, *22*, 1629–1645. [CrossRef]
3. Wang, J.; Gao, Q.; Pan, M.; Fang, Y. Device-Free Wireless Sensing: Challenges, Opportunities, and Applications. *IEEE Netw.* **2018**, *32*, 132–137. [CrossRef]
4. Zhang, W.; Zhou, S.; Yang, L.; Ou, L.; Xiao, Z. WiFiMap+: High-Level Indoor Semantic Inference with WiFi Human Activity and Environment. *IEEE Trans. Veh. Technol.* **2019**, *68*, 7890–7903. [CrossRef]
5. Liu, H.; Hartmann, Y.; Schultz, T. Motion Units: Generalized Sequence Modeling of Human Activities for Sensor-Based Activity Recognition. In Proceedings of the 2021 29th European Signal Processing Conference (EUSIPCO), Dublin, Ireland, 23–27 August 2021; pp. 1506–1510.
6. Liu, H.; Hartmann, Y.; Schultz, T. A Practical Wearable Sensor-based Human Activity Recognition Research Pipeline. In Proceedings of the Proceedings of the 15th International Joint Conference on Biomedical Engineering Systems and Technologies, Online, 9–11 February 2022; pp. 847–856. [CrossRef]
7. Randhawa, P.; Shanthagiri, V.; Kumar, A.; Yadav, V. Human activity detection using machine learning methods from wearable sensors. *Sens. Rev.* **2020**, *40*, 591–603. [CrossRef]
8. Wang, J.; Chen, Y.; Hao, S.; Peng, X.; Hu, L. Deep learning for sensor-based activity recognition: A survey. *Pattern Recognit. Lett.* **2019**, *119*, 3–11. [CrossRef]
9. D'Sa, A.G.; Prasad, B. A survey on vision based activity recognition, its applications and challenges. In Proceedings of the 2019 Second International Conference on Advanced Computational and Communication Paradigms (ICACCP), Gangtok, India, 25–28 February 2019; IEEE: Piscataway, NJ, USA, 2019; pp. 1–8.
10. Zhang, H.B.; Zhang, Y.X.; Zhong, B.; Lei, Q.; Yang, L.; Du, J.X.; Chen, D.S. A comprehensive survey of vision-based human action recognition methods. *Sensors* **2019**, *19*, 1005. [CrossRef]
11. Liu, J.; Teng, G.; Hong, F. Human Activity Sensing with Wireless Signals: A Survey. *Sensors* **2020**, *20*, 1210. [CrossRef]
12. Yi, Z.; Yang, Y.; Xi, Z.; Yan, H.; Jiang, T. Impact of Seasonal Variations on Foliage Penetration Experiment: A WSN-Based Device-Free Sensing Approach. *IEEE Trans. Geosci. Remote Sens.* **2018**, *56*, 5035–5045.
13. Shrestha, A.; Li, H.; Kernec, J.L.; Fioranelli, F. Continuous human activity classification from FMCW radar with Bi-LSTM networks. *IEEE Sens. J.* **2020**, *20*, 13607–13619. [CrossRef]
14. Ding, C.; Hong, H.; Zou, Y.; Chu, H.; Zhu, X.; Fioranelli, F.; Le Kernec, J.; Li, C. Continuous human motion recognition with a dynamic range-Doppler trajectory method based on FMCW radar. *IEEE Trans. Geosci. Remote Sens.* **2019**, *57*, 6821–6831. [CrossRef]
15. Antolinos, E.; García-Rial, F.; Hernández, C.; Montesano, D.; Grajal, J. Cardiopulmonary Activity Monitoring Using Millimeter Wave Radars. *Remote Sens.* **2020**, *12*, 2265. [CrossRef]
16. Gu, T.; Fang, Z.; Yang, Z.; Hu, P.; Mohapatra, P. mmSense: Multi-Person Detection and Identification via mmWave Sensing. In Proceedings of the 3rd ACM Workshop, London, UK, 15 November 2019.
17. Zhong, Y.; Yang, Y.; Zhu, X.; Dutkiewicz, E.; Zhou, Z.; Jiang, T. Device-free sensing for personnel detection in a foliage environment. *IEEE Geosci. Remote Sens. Lett.* **2017**, *14*, 921–925. [CrossRef]
18. Huang, Y.; Zhong, Y.; Wu, Q.; Dutkiewicz, E.; Jiang, T. Cost-effective foliage penetration human detection under severe weather conditions based on auto-encoder/decoder neural network. *IEEE Internet Things J.* **2018**, *6*, 6190–6200. [CrossRef]
19. Wang, H.; Zhang, D.; Wang, Y.; Ma, J.; Wang, Y.; Li, S. RT-Fall: A real-time and contactless fall detection system with commodity WiFi devices. *IEEE Trans. Mob. Comput.* **2016**, *16*, 511–526. [CrossRef]
20. Wang, W.; Liu, A.X.; Shahzad, M.; Ling, K.; Lu, S. Device-free human activity recognition using commercial WiFi devices. *IEEE J. Sel. Areas Commun.* **2017**, *35*, 1118–1131. [CrossRef]
21. Chen, Z.; Zhang, L.; Jiang, C.; Cao, Z.; Cui, W. WiFi CSI based passive human activity recognition using attention based BLSTM. *IEEE Trans. Mob. Comput.* **2018**, *18*, 2714–2724. [CrossRef]
22. Wang, Z.; Jiang, K.; Hou, Y.; Dou, W.; Zhang, C.; Huang, Z.; Guo, Y. A survey on human behavior recognition using channel state information. *IEEE Access* **2019**, *7*, 155986–156024. [CrossRef]
23. Guo, L.; Lei, W.; Liu, J.; Wei, Z. A Survey on Motion Detection Using WiFi Signals. In Proceedings of the International Conference on Mobile Ad-Hoc & Sensor Networks, Beijing, China, 17–20 December 2017.

24. Zheng, Y.; Zhou, Z.; Liu, Y. From RSSI to CSI: Indoor Localization via Channel Response. *ACM Comput. Surv.* **2013**, *46*, 1–32.
25. Zhang, R.; Jing, X.; Wu, S.; Jiang, C.; Yu, F.R. Device-Free Wireless Sensing for Human Detection: The Deep Learning Perspective. *IEEE Internet Things J.* **2020**, *8*, 2517–2539. [CrossRef]
26. Zhong, Y.; Wang, J.; Wu, S.; Jiang, T.; Wu, Q. Multi-Location Human Activity Recognition via MIMO-OFDM Based Wireless Networks: An IoT-Inspired Device-Free Sensing Approach. *IEEE Internet Things J.* **2020**, *8*, 15148–15159. [CrossRef]
27. Yousefi, S.; Narui, H.; Dayal, S.; Ermon, S.; Valaee, S. A survey on behavior recognition using WiFi channel state information. *IEEE Commun. Mag.* **2017**, *55*, 98–104. [CrossRef]
28. Ma, Y.; Zhou, G.; Wang, S. WiFi sensing with channel state information: A survey. *ACM Comput. Surv. (CSUR)* **2019**, *52*, 1–36. [CrossRef]
29. Sen, S.; Radunovic, B.; Choudhury, R.R.; Minka, T. You are facing the Mona Lisa: Spot localization using PHY layer information. In Proceedings of the International Conference on Mobile Systems, Applications, and Services, Low Wood Bay, UK, 25–29 June 2012; pp. 183–196.
30. Yang, J.; Zou, H.; Zhou, Y.; Xie, L. Learning gestures from WiFi: A siamese recurrent convolutional architecture. *IEEE Internet Things J.* **2019**, *6*, 10763–10772. [CrossRef]
31. Trabelsi, C.; Bilaniuk, O.; Zhang, Y.; Serdyuk, D.; Subramanian, S.; Santos, J.F.; Mehri, S.; Rostamzadeh, N.; Bengio, Y.; Pal, C.J. Deep Complex Networks. *arXiv* **2018**,arXiv:1705.09792.
32. Cao, Y.; Lv, T.; Lin, Z.; Huang, P.; Lin, F. Complex ResNet Aided DoA Estimation for NearField MIMO Systems. *IEEE Trans. Veh. Technol.* **2020**, *69*, 11139–11151. [CrossRef]
33. Kingma, D.; Ba, J. Adam: A Method for Stochastic Optimization. *arXiv* **2014**, arXiv:1412.6980.
34. Halperirr, D.; Hu, W.; Sheth, A.; Wetherall, D. Tool release: Gathering 802.11n traces with channel state information. *ACM Sigcomm Comput. Commun. Rev.* **2011**, *41*, 53. [CrossRef]
35. Iandola, F.N.; Han, S.; Moskewicz, M.W.; Ashraf, K.; Dally, W.J.; Keutzer, K. SqueezeNet: AlexNet-level accuracy with 50x fewer parameters and <0.5 MB model size. *arXiv* **2016**, arXiv:1602.07360.
36. Krizhevsky, A.; Sutskever, I.; Hinton, G. ImageNet Classification with Deep Convolutional Neural Networks. *Adv. Neural Inf. Process. Syst.* **2012**, *25*, 1097–1105. [CrossRef]
37. Lu, Y.; Lv, S.; Wang, X. Towards Location Independent Gesture Recognition with Commodity WiFi Devices. *Electronics* **2019**, *8*, 1069. [CrossRef]

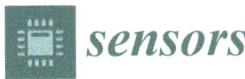

MDPI

Article

Practical and Accurate Indoor Localization System Using Deep Learning

Jeonghyeon Yoon and Seungku Kim *

Department of Electronics Engineering, Chungbuk National University, Cheongju 28644, Korea
* Correspondence: kimsk@cbnu.ac.kr

Abstract: Indoor localization is an important technology for providing various location-based services to smartphones. Among the various indoor localization technologies, pedestrian dead reckoning using inertial measurement units is a simple and highly practical solution for indoor localization. In this study, we propose a smartphone-based indoor localization system using pedestrian dead reckoning. To create a deep learning model for estimating the moving speed, accelerometer data and GPS values were used as input data and data labels, respectively. This is a practical solution compared with conventional indoor localization mechanisms using deep learning. We improved the positioning accuracy via data preprocessing, data augmentation, deep learning modeling, and correction of heading direction. In a horseshoe-shaped indoor building of 240 m in length, the experimental results show a distance error of approximately 3 to 5 m.

Keywords: indoor localization; pedestrian dead reckoning; deep learning; GPS

Citation: Yoon, J.; Kim, S. Practical and Accurate Indoor Localization System Using Deep Learning. *Sensors* **2022**, *22*, 6764. https://doi.org/10.3390/s22186764

Academic Editors: Hugo Gamboa, Tanja Schultz and Hui Liu

Received: 29 July 2022
Accepted: 5 September 2022
Published: 7 September 2022

Publisher's Note: MDPI stays neutral with regard to jurisdictional claims in published maps and institutional affiliations.

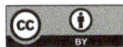
1. Introduction

Recently, with widespread use of smartphones, location-based services (LBS) have gained increasing public attention [1,2]. Navigation and route guidance applications that use GPS are the most representative LBS. In addition, LBS for pedestrians, such as surrounding information search services and evacuation route guidance in the event of a disaster, are currently being actively provided. An indoor localization system is an important technology for providing LBS. This enables the estimation of the location of people in a space in which GPS signals are not provided.

Typical mechanisms for indoor localization use wireless signals or inertial measurement units (IMU). Trilateration, triangulation, and fingerprinting methods using the received signal strength indication (RSSI) or channel state information (CSI) have been widely studied in wireless signal-based indoor localization systems. These methods mainly use radio technologies, such as Wi-Fi, Bluetooth, ZigBee, and ultra-wideband (UWB). The wireless signal-based system can operate only in a space with installed infrastructure. In addition, it is difficult to obtain consistent positioning accuracy because the radio signal is greatly affected by nearby obstacles (e.g., walls, columns, and objects) or interference signals. Indoor localization techniques through trilateration and triangulation calculate the position of the target by measuring the distance or angle between the three coordinates that serve as reference points and the tag that serves as the target [3]. In the case of using Wi-Fi as a radio signal, to measure the distance between the access point (AP) and the tag for transmitting the wireless Wi-Fi signal, the RSSI values are converted into distance information or the time of arrival (ToA), and the location is calculated using triangulation. Indoor localization technology through triangulation uses the angle at which radio signals arrive, i.e., angle of arrival (AoA). Mohammed et al. [4] addressed this problem by identifying the condition of an undetected direct path (UDP), which is a straight path from the transmitter to the receiver and introducing a deep learning model to mitigate it. Michael et al. [5] implemented a more accurate time difference of arrival (TDoA) based indoor position recognition technology through multiband (UWB-wideband) UWB technology and a single-input multiple-output (SIMO) method to address the problem of multipath attenuation of radio signals. Shuai et al. [6] proposed enhanced trilateration localization, which improves localization accuracy through quality evaluation and adaptive selection (IT-QEAS). First, they assess the quality of the distance measurement results among the anchor nodes and select the anchor nodes that have the highest quality. Then, a localization calculation was performed with the selected anchor node. However, although indoor localization systems using triangulation and trilateration have improved through various studies, the use of RSSI or CSI is affected by the irregular signal attenuation characteristics of the radio signal depending on the surrounding environment. In addition, because wireless signals are used, APs for transmitting wireless signals must be preinstalled, and there is a possibility of blind spots that radio signals cannot reach, or that radio signals are blocked by obstacles or walls. In particular, localization solutions that need pre-installation in the infrastructure have reduced practicality.

The fingerprinting method divides the service area into several cells, selects a reference location, and receives a wireless signal sent by the Wi-Fi AP at each cell through a smartphone to measure the RSSI values and create a radio map based on it. Subsequently, the user receives a signal from the AP at a random location, measures the RSSI value, contrasts it with a radio map, and estimates the corresponding cell as the user's location. Yuanchao et al. [7] proposed GradIentFingerprintTing (GIFT) to reduce instability in RSSI values that change over time in indoor environments. Qianwen et al. [8] implemented fingerprinting technology using CSI rather than RSSI and introduced a K-nearest neighbor (KNN) algorithm to increase the accuracy of the final indoor position calculation. Unlike traditional algorithms, Minh et al. [9] introduced a recurrent neural network (RNN) model instead of finding the position of the user one at a time, reducing the instability of the RSSI values that change over time. However, the precise indoor localization of fingerprinting requires a lot of information about the reference locations, that is, cells, used for positioning and the process of collecting RSSI from cells requires service providers to collect them, which is costly. Furthermore, the RSSI value also varies with changes in the surrounding environment as radio maps are pre-written, making it essential to calibrate radio maps over time, and it is impossible to accurately measure RSSI owing to the attenuation of signals caused by interference from adjacent channels. In a relatively static situation, an indoor localization system using fingerprinting can achieve high performance. However, if there are many people and the surrounding environment is very dynamic, it is difficult to expect accuracy because fingerprinting may be hard to implement.

Pedestrian dead reckoning (PDR) is a representative indoor localization method that uses IMU. This uses collected sensor values, such as accelerometers, magnetometers, barometers, and gyroscopes, to estimate the moving distance and direction of movement of people. The positioning accuracy of the PDR is mainly determined by a model or formula that converts the sensor value into moving distance and direction. Various PDR techniques [10–14] have been studied, and they exhibit a position error of several centimeters. However, the models of formulas derived from conventional studies are difficult to generalize under various conditions (e.g., moving patterns, sensor placements, and the surrounding environment). They operate only under specific conditions; therefore, they are difficult to use in practice. PDR is a technology that calculates the next location of pedestrian using sensor data, such as accelerometers, gyroscopes, and magnetometers, from the previous location. The next position of the pedestrian is estimated by estimating the number of steps and stride of pedestrians through acceleration sensors and estimating the pedestrians' orientation using a magnetometer and gyroscope. The PDR is largely divided into two areas according to how the sensor data are used to calculate the next location. First, the pattern of the data collected by the accelerometer is analyzed to calculate the number of steps. Second, the stride is estimated using the value of the accelerometer.

For example, the number of steps can be calculated using a peak detection method based on the accelerometer value of a walking pedestrian. With recent improvements in sensor accuracy and computing power of IMU and smartphones, which are data collection devices, indoor location recognition studies using PDR show an error rate within several centimeters. Godha et al. [15] proposed a PDR system that combines GPS coordinates with sensor values obtained using inertial sensors to achieve reasonable accuracy in indoor and outdoor environments. Ionut et al. [16] introduced a practical system that uses an accelerometer and magnetometer from smartphones, without relying on the Wi-Fi's AP infrastructure, to record pedestrian walking patterns and match them with possible paths on real maps. Kang et al. [17,18] replaced inertial sensors, which are the measuring equipment used in conventional PDR methods, with smartphones to implement indoor position recognition technologies that do not require expensive additional devices or infrastructure. In addition, the number of steps was determined using the accelerometer of the smartphone, and the accuracy of the magnetometer sensor was correlated with the gyroscope to estimate the heading direction. However, it should be considered that the magnetometer sensor is not used as a major data source for estimating the direction of progress for pedestrians because it is greatly influenced by the surrounding environment.

PDR has the advantage that it does not require additional infrastructure. However, there is a significant problem with indoor localization performance, depending on the model and formula that estimates gait information with sensor data. In addition, the selection of the initial position by the user is crucial. The user's next position obtains results from the prior position, the initial position fades over time because fine errors accumulate in the collected sensor data. Another problem is that indoor localization performance varies depending on the user of the PDR system. Different users have different heights, step lengths, gait patterns, and smartphone placements, which can lead to differences in the performance of the model in estimating the moving speed and heading direction.

The other way of using sensor data to calculate the next position is by using deep learning. Deep learning is a technique for predicting the correct answer by learning patterns or characteristics from training data using models based on neural networks. Because the accelerometer data obtained from a walking person has a certain pattern, it is very suitable for applying deep learning. In other words, the accelerometer value of the pedestrian is composed of a training dataset for learning the deep learning model, and the moving speed or distance of the pedestrian is estimated using the trained deep learning model.

Gu et al. [19] proposed a deep learning-based stride estimation method that can adapt to the characteristics of various users, considering that the walking speed and arrangement state of smartphones are different for each pedestrian. After removing noise from the accelerometer and gyroscope data collected from smartphones using a low pass filter (LPF), the sensor data is trained in a supervised learning model that estimates the stride by dividing the sensor data into segments, each segment representing one step. Kang et al. [20] implemented a new technology for indoor localization, using a deep learning model that learns pedestrian walking pattern data collected outdoors. GPS coordinates and accelerometer data were collected outdoors to determine the moving speed of pedestrians using divided signal frames with hybrid multiscale convolutional recurrent neural network models. In addition, traditional PDR methods are proposed to calculate the number of steps and strides of the IMU signal in a passive way; however, in [20], the moving distance is estimated by calculating the average travel rate from the signal frame.

Although the related studies above have increased the accuracy of indoor localization by applying deep learning, the problem of whether they are practical for pedestrians remains. For example, in [19], when mapping training datasets and labels for learning deep learning models, applicants who collected training data counted their own steps, took them as the ground truth, and organized them into labels. This approach has a very impractical drawback in that the user must calculate the label (ground truth) himself and configure the training dataset until the system shows sufficient performance. To solve this problem, [20] proposed a deep learning model that learns sensor data using GPS as a label for the first time; however, only the steps walked on a straight path were evaluated without considering the orientation of pedestrians.

Because users spend most of their time with their smartphones, the location of their smartphones is highly correlated with their location. In addition, smartphones include Wi-Fi, Bluetooth, and diverse sensors that are widely used for indoor localization [21–23]. In this study, we propose a smartphone-based indoor localization system using deep learning. The proposed system operates based on PDR using an accelerometer to estimate the moving speed and a game rotation vector sensor to estimate the heading direction. The data collected by the accelerometer outdoors were used as training data for the deep learning model. The moving speed of the data was labeled using the GPS value. Although the accuracy of the label information decreases owing to the inherent error of GPS, it is very practical because training data can be collected without user intervention. We propose practical solutions and techniques for increasing the positioning accuracy of unspecified smartphone users. The contributions of this study are as follows.

1. Enhancing practicality: Because the moving speed of GPS is used as a data label, anyone can generate training data for supervised learning. The collected accelerometer and gyroscope data were classified according to smartphone placement through unsupervised learning. We derived the required sensor data size for each smartphone placement via empirical experiments and limited the data collection. Using these methods, collecting proper training data for deep learning is possible without user intervention;

2. Improving moving speed estimation: In the data preprocessing step, we removed the noise from the accelerometer and improved the accuracy of the GPS data. Data augmentation using a time-warping scheme expands the collected data size, thereby increasing the accuracy of the deep learning model. Finally, we implemented and compared seven deep-learning models to derive the most accurate model.

The remainder of this paper is organized as follows. Section 2 presents problems that have not been resolved in conventional studies. Section 3 introduces the proposed indoor localization system, and Section 4 evaluates the performance of the proposed system. Finally, conclusions are presented in Section 5.

2. Problem Definition

We studied a PDR-based indoor localization using deep learning. In this section, we describe three major problems of conventional PDR-based indoor localization.

2.1. Low GPS Accuracy

GPS can provide geolocation and time information to a GPS receiver if four or more line-of-sight GPS satellites exist. Using GPS values as training data labels for deep learning may improve the practicality of the indoor localization technology. However, GPS has inherent errors owing to satellite signal blockage and reflection caused by buildings, trees, etc. If the GPS receiver is located in a city center or forest, the quality of the GPS data may be poor. In this case, using GPS data as training data labels is not appropriate because unreliable labels degrade the accuracy of the deep learning models. This affects the performance of indoor localization systems.

We performed an outdoor experiment to analyze the accuracy of the GPS data using a smartphone. The subjects repeatedly moved 75 m in various environments. Figure 1 shows the distance error ratio according to the number of receivable GPS satellites used in the experiment. When the subject moves near high-rise buildings or under a bridge, the smartphone can receive between four and six GPS satellite signals. However, a high distance error ratio of 5.34% to 8.47% was seen in this signal. When the subject moved in the campus playground or field, nine or more GPS satellites could be received. In this case, the distance error ratio was very low (i.e., 0.67–1.72%) compared to the case where the number of receivable GPS satellites is small. In the experiment, we verified that unfiltered GPS data are unsuitable as training data labels for deep learning.

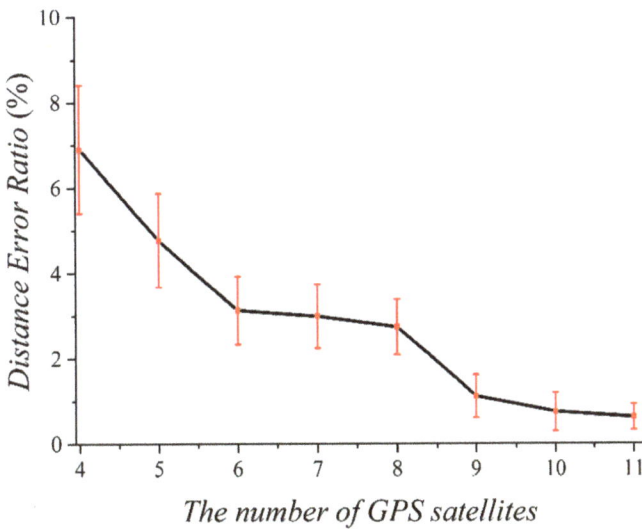

Figure 1. Distance error ratio according to the number of receivable GPS satellites.

2.2. Bias of Sensor Data

An artificial neural network [24] is a statistical learning algorithm constructed by imitating the manner in which nerve cells or neurons are inter-connected in the human brain. Just as human neurons receive and store input values through synapses from several other neurons and then export output values to the next neuron, the artificial neural network model neuron receives multiple inputs and transmits output values to the next neuron in the model. Artificial neural networks are constructed by stacking several neuron models. Deep learning is a type of machine-learning algorithm based on artificial neural networks. Deep learning has been widely used in various applications.

Deep learning refers to a learning model that predicts outcomes by extracting features or patterns from training data. The size and quality of the training data significantly influence the performance of the deep learning model. Thus, it is very important to secure a sufficient amount of high-quality data from which a deep learning model can extract features. A PDR-based indoor localization system mainly uses sensor values, such as data from accelerometers, magnetometers, barometers, and gyroscopes for training. To determine the patterns of movements in daily life, we conducted an outdoor experiment to collect data. In the experiment, a subject collected sensor values every second using a smartphone, while walking freely for 3 h. The moving speed of the subjects was obtained using GPS. Figure 2 shows the distribution of the collected data with respect to the moving speed. As a result, 66.3% of the collected data were distributed between the moving speeds 1.3 m/s and 1.7 m/s. Most of the collected data were within the average human walking speed. Since the number of samples for the speed range 1.3–1.7 m/s is much larger than that for other speeds, the data is biased. If these biased data are used for training deep earning models, it is difficult to expect high accuracy in the case the subject is not walking at an average speed. We do not need to consider data bias, if we can collect huge amounts of data. However, because collecting data is expensive, we assume that data collection is minimized.

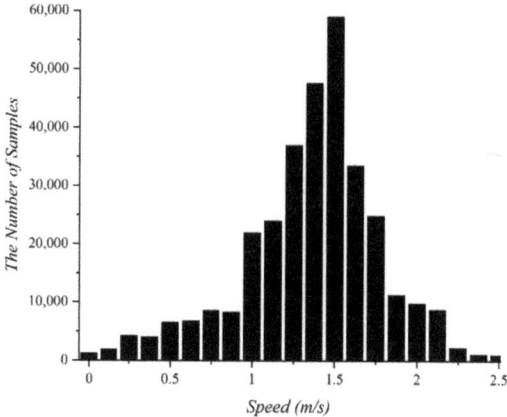

Figure 2. Distribution of the collected data according to moving speed.

2.3. Effect of Magentometer

The heading direction estimation of pedestrians for the indoor localization system is as important as the estimation of the moving distance. Many conventional studies on heading direction estimation use a magnetometer to measure the magnetic north. However, the magnetometer reacts sensitively to the surrounding environment, such as walls, obstacles, and steel, resulting in errors that cannot correctly measure the magnetic north. Android smartphones provide the absolute heading direction through the rotation vector sensor by combining the data obtained from the accelerometer, magnetometer, and gyroscope. Further research is required to estimate a stable heading direction without using a magnetometer that is affected by the surrounding environment.

3. Indoor Localization System

In this section, we introduce a new indoor localization system for pedestrians that uses smartphones. Figure 3 illustrates the structure of the smartphone-based indoor position recognition system using the deep learning method proposed in this study. The proposed system consists of three steps: (1) classifying smartphone placements; (2) estimating the moving speed using deep learning, and (3) estimating the heading direction using game rotation vector sensors. The detailed operation of each step is described in the following subsection.

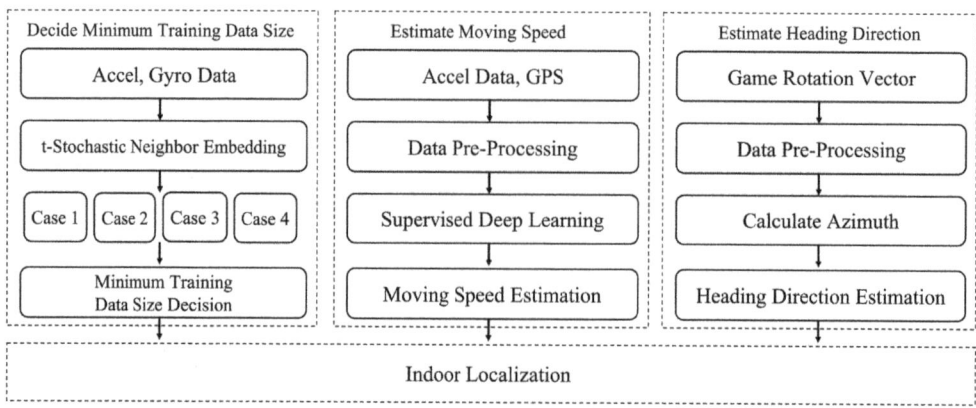

Figure 3. Indoor localization system overview.

3.1. System Overview

The first step was to classify the accelerometer and gyroscope data of pedestrians collected through smartphones as smartphone placements. There are many cases of smartphone placement; however, we assume only the four most representative cases. If it is possible to classify the collected data as smartphone placements, pedestrians can check the amount of data they collect in real-time. In addition, when sufficient pedestrian speed data, enough to achieve good performance, has been collected, the system stops collecting data to minimize battery consumption in smartphones.

The second step involved moving speed estimation using supervised learning. The 3-axis accelerometer data collected from the pedestrians' smartphones and the moving speed labels recorded every 1 s through GPS comprise the training datasets. Before constructing the training dataset, the accelerometer and GPS data were pre-processed. Since the 3-axis accelerometer data change as the smartphone's placement and tilt, regardless of these changes, acceleration data are collected with 3-axes fixed. In addition, accelerometer data are filtered through Kalman and low-pass filters. These filters minimize the impact of the drift of the accelerometer and sudden environmental changes. Because the labels of the deep learning model require high accuracy and reliability, only those GPS coordinates are used as labels and used to calculate the moving speed for which there are more than nine satellite signals that smartphones can receive. As explained in Section 2.2, most of the data were within the average walking speed. To eliminate this bias, additional data on various walking speeds were obtained using time-warping data augmentation technology. The training dataset obtained after these processes is used as an input to a deep learning model that estimates the moving speeds of pedestrians. To find the optimal deep learning model for estimating moving speed, we evaluated the accuracy of moving speed estimation by implementing seven supervised learning models.

In the third step, the heading direction of pedestrians is estimated. Magnetometers are extremely sensitive to the surrounding environment and may have errors, which will affect the estimation of the heading direction. Therefore, we estimated the heading direction using game rotation vector sensors that do not include magnetometers.

3.2. Smartphone Placement Classification

This section describes the technology used for classifying the collected data according to the placements in which pedestrians hold their smartphones. To classify the collected data according to each case, t-stochastic neighbor embedding (t-SNE) [25] unsupervised learning was used. t-SNE is a technique that classifies and visualizes high-dimensional vectors into 2- or 3-dimensional maps humans can understand, while preserving the distance between the data. The t-SNE unsupervised learning model uses accelerometer and gyroscope data as training datasets, and smartphone placements as labels (i.e., cases). Additional gyroscope values were used to increase the accuracy of the classification. Gyroscopes are suitable for data classification because the change in the value, which depends on the placement of the smartphone, is greater than that of the accelerometer. Although the accuracy should be evaluated according to all possible smartphone placements, this study assumes only four of the most commonly used. The four cases are as follows: (1) hand-held, (2) hand swing, (3) in pocket, (4) in a backpack. In this step, pedestrians can check the size of the collected data for each case in real time. In our empirical experiments, we found the proper data size to be 3 h per case (i.e., a total of 12 h) to ensure sufficient accuracy to estimate the moving speed. Thus, the data collection process stopped when the data size was at least 3 h and a total of 12 h to prevent excessive smartphone battery usage. This method allows pedestrians to know the minimum size of the training dataset for learning the deep learning model, thus gaining the practicality that battery consumption can be reduced in the data collection process.

3.3. Moving Speed Estimation

The moving speed estimation step consists of data pre-processing and a supervised learning-based deep learning model. The data needed to estimate the moving speed were the GPS and accelerometer values collected outdoors. Accelerometer data were used to extract the features of pedestrian gait patterns and were used as training datasets for the deep learning models. The moving speed calculated via GPS coordinates was used as a label for the training datasets as in [20].

The accelerometer data collected from the smartphones were pre-processed for use as input to the supervised learning model. The accelerometer data provided by the smartphone were device oriented. As can be seen in Figure 4, when the data are collected by device orientation, there is a problem in that the data show different characteristics depending on the placement and orientation of the smartphone from which they were collected. This means that even when moving in the same direction, the data values of the collected accelerometer vary depending on the tilt and placement of the smartphone. Because pedestrians can place the smartphone anywhere near the body, data should be collected with respect to three axes that are fixed regardless of the tilt and placement of the smartphone. To solve this problem, data pre-processing is used to convert the raw coordinates of the accelerometer (i.e., device-oriented coordinates) into earth-oriented coordinates. Alwin et al. [26] presented a method for converting device-oriented 3-axis accelerometer values into earth-oriented coordinates by multiplying them with rotation vector sensor values. The following Equation (1) represents a formula for transform the device-oriented coordinate to the earth-oriented coordinate.

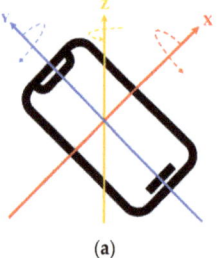 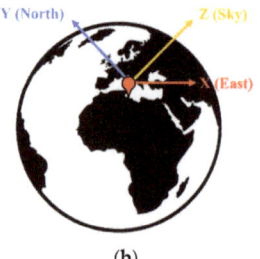

(a)   (b)

Figure 4. Coordinate system (a) Device oriented coordinate (b) Earth oriented coordinate.

$$\begin{bmatrix} A_x \\ A_y \\ A_z \end{bmatrix} = R\begin{bmatrix} a_x & a_y & a_z \end{bmatrix}^T \tag{1}$$

The R in the right term from Equation (1) represents the transform of the rotation vector value obtained through the rotation vector sensor into a rotation matrix, and a_x, a_y and a_z represents the raw value of accelerometer. Both values are obtained through smartphones. Each of A_x, A_y and A_z in the left column represent the value of the three axes of acceleration converted to the earth reference coordinate system. Using this method, accelerometer values can be converted into earth-oriented coordinates to collect data, regardless of smartphone placement. The authors used Kalman filters and low-pass filters for the accelerometer data. Filtering accelerometer data eliminates drift and noise from smartphones.

In this paper, we use the pedestrian moving speed obtained through the GPS as a label for a deep learning model. Labels are correct answers to training data that are input to deep learning models, which affect the performance of deep learning models depending on the accuracy of the labels. In [20], the accuracy of the label is relatively low, because the moving speed was calculated and used as a label regardless of the reliability of GPS. Therefore, in this paper, to increase the reliability of labels on training datasets, we compose the training datasets with only the data collected when the receivable number of satellite signals on smartphones is more than nine. This is a new and novelty method that has not been considered so far. The GPS error rate is inversely proportional to the number of satellite signals that a smartphone can receive, as shown in Figure 1. If the number of satellite signals that can be received is more than nine, high reliability of the label can be expected because the GPS measurement accuracy is approximately 98%. We calculated the moving speed for one second using the GPS coordinates when more than nine satellite signals were received, while collecting the sensor data. Equation (2) represents a formula for obtaining a moving speed of a pedestrian through a distance obtained by collecting GPS coordinates every second.

$$Pedestrian\ Moving\ speed = distance \div 1 \qquad (2)$$

The calculated moving speed and accelerometer values were mapped for a period of one second and used as training data for the supervised learning model. This process can solve the reliability problem for labels collected in the GPS coordinates presented in Section 2.1.

As shown in Figure 2, most of the data collected at the average moving speed are concentrated at a particular moving speed. If the training data do not have sufficient data for all moving speed labels, the deep learning model will fail to estimate the exact moving speed if the pedestrian walks slower or faster than the average moving speed. Thus, to eliminate bias in the collected data, we introduced time-warping to augment the amount of data for various moving speeds. Time warping is a transformation that allows each element value in a sequence to be repeated by an arbitrary number and can compress or expands fixed-length time series data to a particular length. For example, two sequences $S = \{20, 20, 21, 20, 23\}$ and $Q = \{20, 21, 21, 20, 20, 23, 23, 23\}$ may be converted into the same sequence $A = \{20, 20, 21, 21, 20, 20, 23, 23, 23\}$ by time warping. The distance between the two sequences after time warping is defined as a time warping distance. Figure 5 shows the results augmented to data of 24 h by time-warping the original data of 3 h. The black bar graph represents the original data, and the red bar graph represents the data enhanced through time-warping. By augmenting the data through time warping, the data can be constructed to have an even distribution at various moving speeds rather than being concentrated at a specific moving speed. This process solves the data-bias problem presented in Section 2.1.

The data of 12 h are augmented to a size of 96 h through time warping and are used as a training dataset for supervised learning-based deep learning models. The deep learning model derives a result by extracting patterns or features from the accelerometer data of the training dataset and estimating the moving speed for a one-second data segment when learning is completed. Estimation accuracy is the most important indicator of the performance of the deep learning model. One representative way to improve the accuracy of the model is to use an appropriate deep learning model. In this study, performance was evaluated by implementing seven deep learning models: CNN [27], GRU [28], LSTM [29], C-GRU, C-LSTM, GRU-C, and LSTM-C, to find the optimal deep learning model with the highest moving speed estimation accuracy. These models are explained below. A convolutional neural network (CNN) is a useful supervised learning model for identifying patterns to recognize images. CNNs are mainly used to find and learn patterns from training data and then classify new images using learned patterns. It is widely used in object recognition fields, such as self-driving cars and facial recognition. In contrast, the recurrent neural network (RNN), represented by long short-term memory (LSTM) and gated recurrent units (GRU), is a supervised learning model that has strengths in processing sequence data, such as time series and natural language. Because sequence data cannot understand the entire context simply by knowing and understanding only one data segment, LSTM and GRU are models that have improved existing RNNs to identify and learn the context of these sequence data. LSTM and GRU are used in various fields, such as voice recognition and sentence arrangement from listed words. Convolutional GRU (C-GRU) and convolutional LSTM (C-LSTM) refer to deep learning models in which CNN and RNN are combined and are called convolutional recurrent neural networks (CRNNs). Given location and shape data, such as images, the correct answer is estimated by first extracting features from the CNN layer and inputting these features in chronological order into the RNN layer. That is, it is a model that extracts and utilizes time series data from image data. GRU convolutional (GRU-C) and LSTM convolutional (LSTM-C) extract features or patterns from data through convolutional layers and input them into the RNN layer in the same manner as CRNN, but the final output process is different. In the case of the CRNN, the correct answer is estimated by entering the output value of the RNN into several dense layers. However, in the case of LSTM-C and GRU-C, the output value of the RNN is input to one max pooling layer so that the output value of the layer appears as the final estimate. Figure 6 shows the model configuration diagram of the LSTM-C.

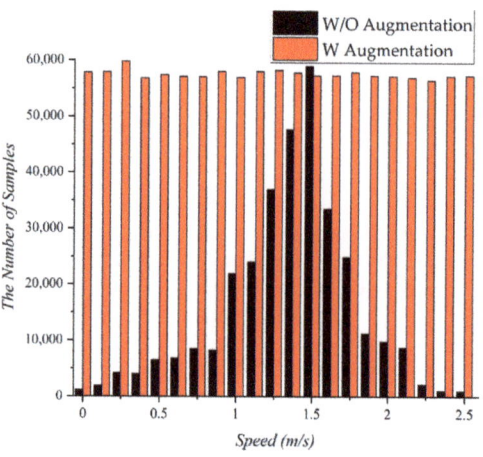

Figure 5. Original (black) and time-warped (red) moving speed data.

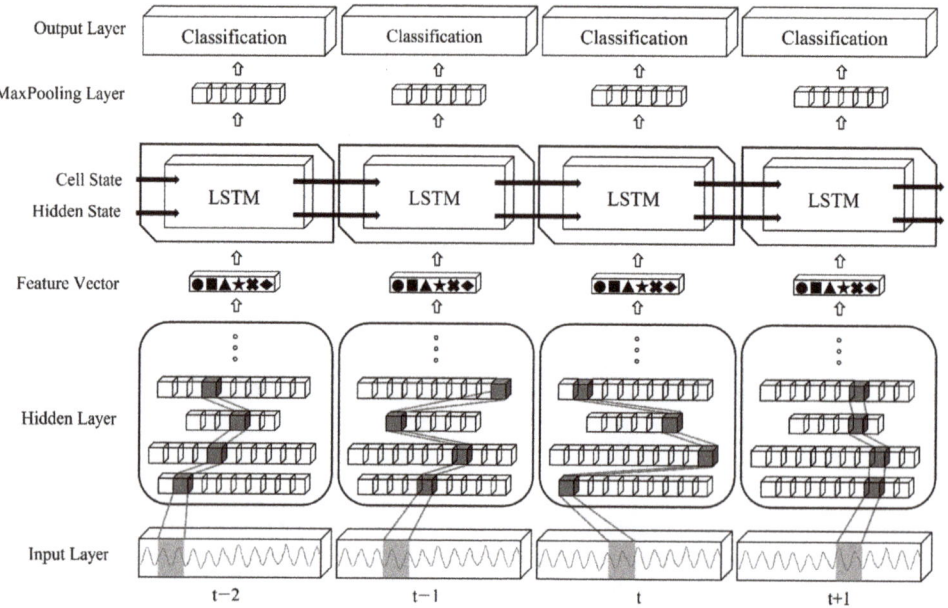

Figure 6. LSTM-C Model.

3.4. Heading Direction Estimation

In the heading direction estimation step, the exact heading direction of the pedestrians was measured. Android smartphones use a rotation vector sensor, including an accelerometer, gyroscope, and magnetometer, to measure the orientation of smartphones [30]. However, obstacles, walls, and steel can affect the magnetometer of the rotation vector sensor, so it can measure the wrong orientation. The other sensor for measuring the orientation is the game rotation vector sensor [31] provided by Android. It is identical to the rotation vector sensor in that it uses an accelerometer and a gyroscope, but it does not use a magnetometer. Hence, the game rotation vector sensor does not provide an absolute heading direction, that is, the magnetic north. Its *y*-axis represents the upward direction of the smartphone, not the north. Therefore, we used game rotation vector sensors instead of rotation vector sensors to measure the orientation. The game rotation vector is a combination of angles and axes in which the smartphone rotates by ψ, θ, and ϕ around the *x*-, *y*-, and *z*-axes, indicating the orientation of the device, as follows:

$$x(\psi) = x \cdot \sin\left(\frac{\psi}{2}\right) \tag{3}$$

$$y(\theta) = y \cdot \sin\left(\frac{\theta}{2}\right) \tag{4}$$

$$z(\phi) = z \cdot \sin\left(\frac{\phi}{2}\right) \tag{5}$$

The three-axis vector value obtained by the game rotation vector sensor is converted to a rotation matrix using quaternion through the getRotationMatricFromVector (getRMFV) function. Subsequently, the getOrientation function allows the rotation matrix acquired from the getRMFV function to be represented by the placement state of the smartphone. Three values are derived. The first value is the azimuth, the angle of rotation on the negative *z*-axis and represents the angle between the *y*-axis of the device and the Earth's Arctic point. The second value is the pitch, which is the angle of rotation on the *x*-axis, and represents the angle between the plane parallel to the screen of the smartphone and the plane parallel to the ground. The third value is the roll, that is, the angle of rotation on the *y*-axis, which represents the angle between the plane perpendicular to the ground and the plane perpendicular to the smartphone screen.

$$q1 = rotationVector[0] \tag{6}$$

$$q2 = rotationVector[1] \tag{7}$$

$$q3 = rotationVector[2] \tag{8}$$

$$q0 = 1 - (q1 * q1) - (q2 * q2) - (q3 * q3) \tag{9}$$

The Rotation Vector [0], [1], and [2] are rotation vector values indicating the tilt of the smartphone same as Equations (3)–(5), respectively. Equations (6)–(9) represent quaternions used to transform the rotation vector value as a rotation matrix. The heading direction of pedestrians can be obtained from the azimuth, and the formula is as Equation (10). The ψ, θ and ϕ each represent an angle at which the smartphone is rotated with respect to the *x*-, *y*-, and *z*-axes, and the angle can be obtained by the rotation vector sensor.

$$\text{Azimuth} = \tan^{-1}((\cos\phi \sin\psi + \sin\phi \cos\theta \cos\psi) - (-\sin\phi \cos\psi - \cos\phi \cos\theta \sin\psi)) \tag{10}$$

Figure 7 shows a graph measuring the azimuth through a rotation vector sensor and a game rotation vector sensor by walking through a straight passage in a building. The black line represents the actual azimuth measured from the north using Google Maps. Because the rotation vector sensor includes a magnetometer, it is difficult to measure a stable azimuth owing to a door or an obstacle made of iron and even an empty space. However, the result of measuring the azimuth angle using the game rotation vector sensor was very stable. Because the azimuth is measured using only accelerometers and gyroscopes, excluding the magnetometer, the results were very similar to the ground truth, except for the shaking caused by the walking of pedestrians.

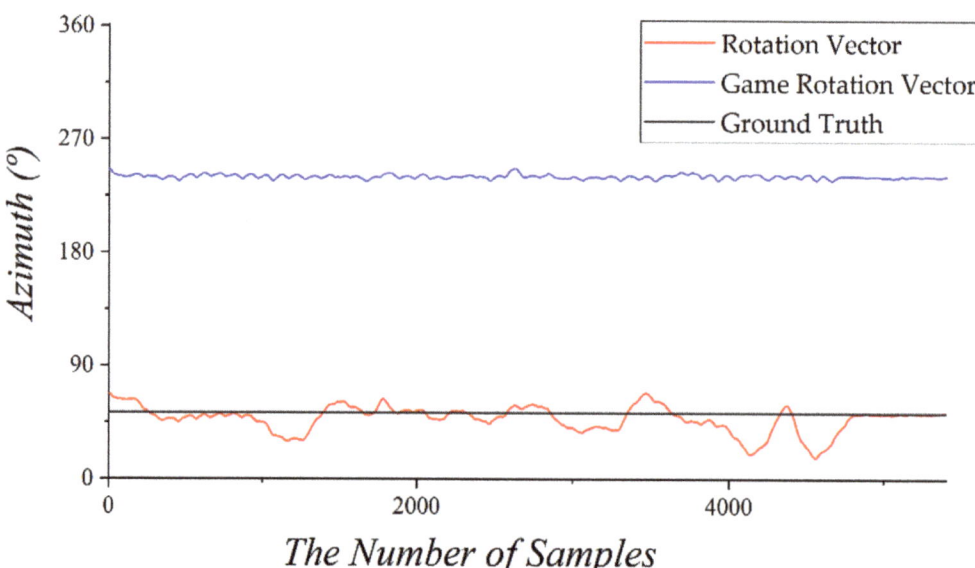

Figure 7. Comparison of each azimuth through rotation vector sensor and game rotation vector sensor.

4. Performance Evaluation

4.1. Evaluation Environments

We evaluated the performance of the proposed system using a computer with the following specifications: Intel i5-6500 CPU, 40 GB RAM and Geforce RTX 2080 GPU. Datasets for supervised and unsupervised learning models were collected through the following processes: As shown in Figure 8, the training data were collected from the playground in Yongam Middle School in Sangdang-ku, Cheongju city, which was approximately 40 m × 90 m area, and had no obstacles or walls. We collected data for four situations. First, hand-held; second, hand-swing; third, in-pocket; and fourth, in a backpack. We collected training data over 10 h for each orientation, for a total of 40 h, as shown in Figure 9. The sampling rate of each sensor is 100 Hz, and the sensors used in this system are an accelerometer, gyroscope, GPS, and a game rotation vector sensor built into the Samsung Galaxy s10. Next, the conditions for collecting data for the validation data set were the same as the training data, except that it was collected inside the E10 building of Chungbuk National University. Table 1 presents the hyperparameters of seven deep learning models implemented to identify which model(s) are optimal for the indoor localization systems proposed in this paper.

Sensors **2022**, *22*, 6764

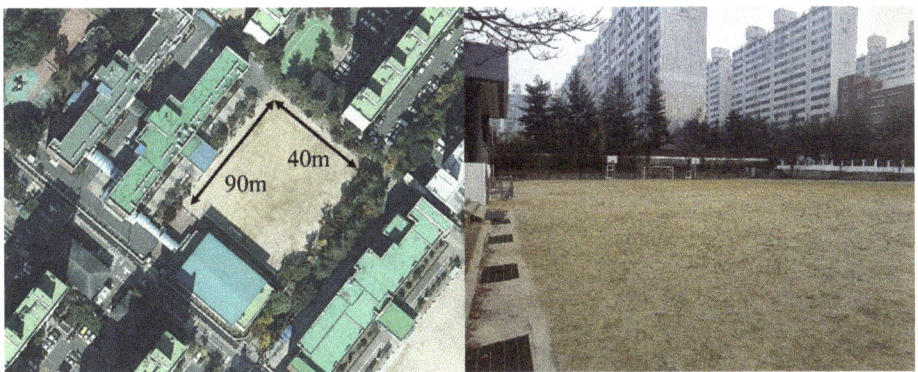

Figure 8. Outdoor data collection environment.

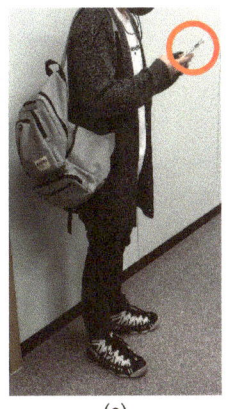 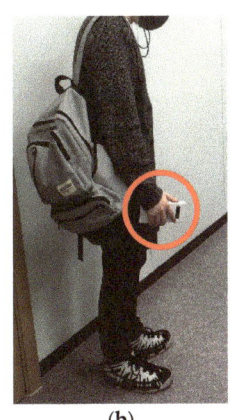 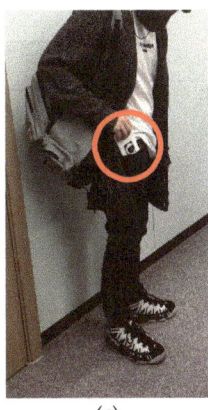 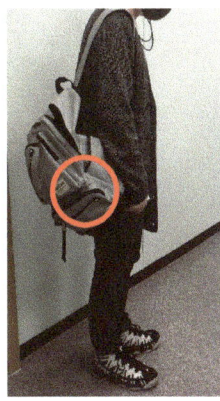

(**a**)   (**b**)   (**c**)   (**d**)

Figure 9. 4 data collect situations (**a**) hand held (**b**) hand swing (**c**) in pocket (**d**) back pack.

Table 1. Deep learning model hyperparameters.

Parameter	CNN	GRU	LSTM	C-GRU	C-LSTM	GRU-C	LSTM-C
Batch Size	128	128	128	128	128	128	128
Activision	ReLu	ReLu	ReLu	ReLu	ReLu	ReLu	ReLu
Optimizer	Adam	Adam	Adam	Adam	Adam	Adam	Adam
Learning Tate	0.001	0.001	0.001	0.001	0.001	0.001	0.001
Epochs	50	50	50	50	50	50	50
Loss Function	Categorical Cross entropy	Categorical Cross entropy	Categorical Cross entropy	Categorical Cross entropy	Categorical Cross entropy	Categorical Cross entropy	Categorical Cross entropy

4.2. Results of Smartphone Placement Classification

Figure 10 shows the confusion matrix of the results from the t-SNE unsupervised learning model. The model was trained using a training data set of 40 h consisting of accelerometer and gyroscope data. The graph resulted from the validation data set of 2 h. The *x*-axis of the Figure 10 represents the results predicted by the unsupervised learning model, and the *y*-axis represents the case in which the actual data belong, that is, the label. For example, in the hand-held case, out of 7200 (half-hour data) samples, the model predicted 6875 data correctly as be hand-held (95.49%). For the remaining 325 data the model failed to classify them as hand held and classified into one of three other cases.

Figure 10 indicates that unsupervised learning using t-SNE can sufficiently classify the data collected in each case.

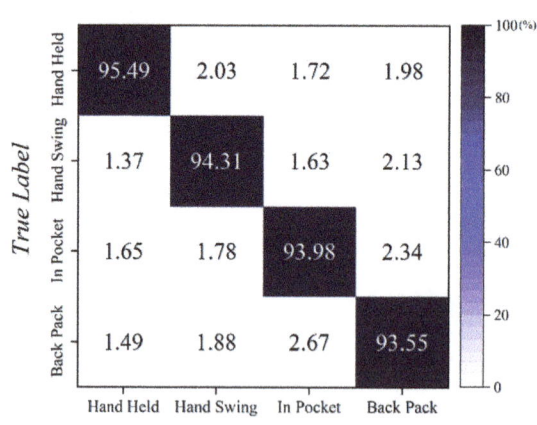

Figure 10. Smartphone placement classification result.

4.3. Results of Moving Speed Estimation

Table 2 shows the results of augmenting data of 12 h to 96 h with time-warping, using them to train seven models, and evaluating the accuracy of each model in estimating the moving speed with a validation data set of 2 h. Of the seven supervised learning models, the best performing model was the LSTM-C model, with approximately 95.6% accurate moving speed estimation. Therefore, the deep learning model to be used in the indoor localization systems proposed in this study was determined to be LSTM-C.

Table 2. Accuracy of deep learning model for data of 12 h.

Models	Evaluation Parameters				
	Distance Error	Accuracy	Precision	Recall	F-1 Score
CNN	11.87	0.908	0.895	0.886	0.890
GRU	9.39	0.919	0.915	0.907	0.911
LSTM	9.39	0.920	0.916	0.909	0.912
C-GRU	9.12	0.931	0.926	0.918	0.922
C-LSTM	8.99	0.935	0.924	0.913	0.918
CRU-C	5.56	0.940	0.932	0.928	0.930
LSTM-C	7.39	0.956	0.950	0.944	0.947

Figure 11 shows the confusion matrix graph of the movement speed estimation of the LSTM-C model. The LSTM-C model was trained using a non-augmented training data set of 40 h. As shown in the Figure 11, the LSTM-C model estimated the data for 1.4 m/s with a high accuracy of 97.6%. However, data belonging to labels other than 1.4 m/s showed relatively low accuracy. These results show that most of the training dataset is densely distributed around 1.4 m/s, as shown in Figure 2, and that the model has not learned enough features for other moving speed labels to classify them correctly. Accordingly, in this study, the training dataset was augmented with time warping to obtain an even distribution across various moving speed labels.

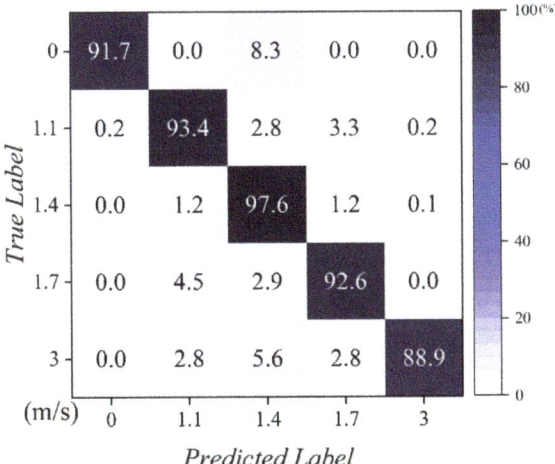

Figure 11. Moving speed estimation using LSTM-C.

Table 3 shows the results of the estimation accuracy of the LSTM-C model, trained by the various training datasets augmented with time warping for moving speed. The TW class represents the number of classes in which the original data is augmented using time-warping. For example, if the TW class is one, the training data are not augmented, if the TW class is three, the training dataset is augmented to three classes, including the original data. With the original data without augmentation, sufficient moving speed estimation accuracy was not achieved. When the TW class was 3, sufficient accuracy in estimating the moving speed for the original data of 16 h and 20 h was observed. However, by checking the loss graph, we found an overfitting problem and did not see high accuracy for various moving-speed labels. Using a confusion matrix, as shown in Figure 11, it was found that the accuracy of the approximately 1.5 m/s label was sufficiently high, but similar accuracy could not be achieved for the other moving speed labels. When the TW class was 5 or 7, sufficient accuracy was achieved, and overfitting problems did not occur. However, the data were not augmented for various moving speed labels; therefore, the model did not show a high accuracy for all labels, as shown in Figure 11.

Table 3. Moving speed estimation accuracy of LSTM-C model according to data size.

TW Class	Data Size (Hours)				
	4	8	12	16	20
1	0.125	0.289	0.597	0.692	0.862
3	0.439	0.804	0.889	0.944	0.951
5	0.669	0.923	0.950	0.953	0.957
7	0.832	0.938	0.953	0.954	0.957
9	0.931	0.945	0.956	0.956	0.958
11	0.931	0.949	0.956	0.963	0.969
13	0.935	0.952	0.961	0.968	0.971

However, when the TW class was more than nine, including the original data, the model showed high accuracy for all labels. If the original data are augmented to more than nine TW classes, the indoor localization system proposed in this study can obtain a high moving speed estimation accuracy for all moving speed classes. However, the larger the total size of the training data set, created by increasing the number of TW classes, the smaller is the increase in accuracy, and the amount of data increases rapidly. For example, the data augmented with 5 and 13 TW classes from 12 h of original data were 60- and

156 hours, respectively, but achieved 95% and 96% accuracy, respectively. In this case, the amount of data increased significantly; however, the accuracy increased only by less than 1%. Of course, it is better to augment and learn the original data into 13 TW classes from the perspective of performance, but this is not practical from a system user perspective. The indoor localization system proposed in this paper categorizes the collected data using unsupervised learning, augments the training dataset with time warping and then learns through the LSTM-C model. These processes require a great deal of time, especially the process of augmenting with time-warping and performing learning of augmented data with deep learning models; the larger the dataset, the more time it takes. Therefore, in this study, the minimum size of the original data required for learning the deep learning model parameters was limited to 3 h for each case, i.e., a total of 12 h, and the number of TW classes was set to nine, including the original data.

Figure 12 shows a CDF graph of the moving speed estimation error rate of an LSTM-C model that learns the training data set augmented to 96 h and applies the improvements proposed in this paper for three different comparators. The red line is a CDF graph of the error rate for estimating the moving speed of the original data of 12 h without augmentation. A marked improvement in accuracy, compared to the other lines, can be seen for the black line, which is the result of applying all the improvements proposed in this study. Furthermore, as shown in Figure 5, time warping eliminates data bias, which increases the estimation accuracy performance for various moving speeds. The blue line is a CDF graph of the moving speed estimation error rate for the test data of 2 h after learning the LSTM-C model by augmenting the collected data of 12 h into nine TW classes, regardless of the number of satellites, to evaluate the reliability of the ground truth information. If data are collected regardless of the number of satellites, the blue line in Figure 12 shows that the exact moving speed cannot be calculated accurately because of the lack of reliability in the moving speed labels, that is, the ground-truth information required for the supervised learning model is not reliable. However, the data collected when the number of satellites is greater than nine are relatively high in accuracy for the moving speed label and show a higher performance. This means that the higher the reliability of the previously mentioned ground-truth information, the better are the deep learning model results. The green line is a CDF graph of the performance of the training dataset collected using device-oriented coordinates. If the data are collected by the device-oriented coordinate system, the sensor value depends on the y-axis of the smartphone. However, when data are collected through an earth-oriented coordinate system, the sensor value does not change depending on smartphone placement. For example, when a smartphone is freely placed at a moving speed of 1.5 m/s for 10 s, the data collected into a device-oriented coordinate system shows significant variations depending on the placement of the smartphone. That is, the 3-axis accelerometer sensor varies with each change in the smartphone placement, but for the earth-oriented coordinate, the values of the 3-axis of the collected accelerometer values do not change even if the smartphone placement changes. It can be seen from the green line in Figure 12 that the device-oriented coordinate data show a large error compared to the data collected through the earth-oriented coordinate. This means that the process of generalizing training data has a significant impact the deep learning model outcome and that the indoor localization system proposed in this paper, which transforms the sensor data collected into earth-oriented coordinates and performs the generalization process and produces improved results.

Sensors **2022**, 22, 6764

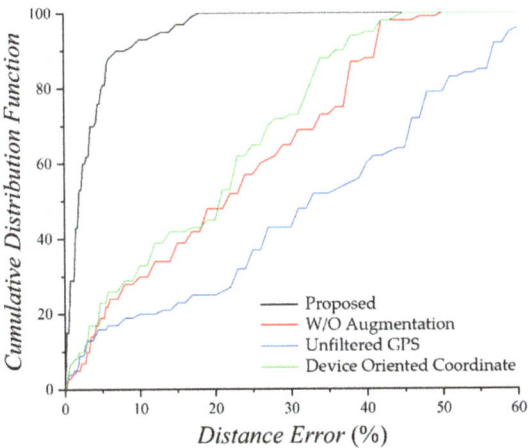

Figure 12. CDF graph of moving speed estimation.

4.4. Results of Indoor Localization System

This section evaluates the performance of path estimation of indoor localization systems by collecting test datasets for routes, including straight paths and rotations in indoor environments. Table 4 lists different versions of the training datasets for evaluating the performance of indoor localization systems. For example, the 'Without augmentation' training dataset refers to a dataset that is composed of data transformed the device-oriented coordinate to the earth-oriented coordinate when the receivable number of satellite signals is more than nine but is not augmented by time-warping. Another example is the 'Unfiltered GPS' training dataset, which is composed of data that transformed the device-oriented coordinate to the earth-oriented coordinate and is augmented by time-warping but is composed in all situations, regardless of the receivable number of satellite signals. Finally, the 'Device oriented coordinate' training dataset that is composed of data collected when the receivable number of satellite signals is more than nine and augmented by time-warping but does not transform the device-oriented coordinate to the earth-oriented coordinate. On the other hand, the 'Proposed' training dataset refers to a dataset with all the techniques proposed in this paper.

Table 4. Parameters for each training dataset.

Parameter	Proposed	Without Augmentation	Unfiltered GPS	Device Oriented Coordinate
Filtered GPS	O	O	X	O
With Augmentation	O	X	O	O
Earth Oriented Coordinate	O	O	O	X

Figure 13 shows the results of the path estimation of the test dataset collected inside a horseshoe-shaped building. The black double line path represents the ground truth information, and the black path with crosses (proposed) is the result of the path estimation of the indoor localization system proposed in this paper. We collected the data, while walking through the black double line, as shown in Figure 13, and the author's smartphone, the Samsung Galaxy s10, was used as the data collection device. In the process of collecting this data, we collected the data, while walking along a path of a total length of 240 m and conducted a total of five-time experiments. In the process of collecting this data, we collected the data, while walking along a path of a total length of 240 m and conducted a total of five time experiments. First, the estimation results of the proposed indoor location recognition system showed a positioning error rate of approximately 3 to 5 m compared to

125

the ground truth. This is a very low error rate compared to other comparators. The blue path (unfiltered GPS) is the result of estimating the path by learning the supervised model with the data collected, regardless of the number of GPS satellites. Regardless of the number of GPS satellites, it is difficult to achieve consistency and high reliability for the collected GPS coordinates. The GPS coordinates collected even when walking at the same speed and path depend on the surrounding environment and the number of satellite signals currently available to the smartphone. The blue path in Figure 13 shows that the errors resulting from the ground truth information significantly influence the overall performance of the system. The red path (without augmentation) is the result of estimating the path by learning 40 h of data without the use of time warping into a supervised learning model. Assuming that the experiment site was a straight path, the distance between the start and end points would not be significantly different from the ground truth. However, after the first right rotation, the red route shows a very large error compared with the ground truth. This is because the deep learning model, which learned training datasets without data augmentation, did not achieve sufficient moving-speed estimation accuracy for various moving-speed labels. Thus, the red route showed unexpected results from accumulated moving speed estimation errors. The green path (device-oriented coordinates) is the result of estimating the path by learning a training dataset that has not converted the device-oriented coordinates into earth-oriented coordinates using a supervised learning model. The data collected with device-oriented coordinates had different characteristics depending on the placement of the smartphone during data collection. As mentioned in Section 2, data that have not been generalized are difficult to use as training datasets for supervised learning models because the 3-axis of the accelerometer varies depending on the tilt or placement of the smartphone. Table 5 represents the positioning error with meters for each supervised learning model that was trained by four different training datasets from a total of five time experiments.

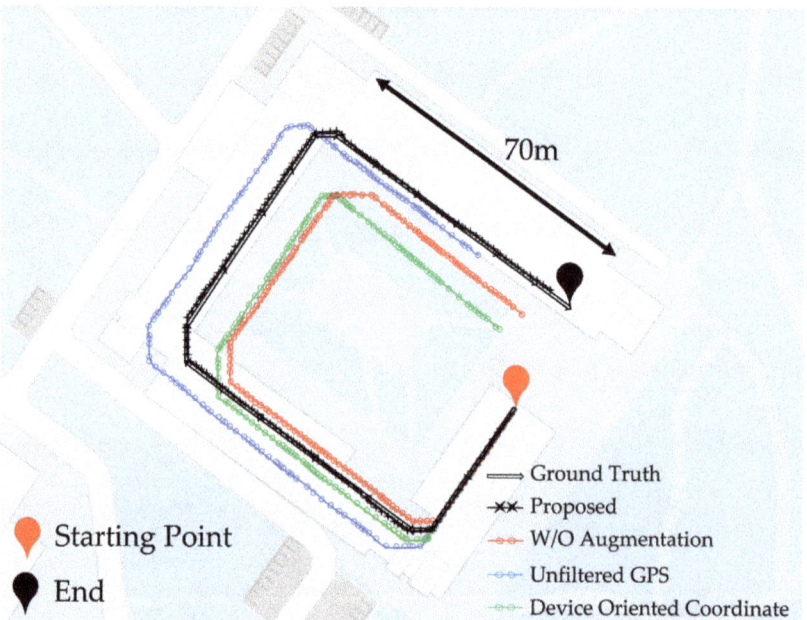

Figure 13. Indoor localization result.

Table 5. Positioning error for each method at every epoch.

Training Dataset	Epoch (Number of Experiments)				
	1	2	3	4	5
Proposed	3.45 m	3.39 m	3.25 m	3.42 m	4.95 m
Without Augmentation	8.72 m	8.12 m	10.05 m	9.42 m	10.15 m
Unfiltered GPS	13.55 m	15.89 m	12.42 m	14.23 m	15.21 m
Device Oriented Coordinate	9.55 m	8.91 m	8.67 m	10.23 m	10.82 m

4.5. Scenario

The smartphone-based indoor localization system using deep learning proposed in this study aims for more practical use by pedestrians by providing on-demand services. Pedestrians can construct a personal indoor localization system exclusively for themselves simply by walking outdoors, while using a smartphone. The virtual scenarios for constructing pedestrian-individual systems are as follows.

Accelerometers, gyroscopes, and GPS data were collected because GPS signals can be received when pedestrians go outdoors. Afterward, when pedestrians enter the indoor environment from the outside and cannot receive GPS signals, data collection is temporarily stopped, but the data collected till then are stored in their smartphones. At this time, we assume that the collected data are valid only when there are nine or more satellite signals that can be received by smartphones, and we exclude the data when there are fewer than nine. Then, the accelerometer and gyroscope data are input into the t-SNE unsupervised learning model to classify the collected data into four cases. The size of the classified data is measured to determine whether the data size reached 3 h for each case. When training data of 3 h or a total of 12 h are accumulated for each case, smartphones stop collecting data outdoors permanently, reducing excessive battery consumption. After the training dataset of 12 h is augmented to a total size of 96 h through time warping, this training dataset is used to learn the LSTM-C model that estimates the pedestrian moving speed. When the learning is completed, pedestrians can check their path in real time by estimating the moving speed and heading direction using only accelerometer data and indoor game rotation vector sensors.

5. Conclusions

In this study, we propose a new smartphone-based indoor localization system using deep learning. The system used the following ideas to increase the practicality for pedestrians: 1. The movement speed calculated using outdoor GPS coordinates was set as the label of the training dataset. 2. A consistent training dataset regardless of the smartphone placement was constructed by converting accelerometer data to earth-oriented coordinates the 3-axis is fixed. 3. An unsupervised learning model was implemented to identify the minimum size of the training dataset in real time to minimize the battery consumption. In addition, the following concepts were proposed to increase the accuracy of estimating the moving speed: 1. Noise was removed to increase the accuracy of GPS and accelerometer data. 2. Data augmentation methods were applied to obtain a uniform distribution of moving speeds of pedestrians. 3. By implementing seven different deep learning models, the optimal deep learning model with the best moving-speed estimation performance was selected. After learning the parameters for the indoor localization system with the data collected outdoors, the proposed system showed a localization estimation error of approximately 3 to 5 m as a result of direct experimentation inside a horseshoe-shaped building compared to the test data of approximately 240 m in length. Compared to existing indoor location recognition studies, the proposed system shows a high location estimation accuracy, and the practicality for pedestrians is also very high. In the future, we plan to develop an in-building floor-recognition technology to provide 3D location information for indoor pedestrians. The three-dimensional location information also allows pedestrians to know which floor of the building they are on, so that they can receive much more diverse location-based services and identify safer evacuation routes in the event of a disaster.

Author Contributions: Conceptualization, S.K.; formal analysis, S.K.; funding acquisition, S.K.; methodology, J.Y. and S.K.; project administration, S.K.; software, J.Y.; supervision, S.K.; validation, J.Y.; visualization, J.Y.; writing—original draft, J.Y.; writing—review & editing, S.K. All authors have read and agreed to the published version of the manuscript.

Funding: This work was supported by the National Research Foundation of Korea (NRF) grant funded by the Korea government (MSIT) (No. 2022R1A5A8026986) and Korea Institute for Advancement of Technology (KIAT) grant funded by the Korea Government (MOTIE) (P0020536, HRD Program for Industrial Innovation).

Institutional Review Board Statement: Not applicable.

Informed Consent Statement: Not applicable.

Data Availability Statement: Not applicable.

Conflicts of Interest: The authors declare no conflict of interest.

References

1. Huang, H.; Gartner, G. Current Trends and Challenges in Location-Based Services. *ISPRS Int. J. Geo-Inf.* **2018**, *7*, 199. [CrossRef]
2. Ghoprade, S.; Zennaro, M.; Chaudhari, B. Survey of localization for internet of things nodes: Approaches, challenges and open issues. *Future Internet* **2021**, *13*, 210.
3. Obeidat, H.; Shuaieb, W.; Obeidat, O.; Abd-Alhameed, R. A Review of indoor localization techniques and wireless technologies. *Wirel. Pers. Commun.* **2021**, *119*, 289–327. [CrossRef]
4. Heidari, M.; Alsindi, N.A.; Pahlavan, K. UDP identification and error mitigation in ToA-based indoor localization systems using neural network architecture. *IEEE Trans. Wirel. Commun.* **2009**, *8*, 3597–3607. [CrossRef]
5. Bocquet, M.; Loyez, C.; Benlarbi-Delai, A. Using enhanced-TDOA measurement for indoor positioning. *IEEE Microw. Wirel. Compon. Lett.* **2005**, *15*, 612–614. [CrossRef]
6. Diao, S.; Luo, Q.; Wang, C.; Ding, J. Enhancing Trilateration Localization by Adaptive Selecting Distances. In Proceedings of the 2021 IEEE 5th Advanced Information Technology, Electronic and Automation Control Conference (IAEAC), Chongqing, China, 12–14 March 2021; IEEE: Piscataway, NJ, USA, 2021; pp. 357–363.
7. Shu, Y.; Huang, Y.; Zhang, J.; Coue, P.; Cheng, P.; Chen, J.; Shin, K.G. Gradient-based fingerprinting for indoor localization and tracking. *IEEE Trans. Ind. Electron.* **2015**, *63*, 2424–2433. [CrossRef]
8. Song, Q.; Guo, S.; Liu, X.; Yang, Y. CSI amplitude fingerprinting-based NB-IoT indoor localization. *IEEE Internet Things J.* **2017**, *5*, 1494–1504. [CrossRef]
9. Hoang, M.T.; Yuen, B.; Dong, X.; Lu, T.; Westendorp, R.; Reddy, K. Recurrent neural networks for accurate RSSI indoor localization. *IEEE Internet Things J.* **2019**, *6*, 10639–10651. [CrossRef]
10. Liu, H.; Hartmann, Y.; Schultz, T. Motion Units: Generalized Sequence Modeling of Human Activities for Sensor-Based Activity Recognition. In Proceedings of the 2021 29th European Signal Processing Conference (EUSIPCO), Dublin, Ireland, 23–27 August 2021; pp. 1506–1510. [CrossRef]
11. Li, Y.; Zhuang, Y.; Lan, H.; Zhou, Q.; Niu, X.; El-Sheimy, N. A hybrid WiFi/magnetic matching/PDR approach for indoor navigation with smartphone sensors. *IEEE Commun. Lett.* **2015**, *20*, 169–172. [CrossRef]
12. Chen, G.; Meng, X.; Wang, Y.; Zhang, Y.; Tian, P.; Yang, H. Integrated WiFi/PDR/Smartphone using an unscented kalman filter algorithm for 3D indoor localization. *Sensors* **2015**, *15*, 24595–24614. [CrossRef] [PubMed]
13. Li, X.; Wang, J.; Liu, C.; Zhang, L.; Li, Z. Integrated WiFi/PDR/smartphone using an adaptive system noise extended Kalman filter algorithm for indoor localization. *ISPRS Int. J. Geo-Inf.* **2016**, *5*, 8. [CrossRef]
14. Zhang, M.; Jia, J.; Chen, J.; Deng, Y.; Wang, X.; Aghvami, A.H. Indoor localization fusing wifi with smartphone inertial sensors using lstm networks. *IEEE Internet Things J.* **2021**, *8*, 13608–13623. [CrossRef]
15. Godha, S.; Lachapelle, G.; Cannon, M.E. Integrated GPS/INS system for pedestrian navigation in a signal degraded environment. In Proceedings of the 19th International Technical Meeting of the Satellite Division of The Institute of Navigation (ION GNSS 2006), Fort Worth, TX, USA, 26–29 September 2006; pp. 2151–2164.
16. Constandache, I.; Choudhury, R.R.; Rhee, I. Towards mobile phone localization without war-driving. In Proceedings of the 2010 Proceedings IEEE INFOCOM, San Diego, CA, USA, 14–19 March 2010; pp. 1–9.
17. Kang, W.H.; Han, Y.N. SmartPDR: Smartphone-based pedestrian dead reckoning for indoor localization. *IEEE Sens. J.* **2014**, *15*, 2906–2916. [CrossRef]
18. Kang, W.H.; Nam, S.; Han, Y.; Lee, S.-J. Improved heading estimation for smartphone-based indoor positioning systems. In Proceedings of the 2012 IEEE 23rd International Symposium on Personal, Indoor and Mobile Radio Communications-(PIMRC), Sydney, Australia, 9–12 September 2012; IEEE: Piscataway, NJ, USA, 2012; pp. 2449–2453.

19. Gu, F.; Khoshelham, K.; Yu, G.; Shang, J. Accurate step length estimation for pedestrian dead reckoning localization using stacked autoencoders. *IEEE Trans. Instrum. Meas.* **2018**, *68*, 2705–2713. [CrossRef]
20. Kang, J.H.; Lee, J.B.; Eom, D.S. Smartphone-based traveled distance estimation using individual walking patterns for indoor localization. *Sensors* **2018**, *18*, 3149. [CrossRef]
21. Li, P.; Yang, Y.Y.; Hao, S.; Niu, Q. Smartphone-based Indoor Localization with Integrated Fingerprint Signal. *IEEE Access* **2020**, *8*, 33178–33187. [CrossRef]
22. Ashraf, I.; Hur, S.; Park, S.; Park, Y. DeepLocate: Smartphone Based Indoor Localization with a Deep Neural Network Ensemble Classifier. *Sensors* **2019**, *20*, 133. [CrossRef]
23. Murata, M.; Ahmetovic, D.; Sato, D.; Takagi, H.; Kitani, K.M.; Asakawa, C. Smartphone-based indoor localization for blind navigation across building complexes. In Proceedings of the IEEE International Conference on Pervasive Computing and Communications (PerCom), Athens, Greece, 19–23 March 2018; pp. 1–10.
24. Jain, A.K.; Mao, J.; Mohiuddin, K.M. Artificial neural networks: A tutorial. *IEEE Comput.* **1996**, *29*, 31–44. [CrossRef]
25. Van Der Maaten, L.; Hinton, G. Visualizing data using t-SNE. *J. Mach. Learn. Res.* **2008**, *9*, 2579–2605.
26. Poulose, A.; Eyobu, O.S.; Han, D.S. An indoor position-estimation algorithm using smartphone IMU sensor data. *IEEE Access* **2019**, *7*, 11165–11177. [CrossRef]
27. Albawi, S.; Mohammed, T.A.; Al-Zawi, S. Understanding of a convolutional neural network. In Proceedings of the International Conference on Engineering and Technology (ICET), Antalya, Turkey, 21–23 August 2017; pp. 1–6.
28. Chung, J.; Culcehre, C.; Cho, K.H.; Bengio, Y. Empirical evaluation of gated recurrent neural networks on sequence modeling. *arXiv* **2014**, arXiv:1412.3555.
29. Xu, Y.; Si, X.; Hu, C.; Zhang, J. A review of recurrent neural networks: LSTM cells and network architectures. *Neural Comput.* **2019**, *31*, 1235–1270.
30. Rotation Vector. Available online: https://source.android.google.cn/devices/sensors/sensor-types#rotation_vector (accessed on 29 July 2022).
31. Game Rotation Vector. Available online: https://source.android.google.cn/devices/sensors/sensor-types#game_rotation_vector (accessed on 29 July 2022).

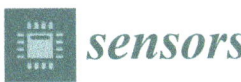

sensors

MDPI

Article

A Customer Behavior Recognition Method for Flexibly Adapting to Target Changes in Retail Stores

Jiahao Wen [1], Toru Abe [2,*] and Takuo Suganuma [2]

[1] Graduate School of Information Sciences, Tohoku University, 6-3-09 Aramaki-Aza-Aoba, Aoba-ku, Sendai 980-8579, Japan
[2] Cyberscience Center, Tohoku University, 6-3 Aramaki-Aza-Aoba, Aoba-ku, Sendai 980-8578, Japan
* Correspondence: beto@tohoku.ac.jp

Abstract: To provide analytic materials for business management for smart retail solutions, it is essential to recognize various customer behaviors (CB) from video footage acquired by in-store cameras. Along with frequent changes in needs and environments, such as promotion plans, product categories, in-store layouts, etc., the targets of customer behavior recognition (CBR) also change frequently. Therefore, one of the requirements of the CBR method is the flexibility to adapt to changes in recognition targets. However, existing approaches, mostly based on machine learning, usually take a great deal of time to re-collect training data and train new models when faced with changing target CBs, reflecting their lack of flexibility. In this paper, we propose a CBR method to achieve flexibility by considering CB in combination with primitives. A primitive is a unit that describes an object's motion or multiple objects' relationships. The combination of different primitives can characterize a particular CB. Since primitives can be reused to define a wide range of different CBs, our proposed method is capable of flexibly adapting to target CB changes in retail stores. In experiments undertaken, we utilized both our collected laboratory dataset and the public MERL dataset. We changed the combination of primitives to cope with the changes in target CBs between different datasets. As a result, our proposed method achieved good flexibility with acceptable recognition accuracy.

Keywords: smart retail; in-store camera; customer behavior recognition; behavior reconstruction

Citation: Wen, J.; Abe, T.; Suganuma, T. A Customer Behavior Recognition Method for Flexibly Adapting to Target Changes in Retail Stores. *Sensors* **2022**, *22*, 6740. https://doi.org/10.3390/s22186740

Academic Editors: Tanja Schultz, Hui Liu and Hugo Gamboa

Received: 31 July 2022
Accepted: 2 September 2022
Published: 6 September 2022

Publisher's Note: MDPI stays neutral with regard to jurisdictional claims in published maps and institutional affiliations.

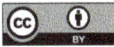
1. Introduction

Smart retail is regarded as an arrangement of the Internet of Things and big data analytics for retail purposes [1]. Usually, it collects data from videos captured by ubiquitous cameras in retail stores. Consequently, we need to extract valuable information collected by videos. Customer behavior (CB) is commonly considered to be a kind of valuable analytic material for business management [2]. As there are an almost infinite number of classes of CBs in retail environments, generally, specific CBs are selected as recognition targets, called target CBs, based on needs. Typically, customer-centric retailing demands different target CBs to analyze the customer decision-making process. Usually, the target CB changes frequently with different products or in-store layouts because of the different customer-product interactions. For instance, trying on clothes in a clothes shop, sitting on a bed in a furniture shop, picking up a bottle from the shelf, picking up an ice cream from a freezer, etc. Accordingly, CB recognition (CBR) methods should be modified to recognize the changed target CBs. In some cases, a current target CB is required to be discriminated, e.g., in the case of "pick a product", discriminating whether a customer is picking a product with one hand or both hands provides information regarding the customer's effort to pick a product. Therefore, a CBR method is expected to be flexible enough to address the issue of frequent changes in the target CB.

As CBR is a branch of human activity recognition (HAR), current CBR methods use machine learning (ML)-based models [3] due to their remarkable accuracy in HAR tasks.

Nevertheless, in contrast to human activity recognition, CBR methods also require flexibility. For frequent target CB changes, to recognize different target CBs, namely, changing the model's output, ML-based models require time-consuming re-collection of training data and training the model. Though transfer learning can be applied in some cases for faster training, the inevitable step of data collection is still time-consuming. This causes current methods to be inflexible when coping with changes in target CBs. Additionally, in existing methods, target CBs are mostly selected arbitrarily according to the training data, instead of business needs, which indicates that change adaptation is not considered in their design. Thus, current CBR methods are not suitable for target CBR tasks in retail environments.

To cope with target changes, we propose a rule-based method to recognize CB by the combination of primitives, each of which is a kind of partitioned unit of CB. Since primitives are allowed to be combined for the customization of various CBs, our proposed method can reuse the primitives to customize the changed target CBs. The number of combinations of primitives increases exponentially as the number of primitives increases linearly. Thus, our method can cover a wide range of CBs with a small number of primitives. As CB analysis focuses on customer-product interaction, we designed the primitive as a unit that describes an object's motion or the relationship between multiple objects.

To conclude, rather than accuracy improvement, we focus on the method's flexibility, which is also important in CBR requirements. Consequently, the main contribution of the paper is the proposal of a flexible CBR method to cope with frequent changes in target CBs.

We evaluated our method on our self-collected laboratory dataset and the public MERL dataset. Compared to the time-consuming collection of data and training of models, our method was able to deal with target changes in a short time, which implies its enhanced flexibility. Moreover, assessment of acceptable recognition accuracy indicated that we did not lose too much accuracy as the cost of achieving a high degree of flexibility.

The remainder of this paper is organized as follows: Section 2 explains the problems of existing methods in terms of their methodology and rationale for selecting target CBs. Section 3 describes our proposal of CB decomposition and the matching of CB patterns in detail. In Section 4, the evaluation of the performance of the proposed method on two different datasets is described. Finally, Section 5 concludes the paper with some final remarks and suggestions for future research.

2. Related Work

In retail environments, we analyze CBs to meet the demands of customer-centric retailing. As a result, CBR tasks should not only address the issues of methodology but also consider the difficulty of application and the customer's experience. Currently, various types of sensors are used in HAR research to acquire data on human movements. In contrast, almost all research on CBR uses visual data. The major reason is that visual data-based approaches can be directly applied to video acquired by surveillance cameras in the store, which makes the application of these approaches hardware-free and avoids active customer participation [2]. In addition, visual data contains much more information than most other types of sensor data.

With the input of videos, existing CBR methods mainly use the pipeline of extracting features from consecutive frames within a certain period and recognizing behavior from the sequenced features using machine-learning-based models, especially the hidden Markov model (HMM). Popa et al. [4] proposed an HMM-based model to recognize customer's buying behavior with optical flow features. Within the next two years, they improved the HMM-based model by partitioning the CB into basic actions [5], which are similar to our proposed primitives. However, they determined the basic actions by optical flow features. Thus, the model is not explainable, which results in it having poor flexibility when dealing with target CB changes. Djamal Merad et al. [6] applied an HMM model for hand movement analysis and an SVM model as eye-tracking descriptors for the classification of a customer's purchasing type. The specific CB classes were not given because the authors conducted CBR indirectly. Moreover, their wearable device was difficult to apply to every customer, and required customers' active participation. However, people are generally reluctant to cooperate without tangible rewards [2].

Apart from HMM models, convolutional neural networks (CNNs) are also widely used due to their excellent performance on spatial feature extraction. Singh et al. [7] used a CNN connected with a long short-term memory (LSTM) [8] model to recognize CBs, such as hand in the shelf, inspecting the products, etc. Using this method, Singh et al. avoided most object occlusions using top-view cameras. Some improved CNN-based models [3,9] have recently been proposed to detect customers and recognize basic customer-product interactions, such as picking up products, returning products back to the shelf, etc. Jingwen Liu et al. [10] employed a dynamic Bayesian network to conduct CBR of six CBs, including turning to shelf, touching, picking, returning, etc., based on hand movements and the orientation of the head and body. Jumpei Yamamoto et al. [11] estimated CB class in a book store based on depth features from a top-view camera and pixel state analysis (PSA) features using a support vector machine (SVM).

In addition, several studies, not using an ML-based model [12,13], implemented a complete CBR system with an RGB-D camera. Basic CBs, such as pick, return, etc., were recognized, based mainly on processing depth information by background subtraction. Unfortunately, since the systems were designed for specific purposes using simple and efficient methods, their flexibility was compromised.

In sum, although the aforementioned ML-based methods achieved improvements in CBR accuracy, they share common limitations with respect to flexibility, as follows:

- Difficulty in adapting to changes in target CBs: The ML models cannot be reused as long as the changed CBs are substantially different from the training data. In this event, time-consuming new training data collection and model re-training are required, which implies inflexibility.
- The model is not explainable: Unexplainable models can only be tuned based on their outputs. This implies poor flexibility during any modifications caused by changes in business needs.

Furthermore, since there are few approaches similar to our method in the field of CBR, we discuss the similarities and differences of several HAR methods with our approach with respect to their application to CBR. Liu et al. [14] proposed an HMM-based method which divides human activity into several phases, called "motion units", analogous to phonemes in speech recognition. Yale et al. [15] proposed interpretable high-level features based on motion units. Different activities sharing the same motion units allow the model to derive more explanatory power from human activities. Although motion units are similar to our proposed primitives, the methods encounter two issues when applied to CBR tasks, which highlight how they differ. Firstly, these methods use data from a smartphone's acceleration sensor. Alhough providing tangible rewards is less of a problem, the methods require the active participation of customers, e.g., downloading an app and agreeing to its terms of service, which increases saliency to customers. Consequently, the rewards increase the cost and the active participation creates privacy issues [2]. Secondly, despite the fairly complete categorization of human activities based on motion units, the methods do not focus on human-item interactions. Since purchase behavior can be easily detected from cashier records, recognizing non-purchase CB becomes one of the objectives of CBR. As the main component of non-purchase CBs, human-item interactions are required in CBR tasks. As an illustration, "picking up a product" and "returning a product" would be practically identical due to their similar hand motions. Nishant Rai et al. [16] divided human activities in indoor living spaces into atomic actions, analogous to the primitives in this paper. The use of both visual and audio data avoided users' active participation, and the training data included human-item interactions. The authors improved recognition accuracy by training the model with annotations of both atomic actions and human activities. In contrast, we concentrated on improving the method's flexibility without sacrificing too much accuracy, as flexibility is one of the important factors for CBR tasks. Romany F.Mansour et al. [17] combined a faster RCNN and a deep Q network for the detection of anomalous entities or human activities in videos. Since this is a typical ML-based HAR method, it requires re-collecting training data and re-training models to adapt to the changed recognition targets, which is inflexible for CBR tasks. In conclusion, the HAR methods described require major modifications before they could be applied to CBR tasks.

3. Proposal

In this paper, we designed a unit, called a primitive, which is a kind of partitioned CB. Our CBR process consists of object tracking, primitive recognition, and CBR by matching recognized primitives with a predefined pattern of primitives. Since the innovative part of our approach is CBR with the combination of primitives, we applied existing methods to object tracking. The workflow of our approach is shown in Figure 1. At the beginning, the existing method tracks objects from the input video captured by in-store cameras. Then, each frame's primitives are recognized based on the object trajectories. We predefine CB as a pattern consisting of primitives. Finally, we match the recognized primitives with the predefined primitive pattern. The matched pattern is regarded as the corresponding CB. This section explains our proposed method in detail, including how we design the primitives, the method for primitive recognition, customizing CB using primitives, and CBR by pattern matching.

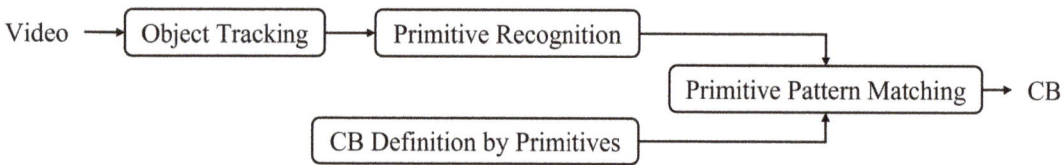

Figure 1. Proposal flow.

3.1. Primitive

The dictionary definition of a behavior is the accomplishment of a thing, usually over a period of time or in stages. We believe that this definition reveals the process by which the human brain recognizes a behavior from visual information. Behavior consists of several stages, and our brains recognize this behavior by checking whether these stages occur in the correct order. In this paper, we refer to these stages as primitives. Thus, CB can be decomposed into primitive(s). Table 1 lists the target CBs in existing methods and the primitives from our subjective decomposition of the target CBs. We did not list a type of CB [18] in Table 1 because they recognize customer's emotion from facial expressions and speech text, which might breach customers' privacy. During the decomposition, we controlled the decomposition granularity to avoid redundancy from over-decomposition. We found that the objects in the target CBs were body parts or products. There are two types of primitives: one describes an object's motion state and the other describes the relationship between two objects. Based on what we have found so far, we can decide what kind of information is in the primitive and how detailed it is.

It is necessary to design an expression format for primitives. Generally, using natural language is considered an efficient method when we need to let others know that we understand a behavior. Therefore, we define the primitive by a sentence with reference to the natural language grammar. The syntax is:

$$subject\ verb\ object\ \text{from}\ where_{start}\ \text{to}\ where_{end}, \tag{1}$$

where italic words are syntax elements which can be replaced by words in the vocabulary below. If $where_{start} = where_{end}$, the syntax can be simplified as *subject verb object where*. As the syntax shows, the primitive consists of *subject*, *verb*, *object* and *where*, each of which has a corresponding vocabulary, as follows:

- *subject*: person, hand, product

- *verb*: move, stay, follow, face to
- *object*: hand, shelf, cart, product
- *where*: in the shelf/cart, out of shelf/cart

Subject and *object* refer to the name of an entity. *verb* describes the movement of *subject* or the relation between *subect* and *object*. *where* means the place where the primitive happens. As our proposed method should cover a wide range of CBs, the vocabulary should be a selection of commonly used words in retail environments. Therefore, these words are selected based on our aforementioned findings from the existing methods in Table 1. Nevertheless, more and more words will be available as our research progresses. There are some constraints and options for the syntax to avoid confusing definition sentences, as below:

- *subject, verb* are required: *subject, verb* should be filled in. *object* is required in relation primitives. *where* is optional.
- Any ignored optional element can be omitted: e.g., if *where* is ignored, we do not care about the value of *where*, the syntax can be simplified as *subject verb object*.
- *subject* ≠ *object*: Same *subject* and *object* is not allowed in logic.
- The logical operator NOT(!) is allowed: It indicates all words except this one.

In sum, the syntax describes what an object does or what happens to it. With some verbs, it could represent two objects' relationship. This design could define motion primitives, the motion of an object, relation primitives, or the relation between two objects. In the case of more than two objects, combining several relation primitives could describe a CB composed of multiple objects.

Table 1. Primitives in target CBs of current approaches.

Target CB	Related Approaches	Primitives ({} = primitive)
Passing by the Shelf	[3,10,12]	{a person is moving in front of the shelf}
Turning to the Shelf	[10]	{a person is turning to face the shelf}
Viewing the Shelf	[5,10,11]	{a person is standing and watching the shelf}
Touch the Shelf	[3–5,10,13]	{one's hand moves to the shelf}, {one's hand moves back from the shelf}
Pick up a Product from the Shelf	[3–5,9,10,12,13]	{one's hand moves to the shelf}, {one's hand moves back from the shelf}, {a product is moving together with one's hand}
Return a Product back to the Shelf	[3,5,10,12,13]	{one's hand moves to the shelf}, {a product is moving together with one's hand}, {one's hand moves back from the shelf}
Put a Product into a Basket/Cart	[10]	{one's hand moves to the cart}, {a product is moving together with one's hand}, {one's hand moves back from the cart}
Holding a Product	[11]	{a product is moving together with one's hand}
Browsing a Product in a Hand	[5,11,13]	{a person is watching his hand}, {a product is moving together with one's hand}

However, though the proposed syntax is enough for our current research, its application range is limited due to the design of *subject, verb, object*, and *where*. Despite the ability to define multi-object interactions theoretically, each sentence only defines two objects' one-to-one relationship. Therefore, the resources for multi-object relationships definition grow exponentially with the number of related objects. Nevertheless, it is currently sufficient for us because there are at most two objects in interaction. Since *where* limits the number of positions only to start and end, it cannot describe complex motion, such as spiral movement.

3.2. Primitive Recognition

In this section, we consider the elements in the syntax from the objects' trajectories. Since most CBs last for a few seconds which implies many frames for a video with 30 fps, this leads to redundancy in the trajectories with the object-tracking method. Consequently, we first perform trajectory segmentation to reduce redundancy in the trajectories. Then, we recognize primitive elements using the results of segmentation.

Trajectory segmentation refers to compressing a trajectory into several segments, which preserve most features of the trajectory. Current approaches [19,20] separate a trajectory based on the moving distance and direction of each vector in the trajectory. Thus, we design an approximate trajectory partitioning (ATP)-based algorithm [19] for trajectory segmentation. However, ATP is sensitive to direction changes. In our case, an object's frequent direction changes over short distances probably refers to idling. We anticipate that the algorithm will only react to change in the moving distance in this case. Hence, we designed a thresholding algorithm based on ATP as shown in Algorithm 1. The algorithm receives two inputs: a list of points $Kpts_{ATP} \leftarrow [p_1, p_2, p_3, ..., p_i, ..., p_N]$ from ATP outputs, where p_i refers to the i-th element in $Kpts_{ATP}$, N is the number of key-points from ATP, and a threshold $threshold_{idle}$ is set to preserve the key-points with a distance longer than $threshold_{idle}$. Since the time complexity of ATP and Algorithm 1 are $O(n)$, the time complexity of the tracjectory segmentation is $O(n^2)$, where n is the length of the trajectory.

Algorithm 1: Thresholding Algorithm for Trajectory Segmentation

Input: List Of Points $Kpts_{ATP} \leftarrow [p_1, p_2, p_3, ..., p_i, ..., p_N]$, Integer $threshold_{idle}$
Output: List Of Points $Kpts$

1   $index \leftarrow 2$;
2   $pt1 \leftarrow p_1$;
3   $idling \leftarrow$ **True**;
4   $Kpts \leftarrow [pt_1]$;
5   **while** $index < N$ **do**
6     $pt_{start} \leftarrow p_{index}$;
7     $pt_{end} \leftarrow p_{index+1}$;
8     $vec \leftarrow p_{end} - p_{start}$;
9     $distance \leftarrow \sqrt{vec.x^2 + vec.y^2}$;
10   **if** $distance \leq threshold_{idle}$ **then**
11   **if** $!idling$ **then**
12        $Kpts.Add(pt_{index-1})$;
13        $pt_{start} \leftarrow pt_{end}$;
14   **end**
15      $idling \leftarrow$ **True**;
16   **else**
17      $Kpts.Add(pt_{index-1})$;
18      $idling \leftarrow$ **False**;
19      $pt_{start} \leftarrow pt_{end}$;
20   **end**
21    $index \leftarrow index + 1$;
22 **end**
23 **if** $!(p_N$ in $Kpts)$ **then**
24   $Kpts.Add(p_N)$;
25 **end**
26 **return** $Kpts$;

In the primitive's syntax, *subject* and *object* are the entity names that can be obtained directly from the trajectory information. The words "in the shelf/cart" and "out of shelf/cart" for *where* can be directly acquired from the coordinates of the trajectory. Therefore, only *verb* needs to be recognized from the trajectories. Algorithm 2 explains the recognition for "move" and "stay". The two words are a pair of antonyms that mean an object is moving faster than a certain speed or staying still. The input segmented trajectory $ST \leftarrow [p_1, p_2, p_3, ..., p_i, ..., p_M]$ contains the trajectory processed by segmentation algorithm, where p_i refers to the i-th point in ST, and M is the number of points of ST. $threshold_{idle}$ is reused in this algorithm to detect whether an object is moving or not. To improve the robustness to noise, we applied a window with length of $len_{window1}$ to filter the noise. The algorithm output $verb_1$ is one of the words "move" and "stay", which means the recognition result for the current frame. The time complexity is $O(n)$, where n is the smaller of the length of the segmented trajectory and $len_{window1}$.

Algorithm 2: Verb Recognition(move, stay)

Input: List Of Points $ST \leftarrow [p_1, p_2, p_3, ..., p_i, ..., p_M]$, Integer $threshold_{idle}$, Integer $len_{window1}$

Output: String $verb_1$

1   $index \leftarrow M$;
2   $results \leftarrow []$;
3   **while** $results.length \leq len_{window1}$ **do**
4     $pt_{start} \leftarrow p_{index}$;
5     $pt_{end} \leftarrow p_{index+1}$;
6     $vec \leftarrow p_{end} - p_{start}$;
7     $distance \leftarrow \sqrt{vec.x^2 + vec.y^2}$;
8   **if** $distance \leq threshold_{idle}$ **then**
9       $results.Add(1)$;
10   **else**
11       $results.Add(0)$;
12   **end**
13    $index \leftarrow index - 1$;
14   **if** $index = 0$ **then**
15   **Break**;
16   **end**
17 **end**
18 $sum \leftarrow 0$;
19 **foreach** *element result of results* **do** $sum \leftarrow sum + result$;
20 ;
21 **if** $sum \leq results.length/2$ **then**
22    $verb_1 \leftarrow$ "stay";
23 **else**
24    $verb_1 \leftarrow$ "move";
25 **end**
26 **return** $verb_1$;

Algorithm 3 shows the recognition for the *verb*, "follow". The word means the *subject* is moving/staying together with the *object*. The inputs are two objects' segmented trajectory $ST1 \leftarrow [p1_1, p1_2, p1_3, ..., p1_i, ..., p1_M]$ and $ST2 \leftarrow [p2_1, p2_2, p2_3, ..., p2_i, ..., p2_M]$, where pj_i refers to the i-th point in the trajectory ST_j, M is the number of points of the segmented trajectory. $threshold_{follow}$ is used to detect whether an object is close to another one or not. Similar to Algorithm 2, a parameter $len_{window2}$ is passed to the algorithm for denoising. The algorithm output $verb_2$ is "follow" or *null*, which means the recognition result for the current frame. The time complexity is $O(n)$. Furthermore, the *verb* "face to" refers to *subject* is facing *object*. Since it requires detecting the orientation of the body or head, which is not currently supported in our method, we intend to omit it in this paper and consider it in future work. The time complexity is $O(n)$, where n is the smaller of the length of the segmented trajectory and $len_{window1}$.

Algorithm 3: Verb Recognition(follow)

Input: List Of Points $ST1 \leftarrow [p1_1, p1_2, p1_3, ..., p1_i, ..., p1_M]$, List Of Points $ST2 \leftarrow [p2_1, p2_2, p2_3, ..., p2_i, ..., p2_M]$, Integer $threshold_{follow}$, Integer $len_{window2}$

Output: String $verb_2$

1   $index \leftarrow M$;
2   $results \leftarrow []$;
3   **while** $results.length \leq len_{window2}$ **do**
4     $pt1 \leftarrow p1_{index}$;
5     $pt2 \leftarrow p2_{index}$;
6     $vec \leftarrow pt2 - pt1$;
7     $distance \leftarrow \sqrt{vec.x^2 + vec.y^2}$;
8   **if** $distance \leq threshold_{follow}$ **then**
9       $results.Add(1)$;
10   **else**
11       $results.Add(0)$;
12   **end**
13    $index \leftarrow index - 1$;
14   **if** $index = 0$ **then**
15   **Break**;
16   **end**
17 **end**
18 $sum \leftarrow 0$;
19 **foreach** *element result of results* **do** $sum \leftarrow sum+result$;
20 ;
21 **if** $sum \leq results.length/2$ **then**
22    $verb_2 \leftarrow null$;
23 **else**
24    $verb_2 \leftarrow$ "follow";
25 **end**
26 **return** $verb_2$;

3.3. Define CB by Primitives

With our designed primitives, we are able to customize a wide range of CBs with a combination of primitives. Since our primitives are designed with reference to target CBs in existing methods, we applied primitives to define those target CBs. The clothes-related CBs are excepted because they are not common in normal retail stores, and because they are too complex for our proposal. We defined CBs in Table 1 by primitives, as shown in Table 2. The symbol "→" defines the primitives' chronological order. Primitives that precede this symbol are assumed to occur first. Since the product is occluded when it is on the shelf in our implementation, a precise definition of "touch the shelf" is difficult to formulate. Therefore, we defined it broadly as the primitive pattern in Table 2.

Table 2. Define target CBs by primitives.

Target CB	Primitive Pattern ({} = Primitive, != Not)
Passing by the Shelf	{person move out of shelf}
Turning to the Shelf	{person !face to shelf} → {person face to shelf}
Viewing the Shelf	{person stay out of shelf}
Touch product in the Shelf	{hand move to in the shelf} → {hand move to out of shelf}
Pick up a Product from the Shelf	{hand move to in the shelf} → {hand move to out of shelf}, {product follow hand}
Return a Product back to Shelf	{hand move to in the shelf}, {product follow hand} → {hand move to out of shelf}
Put a Product into a Basket/Cart	{hand move to in the cart}, {product follow hand} → {hand move to !in the cart}
Holding a Product	{product follow hand}
Browsing a Product in a Hand	{product follow hand}, {person stay}

3.4. Primitive Pattern Matching

The recognized primitives are stored in a sequence to retain their chronological order. Once any primitive has been recognized in the current frame, our method matches the primitive sequence with the predefined primitive patterns. Any matched result is considered as a recognized CB. Algorithm 4 explains the details of the pattern matching. Since forward matching in chronological order consumes a great deal of computational resources to save different matching states for each primitive pattern, it leads to the running speed becoming slow as the running time grows. Therefore, we match recognized primitives in reverse chronological order. In other words, we start matching from the most recently recognized primitives, which saves a great deal of computational resources because there is no need to save the matching states. The algorithm takes the inputs of a sequence, including recognized primitives, a predefined primitive pattern, and a number *timeout*, to stop the algorithm when there are not any matched primitives within the recent *timeout* frames. The output is a Boolean value of whether the corresponding CB is matched or not. The time complexity is $O(n)$, where n is the smaller of the length of P_{seq} and the length of P_{def}.

Algorithm 4: Primitive Pattern Matching

Input: List Of Primitive P_{seq}, List Of Primitive P_{def}, Integer *timeout*
Output: Boolean *matched*

1   $seqIndex \leftarrow P_{seq}$.length;
2   $defIndex \leftarrow P_{def}$.length;
3   $timeoutCounter \leftarrow 0$;
4   **while** $(seqIndex > 0)$ **AND** $(timeoutCounter \leq timeout)$ **do**
5   **if** $P_{seq}[seqIndex] = P_{def}[defIndex]$ **then**
6         $defIndex \leftarrow defIndex - 1$;
7   **if** $defIndex = 0$ **then**
8   **return True**;
9   **end**
10   **else**
11         $timeoutCounter \leftarrow timeoutCounter + 1$;
12   **end**
13      $seqIndex \leftarrow seqIndex - 1$;
14   **end**
15   **return False**;

---

4. Evaluation

4.1. Experiment Settings

Our proposed method can be flexibly modified to recognize different target CBs to cope with frequently changing target CBs in smart retail solutions. To evaluate our proposed method, we used our collected laboratory dataset [21] and the public MERL dataset [7]. Our proposed method recognizes target CBs in input videos and calculates their f1-score as the accuracy metric. Since videos in two datasets were taken in different environments, it can be considered a change in retail environments to some extent. To recognize different target CBs in the two different datasets, we only changed a few parameters of our designed algorithms and predefined primitive patterns. By observing the accuracy of our method on different datasets, and considering only a few modifications when changing datasets, we could infer our method's flexibility to some degree.

The inputs of our method are the trajectory coordinates, which need to be obtained using object detection and a tracking model. However, wrong tracking results obtained by other models mean wrong inputs to our method, which probably leads to wrong outputs. To eliminate the influence of different object detection models on our evaluation results, we track the annotated bounding boxes with a Kalman-filter and Hungarian algorithm [22] to obtain the input trajectories for our method. In addition, although some tracking models can predict the trajectories of occluded objects, the occluded trajectories are not annotated in the evaluation. Regarding the output CB annotations, we annotated the target CB in each frame for our laboratory dataset. As the MERL dataset is public, we used its original CB annotations. For the experiments on both datasets, we implemented our method in the same Windows 11 device with RAM of 16 GB. The CPU was an Intel i7-12700K (3.6 GHz). The GPU was an NVIDIA GeForce RTX 3060 Ti (8 GB). The program was written in Python 3.9. The ML framework was PyTorch 1.12. The third-party libraries used included numpy 1.22 and scipy 1.8.

4.2. Our Laboratory Dataset

This is a dataset we collected at a public activity, where the randomly selected 19 participants were requested to simulate shopping in front of the shelf one-by-one. The dataset includes 19 top-view videos of 19 subjects with a resolution of 640×480. Each video was about 30–60 s with 10 FPS and only one subject. Figure 2 shows some examples of the annotated target CBs in the dataset. We built a laboratory retail environment and installed an RGB top-view camera to obtain an occlusion-free view. Each participant in the videos was asked to interact with the products on the shelf. The participant were required to take at least one product from the shelf. There were four products of different shapes and sizes, including a boxed juice, a deodorant spray, a stainless steel bottle, and a wet-tissue. The products were not visible when they were on the shelf. Our data was collected when our proposed method was demonstrated in a public activity. The videos were collected without requiring the participants to sign any confidentiality agreement, and the participants' faces were exposed to the cameras. Unfortunately, as a result, we cannot publish our collected dataset until all the private information has been removed, such as by masking the faces.

Since the innovative part of our proposed method involves the receipt of trajectory coordinates as inputs, we annotated the bounding box of person, hand, and four products in each frame. Then, we used a tracker with a Kalman-filter and Hungarian algorithm [22] to obtain the object's trajectory as input. Regarding the output CBs, we selected eight CBs as listed in Table 3. Among them, the first six CBs included most target CBs used in existing methods. However, with the annotation of the first six CBs, we found that many frames still remained without annotation. Thus, we added two CBs to fill the frames without annotations. We used some approximate definitions for some CBs, such as "browse", because the approximate definition enabled reuse of primitives with nearly no loss of accuracy.

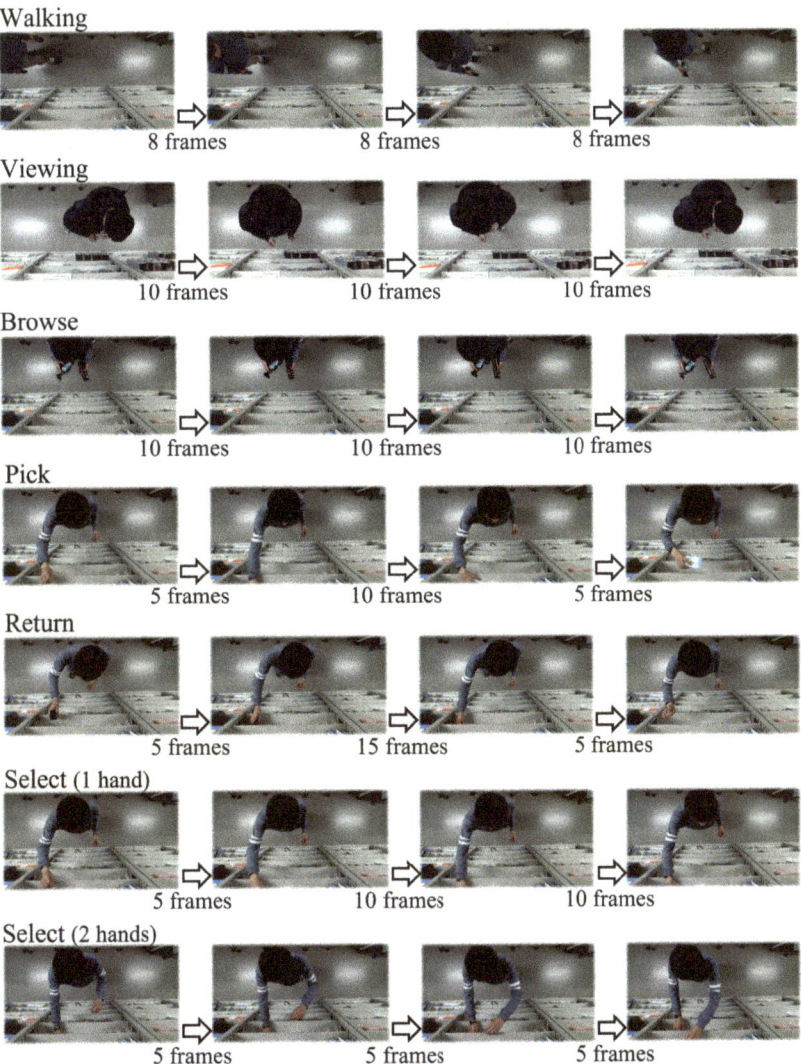

Figure 2. Example of annotated CB in our laboratory dataset.

Figure 3 shows the confusion matrix of our laboratory dataset. Each CB's column includes two columns of frame count and each row's frame count percentage. Figure 4 shows the f1-score and some statistics for our laboratory dataset. The total average is the average value of the column calculated using the sum of the product of the frame percent and each row's value. The total average f1-score of our method was 89.35%, which is an acceptable result. The f1-score for most CBs was also acceptable, except for "viewing," "walking," and "touch". In terms of "viewing", the confusion matrix revealed the reason with 68.18% precision. Some "viewing" frames were recognized as "select" and "browse." The ambiguous boundary caused the wrong prediction of "select". The different definition of "viewing" between annotation and CB definition led to the wrong prediction of "browse". As our proposed method cannot recognize the target's orientation or track the target's eyes currently, our CB definition approximately defines "viewing" as stay static out of the shelf, while the annotation of "viewing" means the target is standing still and looking at the shelf. The low recall of "viewing" indicates that most frames of "browse" were recognized as "viewing". The difference in CB definition is whether the target is holding a product or not. Products are usually occluded in the "browse" frames, which caused the wrong recognition output for "viewing".

Table 3. Primitive patterns in our laboratory dataset.

Name	Description	Primitive Pattern ({}= Primitive, != Not)
Walking	one is walking along the shelf	{person move out of shelf}
Viewing	one is standing in front of the shelf	{person stay out of shelf}
Browse	one is holding and watching a product without moving	{product follow hand}, {person stay}
Pick	one picks up a product from the shelf	{hand move to in the shelf} → {hand move to out of shelf}, {product follow hand}
Return	one returns a product back to the shelf	{hand move to in the shelf}, {product follow hand} → {hand move to out of shelf}
Touch	one hand into the shelf without taking any product out	{hand move to in the shelf} → {hand move to out of shelf}
Select (1 hand)	one hand is selecting products in the shelf	{hand in the shelf}, {hand out of shelf}
Select (2 hands)	both hands are used to select products in the shelf	{hand out of shelf}

Truth		Predicted (frame count | row percentage)														
	A		B		C		D		E		F		G		H	
select(1 hand) = A	496	94.7%	2	0.4%	21	4.0%	4	0.8%	0	0.0%	0	0.0%	0	0.0%	1	0.2%
select(2 hands) = B	2	3.3%	54	90.0%	2	3.3%	0	0.0%	1	1.7%	1	1.7%	0	0.0%	0	0.0%
browse = C	30	1.4%	8	0.4%	1896	88.2%	136	6.3%	21	1.0%	2	0.1%	56	2.6%	0	0.0%
viewing = D	15	11.4%	0	0.0%	25	18.9%	90	68.2%	2	1.5%	0	0.0%	0	0.0%	0	0.0%
return = E	3	1.3%	1	0.4%	5	2.2%	3	1.3%	208	91.6%	5	2.2%	2	0.9%	0	0.0%
pick = F	1	0.3%	0	0.0%	11	3.4%	0	0.0%	0	0.0%	291	90.1%	0	0.0%	20	6.2%
walking = G	0	0.0%	0	0.0%	26	32.5%	0	0.0%	0	0.0%	0	0.0%	54	67.5%	0	0.0%
touch = H	0	0.0%	0	0.0%	0	0.0%	0	0.0%	0	0.0%	0	0.0%	0	0.0%	6	100.0%

Figure 3. Confusion matrix of our laboratory dataset.

	total frames	frame percent	happen times	precision	recall	f1-score	
select(1 hand)	524	14.97%	27	94.66%	90.68%	92.62%	100%
select(2 hands)	60	1.71%	4	90.00%	83.08%	86.40%	
browse	2149	61.38%	54	88.23%	95.47%	91.70%	80%
viewing	132	3.77%	9	68.18%	38.63%	49.32%	60%
return	227	6.48%	31	91.63%	89.66%	90.63%	
pick	323	9.23%	47	90.09%	97.32%	93.57%	40%
walking	80	2.29%	8	67.50%	48.21%	56.25%	
touch	6	0.17%	1	100.00%	22.22%	36.36%	20%
Total Average				88.40%	90.98%	89.35%	0%

Figure 4. Results of F1-score of our laboratory dataset.

With respect to "walking", some of its frames were recognized as "browse". When the target is walking while holding a product, it is difficult to determine the ambiguous boundary between "browse" and "walking". The CB definition in Table 3 recognizes them by distinguishing whether the target is moving while holding a product. "Browse" refers to holding a product while staying static. We used a single threshold to divide the object's moving speed to detect move or stay, which was not sufficiently accurate for totally correct detection. Some frames were detected as staying static, which led to the wrong recognition. This also applied to the low recall of "walking".

In the case of "touch", there was only one case in the dataset. It was defined as a customer putting their hand inside the shelf but taking nothing out of it. Some wrong recognition of "pick" results in the low recall occurred because the picked object was occluded. In addition, Figure 3 shows that most video frames were "browse" and occurred more frequently than any other CBs. Thus, we considered discriminating within "browse" to make the distribution of CBs more uniform.

According to the above results, our method showed acceptable accuracy for the laboratory dataset. Some individual CBs with low f1-score are anticipated to be improved by changing the CB definitions into more accurate definitions. To evaluate our proposed method's ability to discriminate CB, we predefined different primitive patterns to discriminate the CB "select" according to whether one hand or both hands were used. This indicates that our proposed method is able to deal with CB discrimination to some extent. Concerning the evaluation of flexibility, we measured the time required by our method when applied to different datasets. For the collected laboratory dataset, we spent about an hour tuning the five parameters in the three designed algorithms and two to three hours defining the primitive patterns in Table 3. Then, we annotated the CBs in each frame for about five hours per day. The annotations took about one week in total. Since annotation is not required during the application of our method, the time for annotation is considered as a reference for the ML-based methods' modification time.

4.3. MERL Dataset

The MERL shopping dataset [7] is a public dataset consisting of 106 top-view videos with a resolution of 920×680, each of which is about two minutes long with 30FPS. All 41 subjects were asked to do shopping in a retail store setting. Figure 5 presents some examples of the annotated CBs in the dataset. With regard to the input trajectory coordinates, we annotated the bounding box of person and hand in each frame based on the results from the pose estimation model Higher HRNet [23] pretrained on the COCO dataset [24]. We manually annotated the product's bounding box in each frame. Due to the limited time, we only finished the object's bounding box annotations in 46 videos for evaluation. Similar to the process for the laboratory dataset, we used the same tracker with a Kalman-filter and Hungarian algorithm [22] to obtain the input trajectories.

For the output CBs, we used the CB annotations included in the dataset. This provided five CBs' annotation, and we defined them using our proposed method, presented in Table 4. Among the five CBs, we excluded the CB "hand in shelf" from the evaluation because many ground truths were not annotated during our random check of the annotations.

Table 4. Primitive Patterns in MERL dataset.

Name	Description	Primitive Pattern ({}= Primitive)
Reach To Shelf	reach one's hand to shelf	{hand move out of shelf} → {hand move in the shelf}
Retract From Shelf	retract hand from shelf	{hand move in the shelf} → {hand move out of shelf}
Hand In Shelf	extended period with hand in the shelf	{hand in the shelf}
Inspect Product	inspect product while holding it in hand	{product follow hand}
Inspect Shelf	look at shelf while not touching and reaching for the shelf	{person stay out of shelf}

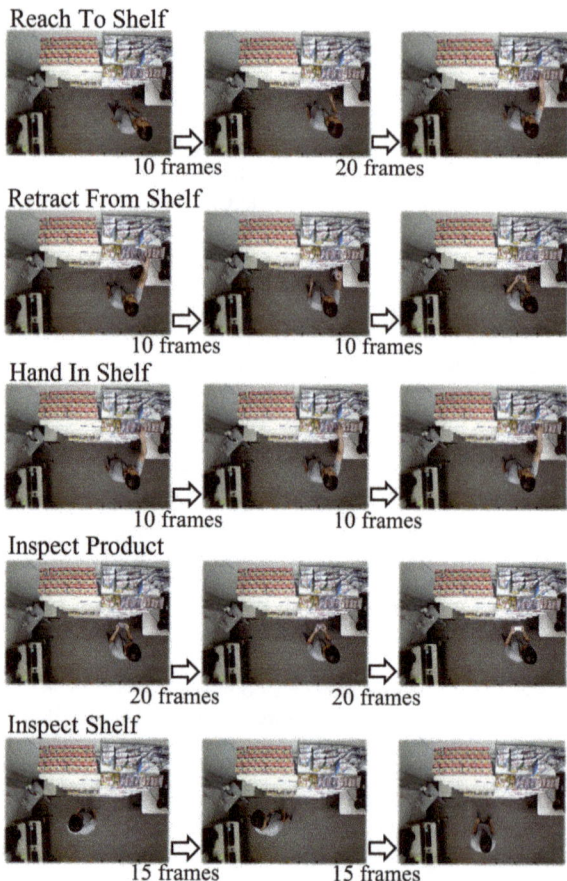

Figure 5. Example of annotated CB in MERL dataset.

Figure 6 shows the confusion matrix of the MERL dataset. Each CB's column includes two columns of frame count and each row's frame count percentage. Figure 7 shows the f1-score and statistics for the MERL dataset. The calculation of the total average was the same as in Figure 4. The average f1-score of our method was 79.66%, which is acceptable for our proposed method with only a change in CB definitions. Among the four target CBs, our method achieved only about 60% precision for "reach to shelf" and "retract from shelf". We found that this was caused by the different boundary in the definition. Specifically, there was a difference between our definition of "reach to shelf" and the definition in the MERL dataset. We defined the CB's boundary using a threshold of moving speed. Therefore, our method started to recognize "reach to shelf" from the frame in which the hand was already moving. The MERL dataset defines the start of "reach to shelf" as when one intends to "reach to shelf", when one's hand has not yet moved. Thus, our recognition results always differed from the annotations by a few frames. For "retract from shelf", this accounted for the low precision. The errors for "reach to shelf" and "retract from shelf" were caused by different definitions. We consider our method to have been successful in recognizing every "reach to shelf" and "retract from shelf" CB with a few frames' difference. This implies that we could improve our method by recognizing intention in our future research.

Truth	Predicted (frame count | row percentage)							
	A		B		C		D	
reach to shelf = A	12254	61.7%	0	0.0%	731	3.0%	7152	35.3%
retract from shelf = B	0	0.0%	14061	63.3%	1423	6.3%	7364	30.4%
inspect shelf = C	1007	2.7%	36	0.2%	33621	80.9%	4147	16.2%
inspect product = D	0	0.0%	0	0.0%	0	0.0%	36368	100.0%

Figure 6. Confusion matrix of MERL dataset.

	total frames	frame percent	happen times	precision	recall	f1-score
reach to shelf	20145	17.17%	918	63.49%	87.50%	73.59%
retract hand from shelf	23552	20.07%	928	61.85%	90.97%	73.64%
inspect shelf	32674	27.84%	836	83.60%	86.98%	85.26%
inspect product	40984	34.92%	302	95.93%	71.06%	81.64%
Total Average				80.09%	82.31%	79.66%

Figure 7. Results of F1-score of MERL dataset.

Except for recognition accuracy, Table 5 compares the required modifications and the estimated required time when applying our approach and the machine learning-based approach to different datasets. Our proposed method changed the five parameters ($threshold_{idle}$, $len_{window1}$, $threshold_{follow}$, $len_{window2}$, $timeout$) in the three algorithms we designed in Section 3. They were mainly used to cope with change in the person's scale in the video frames. We also re-defined the primitive patterns for the new target CBs. As shown in Table 5, in our experiments, all the modifications took about 3–4 h.

Table 5. Flexibility: Modifications for dataset change adaptation.

Method	Modifications	Estimated Required Time
Our proposed method	5 parameters for our designed 3 algorithms	1 h
	Re-define primitive patterns	2–3 h
ML-based methods	Re-collecting video data	no reference data
	Re-annotating collected data	a week (our dataset) 3 months (MERL)
	Training and tuning model(s)	no reference data

For the ML-based methods, the main modification was re-annotation. Since the required time for data re-collection and model tuning varied greatly when dealing with changes of datasets, we currently lack sufficient reference data to estimate its required time. However, regarding the time spent on re-annotation, as we annotated both datasets for the purpose of accuracy calculation, the required time for modification was estimated to be about 2–3 months.

In conclusion, since our method cannot be fine-tuned as ML-based methods are, our proposed method sacrifices accuracy to obtain flexibility. Nonetheless, the huge difference in modification time indicates that the trade-off is justified. The considerably enhanced flexibility could have application value in the context of CBR.

5. Conclusions

Smart retail solutions usually require the recognition of a wide range of CBs from captured video in stores. The CBs that are selected as recognition targets are called target CBs. Target CBs frequently change with changes in needs, environments, etc. To achieve flexible target CB change adaptation, we proposed a flexible CBR approach. Our main idea is recognizing CB using a combination of primitives, which are a kind of partitioned CB. Since different CBs share the same primitives; the primitives can be reused when adapting to target CB changes, which avoids time-consuming steps, such as re-collecting training data and re-training the recognition models. Consequently, our method can flexibly adapt to changes in target CB by changing the combinations of primitives only. In addition, we designed a syntax based on natural language grammar to define primitives. The readable syntax improves the explanatory power of our method. Therefore, the usage of primitives and our proposed syntax can enable a high degree of flexibility in target CB change adaptation. Evaluation experiments undertaken demonstrated that our method achieved an acceptable level of accuracy for different datasets, and great flexibility across different datasets.

Nevertheless, the experiments also revealed some limitations of our proposed method. Since our method is difficult to fine-tune to fit some individual situations, the recognition accuracy is decreased compared to ML-based methods. A possible solution would be to replace the current pattern matching algorithm with a probabilistic model. In addition, because the element *where* in the primitive syntax limits the number of positions, the syntax cannot represent complex movement, such as spiral movement. This leads to a limited cover range of CB. Increasing the vocabulary of *where* could improve the model's expressive power to represent complex movement. Furthermore, though the syntax element *face to* includes orientation information, the orientation detection is currently not applied. These limitations may be addressed in future work.

Author Contributions: Conceptualization, J.W. and T.A.; data curation, J.W.; formal analysis, J.W.; investigation, J.W.; methodology, J.W. and T.A.; project administration, J.W. and T.A.; resources, T.A. and T.S.; software, J.W.; supervision, T.A. and T.S.; validation, J.W.; visualization, J.W.; writing—original draft, J.W.; writing—review and editing, J.W., T.A. and T.S. All authors have read and agreed to the published version of the manuscript.

Funding: This research received no funding.

Institutional Review Board Statement: Not applicable.

Informed Consent Statement: Not applicable.

Data Availability Statement: Not applicable.

Conflicts of Interest: The authors declare no conflict of interest.

Abbreviations

The following abbreviations are used in this manuscript:

CB	Customer behavior
CBR	Customer behavior recognition
HAR	Human activity recognition
ML	Machine learning

References

1. Data Bridge Market Research. Global Smart Retail Market—Industry Trends and Forecast to 2029. 2022. Available online: https://www.databridgemarketresearch.com/reports/global-smart-retail-market (accessed on 18 June 2022).
2. Hernandez, D.A.M.; Nalbach, O.; Werth, D. How computer vision provides physical retail with a better view on customers. In Proceedings of the 2019 IEEE 21st Conference on Business Informatics, Moscow, Russia, 15–17 July 2019; pp. 462–471. [CrossRef]
3. Paolanti, M.; Pietrini, R.; Mancini, A.; Frontoni, E.; Zingaretti, P. Deep understanding of shopper behaviours and interactions using RGB-D vision. *Mach. Vision Appl.* **2020**, *31*, 1–21. [CrossRef]
4. Popa, M.C.; Gritti, T.; Rothkrantz, L.J.M.; Shan, C.; Wiggers, P. Detecting customers' buying events on a real-life database. In Proceedings of the 14th International Conference on Computer Analysis of Images and Patterns, Seville, Spain, 29–31 August 2011; pp. 17–25. [CrossRef]
5. Popa, M.C.; Rothkrantz, L.J.M.; Wiggers, P.; Shan, C. Shopping behavior recognition using a language modeling analogy. *Pattern Recognit. Lett.* **2013**, *34*, 1879–1889. [CrossRef]
6. Merad, D.; Drap, P.; Lufimpu-Luviya, Y.; Iguernaissi, R.; Fertil, B. Purchase behavior analysis through gaze and gesture observation. *Pattern Recognit. Lett.* **2016**, *81*, 21–29. [CrossRef]

7. Singh, B.; Marks, T.K.; Jones, M.; Tuzel, O.; Shao, M. A multi-stream bi-directional recurrent neural network for fine-grained action detection. In Proceedings of the 2016 IEEE Conference on Computer Vision and Pattern Recognitiont, Las Vegas, NV, USA, 27–30 June 2016; pp. 1961–1970. [CrossRef]
8. Hochreiter, S.; Schmidhuber, J. Long short-term memory. *Neural Comput.* **1997**, *9*, 1735–1780. [CrossRef] [PubMed]
9. WaqasMaria; NasirMauizah; Hussain, S.; NazHabiba; TanveerMaheen. Customer Activity Recognition System using Image Processing. *Int. J. Comput. Sci. Netw. Secur.* **2021**, *21*, 63–66.
10. Liu, J.; Gu, Y.; Kamijo, S. Customer behavior recognition in retail store from surveillance camera. In Proceedings of the 2015 IEEE International Symposium on Multimedia (ISM), Miami, FL, USA, 14–16 December 2015; pp. 154–159. [CrossRef]
11. Yamamoto, J.; Inoue, K.; Yoshioka, M. Investigation of customer behavior analysis based on top-view depth camera. In Proceedings of the 2017 IEEE Winter Applications of Computer Vision Workshops, Santa Rosa, CA, USA, 24–31 March 2017; pp. 67–74. [CrossRef]
12. Frontoni, E.; Raspa, P.; Mancini, A.; Zingaretti, P.; Placidi, V. Customers' activity recognition in intelligent retail environments. In Proceedings of the 2013 Image Analysis and Processing, Naples, Italy, 9–13 September 2013; pp. 509–516. [CrossRef]
13. Liciotti, D.; Contigiani, M.; Frontoni, E.; Mancini, A.; Zingaretti, P.; Placidi, V. Shopper analytics: A customer activity recognition system using a distributed RGB-D camera network. In Proceedings of the International Workshop on Video Analytics for Audience Measurement in Retail and Digital Signage, Stockholm, Sweden, 24 August 2014; pp. 146–157. [CrossRef]
14. Liu, H.; Hartmann, Y.; Schultz, T. Motion Units: Generalized Sequence Modeling of Human Activities for Sensor-Based Activity Recognition. In Proceedings of the 2021 29th European Signal Processing Conference (EUSIPCO), Dublin, Ireland, 23–27 August 2021; pp. 1506–1510. [CrossRef]
15. Hartmann., Y.; Liu., H.; Lahrberg., S.; Schultz., T. Interpretable High-level Features for Human Activity Recognition. In Proceedings of the 15th International Joint Conference on Biomedical Engineering Systems and Technologies—BIOSIGNALS, Online, 9–11 February 2022; pp. 40–49. [CrossRef]
16. Rai, N.; Chen, H.; Ji, J.; Desai, R.; Kozuka, K.; Ishizaka, S.; Adeli, E.; Niebles, J.C. Home Action Genome: Cooperative Compositional Action Understanding. In Proceedings of the IEEE/CVF Conference on Computer Vision and Pattern Recognition, Nashville, TN, USA, 20–25 June 2021.
17. Mansour, R.F.; Escorcia-Gutierrez, J.; Gamarra, M.; Villanueva, J.A.; Leal, N. Intelligent video anomaly detection and classification using faster RCNN with deep reinforcement learning model. *Image Vis. Comput.* **2021**, *112*, 104229. [CrossRef]
18. Generosi, A.; Ceccacci, S.; Mengoni, M. A deep learning-based system to track and analyze customer behavior in retail store. In Proceedings of the 2018 IEEE 8th International Conference on Consumer Electronics, Berlin, Germany, 2–5 September 2018; pp. 1–6. [CrossRef]
19. Lee, J.G.; Han, J.; Whang, K.Y. Trajectory clustering: A partition-and-group framework. In Proceedings of the 2007 ACM SIGMOD International Conference on Management of Data, Beijing, China, 12–14 June 2007; pp. 593–604. [CrossRef]
20. Leal, E.; Gruenwald, L. DynMDL: A parallel trajectory segmentation algorithm. In Proceedings of the 2018 IEEE International Conference on Big Data, Seattle, WA, USA, 10–13 December 2018; pp. 215–218. [CrossRef]
21. Wen, J.; Guillen, L.; Abe, T.; Suganuma, T. A Hierarchy-Based System for Recognizing Customer Activity in Retail Environments. *Sensors* **2021**, *21*, 4712. [CrossRef] [PubMed]
22. Bewley, A.; Ge, Z.; Ott, L.; Ramos, F.; Upcroft, B. Simple Online and Realtime Tracking. *arXiv* **2016**, arXiv:1602.00763.
23. Cheng, B.; Xiao, B.; Wang, J.; Shi, H.; Huang, T.S.; Zhang, L. Bottom-up Higher-Resolution Networks for Multi-Person Pose Estimation. Available online: https://www.catalyzex.com/paper/arxiv:1908.10357 (accessed on 12 July 2022).
24. Lin, T.Y.; Maire, M.; Belongie, S.; Bourdev, L.; Girshick, R.; Hays, J.; Perona, P.; Ramanan, D.; Zitnick, C.L.; Dollár, P. Microsoft COCO: Common Objects in Context. In *Computer Vision—ECCV 2014*; Springer: Cham, Switzerland, 2014.

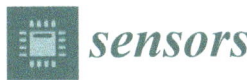

sensors

Article

How Validation Methodology Influences Human Activity Recognition Mobile Systems

Hendrio Bragança [†], Juan G. Colonna, Horácio A. B. F. Oliveira and Eduardo Souto [*,†]

Institute of Computing, Federal University of Amazonas, Manaus 69067-005, Brazil;
hendrio.luis@icomp.ufam.edu.br (H.B.); juancolonna@icomp.ufam.edu.br (J.G.C.);
horacio@icomp.ufam.edu.br (H.A.B.F.O.)
* Correspondence: esouto@icomp.ufam.edu.br
† These authors contributed equally to this work.

Abstract: In this article, we introduce explainable methods to understand how Human Activity Recognition (HAR) mobile systems perform based on the chosen validation strategies. Our results introduce a new way to discover potential bias problems that overestimate the prediction accuracy of an algorithm because of the inappropriate choice of validation methodology. We show how the SHAP (Shapley additive explanations) framework, used in literature to explain the predictions of any machine learning model, presents itself as a tool that can provide graphical insights into how human activity recognition models achieve their results. Now it is possible to analyze which features are important to a HAR system in each validation methodology in a simplified way. We not only demonstrate that the validation procedure k-folds cross-validation (k-CV), used in most works to evaluate the expected error in a HAR system, can overestimate by about 13% the prediction accuracy in three public datasets but also choose a different feature set when compared with the universal model. Combining explainable methods with machine learning algorithms has the potential to help new researchers look inside the decisions of the machine learning algorithms, avoiding most times the overestimation of prediction accuracy, understanding relations between features, and finding bias before deploying the system in real-world scenarios.

Keywords: human activity recognition; validation methodology; leave-one-subject-out cross-validation; explainable methods; Shapley additive explanations; machine learning

Citation: Bragança, H.; Colonna, J.G.; Oliveira, H.A.B.F.; Souto, E. How Validation Methodology Influences Human Activity Recognition Mobile Systems. *Sensors* **2022**, *22*, 2360. https://doi.org/10.3390/s22062360

Academic Editors: Tanja Schultz, Hui Liu and Hugo Gamboa

Received: 12 February 2022
Accepted: 15 March 2022
Published: 18 March 2022

Publisher's Note: MDPI stays neutral with regard to jurisdictional claims in published maps and institutional affiliations.

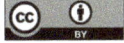

1. Introduction

Human Activity Recognition (HAR) is an emergent research area for autonomous and real-time monitoring of human activities and has been widely explored because of its good practical applications, such as behavior detection, ambient assisted living, elderly care, and rehabilitation [1–8]. Individuals express their routines through activities that are performed in particular situations and understanding these situations enables people to improve their daily lives. Physical activities performed by an individual (e.g., walking and running) can create recommendations and avoid the negative impacts of illness. For instance, the time spent sitting is associated with an increased risk of becoming obese and developing diabetes and cardiovascular diseases [3]. A HAR system can observe elderly people by analyzing data from a smart wearable and improve their lifestyle by warning them about forthcoming unprecedented events such as falls or other health risks [9].

Smartphones have been used to monitor everyday activities automatically through a variety of embedded sensors such as accelerometers, gyroscopes, microphones, cameras and GPS units [1,10]. Understanding how individuals behave by analyzing smartphone data through machine learning is the fundamental challenge in the human activity recognition research area [11].

To recognize physical activity from reading data from sensors, most proposed solutions rely on the Activity Recognition Process (ARP) protocol: Data acquisition, preprocessing/segmentation, feature extraction, classification and evaluation [10,12–14]. Several parameters in each one of these stages (sample size, experimental methodology, cross-validation settings and type of application) can affect the overall recognition [15]. Even when these parameters are well adjusted, the final evaluation of the system may not reflect the true accuracy when recognizing data from new individuals. The main reason for this is that, in most cases, the methodology used to validate the results does not consider the label that identifies the individuals.

The most commonly adopted validation strategy in Machine Learning (ML) literature is the k-fold cross-validation (k-CV) [16]. The k-CV splits a dataset into two subsets: One for training the ML algorithm and one for testing the performance, repeating this process k times. The k-CV procedure does not consider whether all samples belong to the same subject (i.e., individual). This is usually because of the windowing step used to segment the time series during the pre-processing stage. Therefore, in a HAR application that aims for generalization, randomly partitioning the dataset becomes a problem when samples of one subject are in both training and test sets at the same time. As a result, an information leak appears, artificially increasing the classifier's accuracy. We can confirm this observation in several studies in the literature [7,17–22].

In practice, the introduction of illegitimate information in the evaluation stage is unintentional and facilitated by most data partitioning processes, making it hard to detect and eliminate. Even then, identifying this situation as the reason for the overestimated results might be non-trivial [18,23].

In this article, we use the explainable artificial intelligence (XAI) tools' capacity to detect and address bias and fairness issues when choosing different validation methodologies. This is a critical topic that has grown rapidly in the community because the decisions of machine learning models can reproduce biases in historical data used to train them [24]. A variety of reasons, like lack of data, imbalanced datasets and biased datasets, can affect the decision rendered by the learning models. We found it is possible to explain model behavior and its capability in a simple way. Machine learning engineers can use this information to suggest modifications needed in the system to reduce critical issues linked to bias or fairness.

Our work aims to discover bias problems that overestimate the predictive accuracy of a machine learning algorithm because of an inappropriate choice of validation methodology. We examine how different HAR system approaches make generalizations based on a new subject(s) by using k-fold cross-validation, holdout and leave-one-subject-out cross validation. In particular, we show how the SHAP (Shapley additive explanations) framework presents itself as a tool that provides graphical insights into how human activity recognition models achieve their results. This is important because it allows us to see which features are relevant to a HAR system in each validation method.

We can summarize the main contributions of this work as follows:

(1) We evaluate three different approaches for building a HAR system: Personalized, universal and hybrid. Our experiments reveal pitfalls caused by incorrectly dividing the dataset, which can lead to unnoticed over-fitting. We show that k-CV achieves an average accuracy of 98% on six human activities, whereas with leave-one-subject-out cross-validation the accuracy drops to 85.37%. We achieved the results by merging three widely used datasets, SHOAIB [2], WISDM [25] and UCI-HAR [26], which have human activities performed by 59 different subjects.

(2) We propose a new approach by using XAI methods to show how machine learning models choose different features to make its prediction based on the selected validation strategy. We performed several experiments that allowed us to measure the impacts of each of these methodologies on the final results. With this, we could quantify the importance of choosing the correct evaluation methodology of a HAR system.

The remainder of this paper is organized as follows. Section 4 presents the most common procedures for building a HAR system. Section 5 presents a discussion of a fair evaluation for HAR systems. Section 6 introduces explainable algorithms used to interpret the predictions of machine learning models. Section 7 presents the experimental protocol and Section 8 the results of our evaluation scenarios. Section 3 presents the work related to this research. Finally, Section 9 presents the conclusions of this work.

2. Human Activity Recognition

Smartphones are devices capable of monitoring everyday activities automatically through a variety of built-in sensors such as accelerometers, gyroscopes, microphones, cameras and GPS units [10]. Human activity recognition involves complicated tasks which often require dedicated hardware, sophisticated engineering and computational and statistical techniques for data pre-processing and analysis [7].

To find patterns in sensors data and associate them to human activities, the standard pipeline used in most works follows the Activity Recognition Process (ARP) protocols [7,11,13,27–30]. As depicted in Figure 1, ARP consists of five steps, acquisition, preprocessing, segmentation, feature extraction and classification [7]. Our work also includes the evaluation phase in the ARP pipeline to present in detail how validation methodology impacts the general performance of a HAR system. We can find in literature extensions of the standard pipeline with specific stages such as annotation and application stage [31], or even privacy and interpretability [32,33].

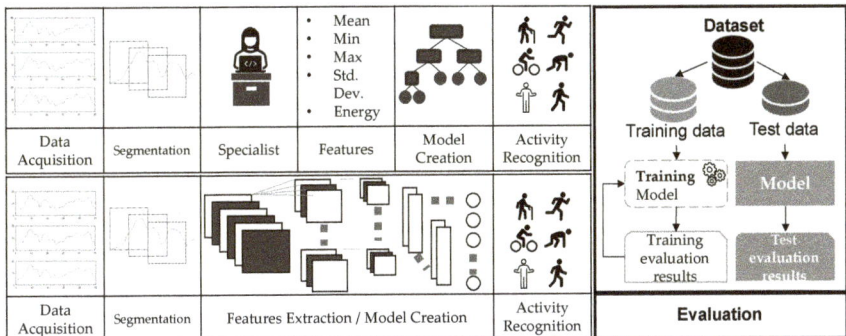

Figure 1. The common methodology used in HAR: Data acquisition, segmentation, feature extraction, classification and evaluation.

2.1. Data Acquisition

In the data acquisition phase, motion sensors are used to gather data, such as angle, vibration, rotation and oscillation from the smartphone. The individual actions are reflected in the sensor data or linked to the physical environment in which the device is located. For this reason, choosing suitable sensors is crucial. Currently, the accelerometer sensor is mostly used in HAR systems because it is built-in in most smartphones and wearable devices and also has shown superior results concerning representing activities if compared with other inertial sensors. The combination of accelerometer and gyroscope allows HAR systems to find patterns in the sensor signals and associate them with the activities performed, such as activity of daily living (ADL) and sports. However, finding such patterns is not trivial, since smartphones are often held near different parts of the user's body and each subject may have a personal signature of activity [11,13,28].

2.2. Pre-processing and Segmentation

After data acquisition, the raw data collected by motion sensors may contain noises and must be processed, adapted into a readable format and segmented to be used by future stages of the HAR applications. The segmentation phase comprises dividing the signals that are recorded continuously into smaller segments. Choosing smaller segments allows the detection of activities faster, since the wait to mount the segment is smaller and the resource requirements in the process are also reduced. Using larger segments allows more complex activities to be recognized, but an additional amount of time will be required to assemble and process the segment. The HAR community have used different sizes of segments in the literature with the use of segment sizes ranging from 1 s to 10 s, with a recognition rate above 90% [7,25,34,35].

2.3. Feature Extraction Process

The feature extraction phase aims to find a high-level representation from each activity segment. For sensor-based activity recognition, feature extraction is more difficult because there is inter-activity similarity. Different activities may have similar characteristics (e.g., walking and running). Therefore, it is difficult to produce distinguishable features to represent activities uniquely [32].

Many HAR systems are based on shallow approaches. Features are handcrafted by a domain specialist that transform data gathered from sensors into a high-level representation. The handcraft features can be divided into three domains: Time, frequency and symbolic [11,13,14,26,27,35].

The time-domain features are obtained by simple statistical calculations, such as average, median and standard deviation. These features are simple to calculate and understand and have low computational complexity when compared to other feature extraction processes, such as those based on deep neural networks [12,36]. The frequency-domain features are used to capture natural repetitions by decomposing the time series into a set of real and imaginary values representing wave components, through the use of Fourier or Wavelet transforms, for example. The symbolic domain features represent the sensor signals in a sequence of symbols obtained through a discretization process, allowing data to be compressed into a smaller space than the original data [11,27].

The low computational complexity and its simple calculation process make handcrafted features still practicable. The major disadvantage is that resources created or selected manually are time consuming, domain specific and require specialized knowledge.

2.4. Human Activity Classification

A machine learning algorithm can automatically detect patterns in a dataset and can be used to make decisions in situations of uncertainty. There are several supervised learning algorithms such as decision tree, naive Bayes, support vector machine (SVM), artificial neural networks (ANN), logistic regression and KNN (K-Nearest Neighbors) [37]. For these methods, it is essential that the sensors data be converted into a high-level representation, since machine learning models do not work very well if they are applied directly to the raw data [25].

More recently, deep learning models reach human-level performance in various domains, including HAR. This approach can automatically learn abstract features from sensors' data and thus eliminating the need for a dedicated feature extraction phase because the entire process is performed within the network hidden layers. Moreover, it outperforms in performance when applied to large masses of data if compared with traditional ML algorithms.

For HAR, the most common solutions found in the literature are based on Convolutional Neural Networks (CNN) and Long-Short-Term Memory Recurrent (LSTMs) [28,36,38,39]. Unfortunately, one of the main drawbacks of deep learning algorithms is related to their high computational cost which could make its implementation unsuitable for creating real-time HAR applications implemented on devices with low computational power [36,39].

A crucial stage of the classification process is to assess the performance of the trained machine learning algorithm. The next section presents the most common evaluation metrics used to estimate the future performance of a classifier.

2.5. Evaluation Metrics for HAR Systems

The performance of the classification model is evaluated by a set of metrics that shows how reliable is the model under evaluation, in mathematical terms [16,40]. The evaluation metrics commonly used in the smartphone-based HAR literature are accuracy, recall (sensitivity), specificity, precision and *F*-measure [15,41]. In HAR, accuracy is the most popular and can be calculated by dividing the number of correctly classified activities and the total number of activities. Accuracy gives a general idea of classification models' performance. However, this metric treats all classes as equally important in a dataset. This leads to an unreliable metric in unbalanced databases, strongly biased by dominant classes, usually the less relevant background class [15,42]. To avoid unreliable results in unbalanced datasets, there are other metrics that evaluate classes separately, such as precision and recall, as shown in Table 1.

The precision metric is the ratio of true positives and the total positives. If the precision value is equal to "1", it means that the classifier correctly predicts all true positives and is able to correctly classify between correct and incorrect labeling classes. The recall metric analyzes the true positive (*TP*) rate to all the positives. A low recall value means that the classifier has a high number of false negatives. Finally, *F*-measure deals with a score resulting from the combination of precision and recall values to provide a generic value that represents these two metrics. High *F*-measure values imply both high precision and high recall. It gives a balance between precision and recall, which is suitable to imbalanced classification problems, including HAR.

Table 1. Summarization of accuracy, recall, precision and F-measure. *TP* means true positives, *TN* true negatives, *FP* false positives and *FN* means false negatives.

Metric	Equation	Description
Accuracy	$\frac{TP+TN}{TP+TN+FP+FN}$	Accuracy is the ratio of correct predictions divided by the total predictions.
Precision	$\frac{TP}{TP+FP}$	*Precision* is the ratio of true positives and total positives predicted.
Recall	$\frac{TP}{TP+FN}$	*Recall* is the ratio of true positives to all the positives in ground truth.
F Measure	$2 \times \frac{Precision \times Recall}{Precision+Recall}$	The *F*-measure is the harmonic mean of *Precision* and *Recall*.

Different from most works that comprise all ARP stages, our focus in this article relies on the evaluation process and validation methodologies. By looking deep into the evaluation stage, we aim to understand how human activity recognition models achieve their results according to validation methodology.

3. Related Works

Many works in the literature alert researchers to the correct assessment of activity recognition models and, although this problem is widely known, it is often overlooked. Hammerla and Plötz [43] found inappropriate use of *k*-CV by almost half of the retrieved studies in a systematic literature review that used accelerometers, wearable sensors or smartphones to predict clinical outcomes, showing that record-wise (segmentation over the same user data) cross-validation often overestimates the prediction accuracy. Nevertheless, HAR system designers often either ignore these factors or even neglect their importance. Widhalm et al. [22] also has pointed unnoticed over-fitting because of autocorrelation (i.e., dependencies between temporally close samples). Hammerla and Plötz [43] showed that the adjacent overlapping frames probably record the same activity in the same context and, therefore, they share the same information. These adjacent segments are not statistically independent.

Dehghani et al. [29] extend the work of Banos et al. [44] by investigating the impact of Subject Cross-Validation (Subject CV) on HAR, both with overlapping and with non-overlapping sliding windows. The results show that *k*-CV increases the classifier performance by about 10%, and even by 16% when overlapping windows are used. Bulling et al. [15] provide an educational example, demonstrating how different design decisions in the HAR applications impact the overall recognition performance.

Gholamiangonabadi et al. [45] examine how well different machine learning architectures make generalizations based on a new subject(s) by using Leave-One-Subject-Out (LOSO) in six deep neural networks architectures. Results show that accuracy improves from 85.1% when evaluated with LOSO to 99.85% when evaluated with the traditional 10-fold cross-validation.

In contrast to the reviewed works related that deal with validation methodologies, our study examines bias problems that overestimate the predictive accuracy of a machine learning algorithm using graphical insights obtained from SHAP framework to understand how human activity recognition models achieve their results according to validation methodology. While there are works that make use of explainable methods in HAR context [9,33,46,47], most of the methods for explainability focus on interpreting and making the entire process of building an AI system transparent. The finds focused on validation methodology are important because it allows us to see which features are relevant to a HAR system in each validation method. We examine how different HAR systems approaches make generalizations based on a new subject(s) by using k-fold cross-validation, holdout and leave-one-subject-out cross-validation.

4. Evaluation Procedures

A common practice for computing a performance metric (e.g., accuracy), when performing a supervised machine learning experiment, is to hold aside part of the data to be used as a test set [16]. Splitting data into training and test sets can be done using various methods, such as hold-out, k-fold cross-validation (*k*-CV), leave-one-out cross-validation (LOOCV) and leave-one-subject-out (LOSO). Then, the classifier is trained on the training set, while its accuracy is measured on the test set. Thus, the test set is seen as new data never seen by the model before [16]. We briefly explained these methods in the following sections.

4.1. Hold-Out

The hold-out is the simplest form of splitting data and relies on a single split of the dataset into two mutually exclusive subsets called training set and a test set [16,42]. A common dataset split uses 70% or 80% for training and 30% or 20% for testing. The advantage of this method is the lower computational load. The hold-out is a pessimistic estimator because the classifier is trained only with part of the samples. If more data is left for the test, the bias of the classifier will be higher, but if only a few samples are used for the test, then the confidence interval for accuracy will be wider [42]. It has lower computational costs because it needs to run once but if the data are split again, the results of the model probably will change. This means that the accuracy depends on the subject(s) selected for the evaluation [45].

4.2. K-fold Cross-Validation (k-CV)

The *k*-CV consists of averaging several hold-out estimators corresponding to different data splits [16,37,40]. This procedure randomly divides the dataset (from one subject or all subjects) into *k* disjoint folds with approximately equal size, and each fold is in turn used to test the classification model induced from the remaining $k - 1$ folds. Then, the overall performance is computed as the average of the *k* accuracies resulting from *k*-CV [40,42]. The disadvantage of using this strategy is its computational cost when the values of k are relatively high for large samples. In addition, no single cross validation procedure is universally better but it should focus on the particular settings [16].

4.3. Leave-One-Subject-Out Cross-Validation (LOSO)

The LOSO (Leave-One-Subject-Out Cross-Validation) strategy aims at finding out whether a model trained on a group of subjects generalizes well to new, unseen subjects. It is a variant of the *k*-fold cross-validation approach but with folds consisting of a subject [45]. To measure this, we have to ensure that all of the samples in the test fold come from subjects that are not represented at all in the paired training fold.

The LOSO strategy uses a subset of size p for testing and $n - p$ for training, where p keeps all of the samples from a single subject together. This procedure ensures that the same subject is not represented in both testing and training sets at the same time. This configuration allows evaluating the generalization of the model based on data from new subjects; otherwise, if the model learns person-specific features, it may fail to generalize to new subjects.

When the number of subjects in a dataset is small, it is common to adopt LOSO to evaluate the performance of a classification algorithm. The LOSO is an extreme case of *k*-CV, where the number of folds is equal to the number of subjects on the dataset. It has a high variability as only one subject is used as the validation set to test the model prediction. This exhaustive procedure should be used when the random partition in *k*-CV has a large impact on performance evaluation [40,42].

4.4. Types for HAR Systems

The main goal of machine learning algorithms is to develop models that work not only on the specific dataset for which they were trained but also on new and unseen data. However, what does new data mean in human activity recognition problems? To answer this question, we need to know the purpose for which the algorithm is being developed. If we developed specifically for one subject, new data means new samples, or records, from the same subject. This falls into the category of personal systems. However, if the goal is to develop universal systems that can classify activities from a new subject, new data means new subjects.

Each type of HAR system addresses a slightly different learning problem and makes different assumptions about how the learning algorithm is applied [45,48]. There are three types of HAR systems [45,49,50], as shown in Figure 2: Universal or generalized, personal or personalized and hybrid.

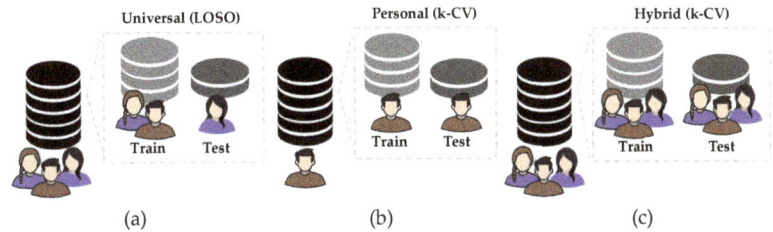

Figure 2. Visualization of each procedure used to build the model types for HAR systems. To build universal models, the LOSO procedure (**a**) separates train and test by subjects. For personalized models (**b**), the *k*-CV is used with samples of only one subject. Finally, for hybrid models (**c**), the *k*-CV is also used, but in this case, for a group of subjects, data are split by samples into the training and test set.

Universal systems must be capable of generalizing patterns of any subject. The most common validation procedure used in this context is the leave-one-subject-out cross-validation (LOSO) [45,51]. The LOSO considers the subject information when splitting the training and test set. This information is useful for preventing data from the same subject being present in both sets, as shown in Figure 2a.

Personalized systems aim at creating models that are experts in recognizing patterns from the same subject. This is called personalized validation [8,34,49,50,52]. In personalized systems, the selected machine learning algorithm is trained and tested with data from only one subject. Thus, the samples from this subject are divided between training and testing, as shown in Figure 2b.

Most studies in HAR use hybrid systems to validate the model performance with k-CV as validation methodology. It is hybrid because all sample data from over one subject are mixed and data from the same subject can be in the training and test sets, as shown in Figure 2c [25].

Each system has a specialization and this determines how training and test data are partitioned for evaluation. The next section presents a discussion about the correct evaluation that systems designers should consider in each model type.

5. A Fair Evaluation for Human Activity Recognition Systems

Most machine learning algorithms need Independent and Identically Distributed (i.i.d.) data [40]. If the recruitment process used is i.i.d., the subjects will be a representative sample of the overall population. Otherwise, if the i.i.d. is not assured, such as recording activities in which several samples are collected from each subject, the sampling process might generate groups of dependent samples. Therefore, k-CV is not a good procedure for validating universal models because of the temporal dependency among samples from the same subject. This means that the model trained using k-CV procedure knows the activity patterns of a specific subject, shared in both training and test sets. This situation may lead a model to learn a biased solution, where the machine learning algorithm can find a strong association between unique features of a subject (e.g., walking speed), artificially increasing its accuracy on the test set [20,45]. It explains why some systems report high accuracies.

To minimize the problem of weak generalization, the data should be adequate for a fair validation procedure according to the application purpose. This means that the application of the k-CV to new samples or new subjects does not measure the same thing and it should be determined by the application scenario, not by the statistics of the data. For instance, if the generative process has some kind of group structure, such as samples collected from different subjects, experiments or measurement devices, it is more appropriate to use cross-validation by subject or by a group. In this procedure, the preservation of independence means that full subjects' information must be left out for CV. For applications that aim at a personalized classification model, the traditional k-CV is an acceptable procedure.

6. Explainable Algorithms for Creating Fairer Systems

Explaining the decisions made by a machine learning model is extremely important in many applications. Explainable models can provide valuable information on how to improve them and also help to better understand the problem and the information provided by the input variables [53].

Identifying issues like biased data could allow systems design to select sensitive attributes that they want to focus their evaluations on. This is a key feature for explainability that has a clear purpose for evaluating fairness, as well as in non-fairness-related explanations where certain features should be weighed more or less heavily in class selection than others. Mitigating the bias and unfairness within the training data is a necessity, both out of ethical duty and because of the impact that perceived inaccuracies have on user trust [54–56].

More recently, XAI methods have been proposed to help interpret the predictions of machine learning models, as example, LIME [57], Deep Lift [58] and SHAP [59]. XAI methods have been used in HAR context to understand the rationale behind the predictions of the classifier [9,33,46,47]. In this work, we choose a unified framework for interpreting model predictions, called SHAP (Shapley additive explanations), to explain graphically and intuitively the results of different validation methodologies used in HAR systems.

The SHAP (Shapley additive explanations) [59] is based on a game-theoretic approach extensively used in literature to explain the predictions of any machine learning model. The Shapley values acted as a unified measure of feature importance. It aims to explain the prediction of an instance x by computing the contribution of each feature to the prediction. In summary, the Shapley values give each feature a score that is distributed across the features of that instance.

The Algorithm 1 shows the pseudo-code to approximate Shapley estimation for single feature value [60]. First, select an instance of interest x, a feature j and the number of iterations M. For each iteration, a random instance z is selected from the data and a random order of the features is generated. Two new instances are created by combining values from the instance of interest x and the sample z. The instance x_{+j} is the instance of interest, but all values in the order after feature j are replaced by feature values from the sample z. The instance x_{-j} is the same as x_{+j}, but in addition has feature j replaced by the value for feature j from the sample z. The difference in the prediction from the black box is computed by $\phi_j^m = \hat{f}(x_{+j}^m) - \hat{f}(x_{-j}^m)$ and all differences are averaged, resulting in $\phi_j(x) = \frac{1}{M} \sum_{m=1}^{M} \phi_j^m$. Averaging implicitly weighs samples by the probability distribution of X. The procedure has to be repeated for each of the features to get all Shapley values.

Algorithm 1 SHAP basic algorithm

1: **Required**: **M**: Number of interactions; **x**: Instance of interest; **j**: Features index; **X**: Data matrix; **f**: Machine learning model.
2: **procedure** $\text{SHAP}(M, x, j, X, f)$
3:     **for** m=1 in M **do**
4:         Draw random instance z from the data matrix X
5:         Choose a random permutation o of the feature values
6:         Order instance x: $x_0 = (x_{(1)}, ..., x_{(j)}, ..., x_{(p)})$
7:         Order instance z: $z_0 = (z_{(1)}, ..., z_{(j)}, ..., z_{(p)})$
8:         Construct two new instances
9:         Compute marginal contribution $\phi_j^m = \hat{f}(x_{+j}) - \hat{f}(x_{-j})$
10:    **end for**
11:    Compute Shapley value as the average $\phi_j(x) = \frac{1}{M} \sum_{m=1}^{M} \phi_j^m$
12: **end procedure**

The Shapley values can be combined into global explanations [59,60] by running SHAP algorithm for every instance to obtain a matrix of Shapley values, one row per data instance and one column per feature. We can interpret the entire model by analyzing the Shapley values in this matrix. The idea behind SHAP feature importance is simple: Features with large absolute Shapley values are important. Since we want the global importance, we average the absolute Shapley values per feature across the data.

In this sense, SHAP framework can understand the decision-making of a classification model globally by summarizing how a model generates its outputs. Global explanations are beneficial as they might reveal biases and help diagnose model problems [61]. They can also explain model predictions at the instance level once each observation gets its own set of SHAP values. This greatly increases its transparency.

We have used a specific method for local explanations of tree-based models, called TreeExplainer [59,62], which provides fast and accurate results by calculating the SHAP values for each leaf of a tree.

7. Experimental Protocol

This section describes the experimental protocol, considering four evaluation scenarios. We detail the datasets used in this study, the baselines that are built with time and frequency domain features and the performance metrics.

7.1. Datasets

The physical activity data used in this work were obtained from three publicly available datasets: SHOAIB (SH) [2], WISDM [25] and UCI [26]. Table 2 presets a summarization of the datasets used in our study [11].

Table 2. Summarization of SHOAIB (SH) [2], WISDM [25] and UCI [26] datasets. Items marked with (*) were not used in the experiment.

Dataset	SHOAIB SH	WISDM	UCI
Individuals	10	19 (36)	30
Hz	50	20	50
Segment length	2.5 sec	2.5 sec	2.5 sec
Sensors	Accelerometer, Gyroscope *, Magnetometer *	Accelerometer	Accelerometer, Gyroscope *
Location	Belt, Left Pocket, Right Pocket, Upper Arm, Wrist	Belt	Belt
Activities used	Walking, Running, Sitting, Standing, Walking Upstairs, Walking Downstairs, Jogging *, Biking *	Walking, Jogging, Sitting Standing, Walking Upstairs, Walking Downstairs	Walking, Lying Down, Sitting, Standing, Walking Upstairs, Walking Downstairs

In our experiments, we use only accelerometer data. For the WISDM dataset, we chose users who performed all activities, totaling 19 individuals. For the SHOAIB dataset, we selected the six most similar activities with WISDM and UCI datasets, so that all datasets had the same number of classes to compare results. We removed the Jogging and biking activities from our experiments because of this. The SHOAIB dataset contains data collected from five different body positions merged to run our experiments. Moreover, SHOAIB is balanced and should represent a fairer evaluation. This means a reduction in bias caused both by individuals with more activity or unbalanced class labels.

7.2. Baselines

The baselines are shallow approaches based on traditional machine learning algorithms such as Random Forest (RF), Naive Bayes (NB), K-Neighbors (KNN) with $k = 1$ and Simple Logistic (SL). We trained each algorithm with a set of handcraft features extracted from the time and frequency domain. Table 3 presents a list of mathematical functions used for creating the features used by the baselines [7,11,27]. The experiments were executed in the WEKA library (Waikato Environment for Knowledge Analysis) [63].

While we know the benefits of using complex models, especially in dealing with large masses of data, in our HAR context, we are adopting simple models, such as random forest, mainly because of speed, good performance and easy interpretation. Our focus is not on evaluating the best model for recognizing human activities but discovering bias problems that overestimate the predictive accuracy because of an inappropriate choice of validation methodology.

Table 3. List of all features used in the experiments with the baseline classifiers.

Domain	Features
Time	min, max, amplitude, amplitude peak, sum, absolute sum, Euclidian norm, mean, absolute mean, mean square, mean absolute deviation, sum square error, variance, standard deviation, Pearson coefficient, zero crossing rate, correlation, cross-correlation, auto-correlation, skewness, kurtosis, area, absolute area, signal magnitude mean, absolute signal magnitude mean, magnitude difference function.
Frequency	Energy, energy normalized, power, centroid, entropy, DC component, peak, coefficient sum.

7.3. Evaluation Scenarios

The experiments are based on the three model types commonly found in literature: Personalized, universal and hybrid.

1. Universal model: This scenario evaluates the model's generalization capacity using LOSO. We separated the data set in training and testing and there is a guarantee that these two sets are not mixed.
2. Personalized model: This scenario evaluates the model personalization capacity using k-CV. We partition the data from a single subject into two sets of samples. The validation process is based on 10-CV.
3. Hybrid model: This scenario evaluates a hybrid model that combines all subject data from the universal model using the validation process of the personal model.

In addition, we use SHAP explanation method to understand how machine learning models tend to select different features based on the validation methodology. For this experiment, we have used UCI dataset with a 561-feature vector with time and frequency domain variables [26] using holdout and cross-validation to analyze how model select different features to make its predictions. We select the Random forest algorithm to conduct this experiment. In Section 8.1 we also provide explanations of individual predictions using shap values based on subject number 9 of UCI dataset.

7.4. Performance Metrics

To measure the performance metrics of universal, hybrid and personal models, we use standard metrics such as accuracy, precision, recall and F-measure (or F-Score) [1,45] obtained from confusion matrix analysis. We used other metrics, besides accuracy, since it alone may not be the most reliable way to measure the actual performance of a classification algorithm, mainly because class imbalance can influence the results. Our research employs the metrics summarized in Table 1 (Section 2).

8. Results

This section presents a comparative analysis of different validation procedures based on the machine learning results and the interpretable methods. We divide results into four different setups. First, we deal with the validation of personalized models. Second, we deal with the valuation of universal models. The third scenario deals with the validation of a hybrid model. The performance results of five classifiers are presented using accuracy as the main metric for universal models (Figure 3), personalized models (Figure 4) and hybrid models (Figure 5). Finally, we present the insights based on Shapley values that give us an alternative manner to analyze and understand results.

The results presented in Figures 3–5 show that, for all classification algorithms, the personal models perform very well, the hybrid models perform similarly and the universal models have the worst performance. The main reason for this result is that different people may move differently and universal models cannot effectively distinguish between some activities which are highly related to the respective user and, consequently, it will have low performance on classification and a high confidence interval because of the variance in the population.

The hybrid models have performed much closer to personal models. Most HAR studies use cross-validation (k-CV) to evaluate and compare algorithms' performance. The mixture between the train and test sets results in a classification model that already knows part of its test set. In other words, the model trained using the k-CV can associate activity patterns of a specific subject on both train and test sets. The result of this process is the creation of models with higher classification accuracy. However, they do not reflect reality. If we insert new subjects into the domain, the model will have difficulties recognizing them.

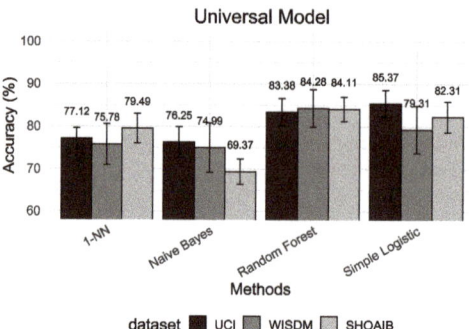

Figure 3. Accuracy results based on universal model for the classifiers 1-NN, Naive Bayes, Random Forest and Simple Logistic.

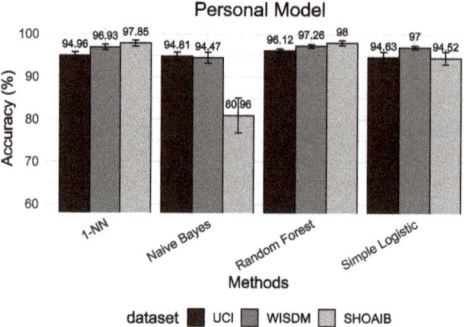

Figure 4. Accuracy results based on personalized model for the classifiers 1-NN, Naive Bayes, Random Forest and Simple Logistic.

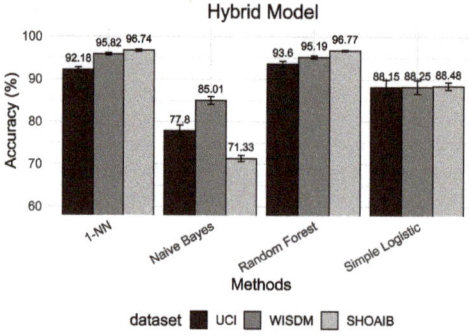

Figure 5. Accuracy results based on hybrid model for the classifiers 1-NN, Naive Bayes, Random Forest and Simple Logistic.

Tables 4 and 5 analyze the performance of the best model (random forest) on individual subjects for universal and personalized scenarios using SHOAIB dataset. In Table 4 the rows for subjects 1 to 10 represent the folds of the subject cross-validation. For subject 1 row, the model is trained using subjects 2–10 and evaluated on subject 1 and so on. In Table 5 the rows represent subjects 1 to 10. For subject 1 row, the model is trained using only data of subject 1, subject 2 using data of subject 2 and so on.

As can be observed in Table 4 the accuracy of the same model varies greatly among subjects as opposed to *k*-CV used in the personalized model (Table 5) in order to capture variability among subjects. Moreover, the standard deviation is higher for the universal model than for the personalized model. This shows that if a single generic model will be used for all users, the standard deviation should be considered when selecting the model.

The Figure 6 allows us to compare the universal model (LOSO) and personal model (*k*-CV) using the Random Forest algorithm. As it can be noticed from the confusion matrix, most of classes are correctly classified with very high accuracy. However, the universal model has difficulty in differentiating the walking class from upstairs and downstairs classes. This is expected as these three are very similar activities so the underlying data may not be sufficient to accurately different them. For stationary classes, such as standing and sitting, the misclassification is very low, demonstrating that distinction between those classes generalizes well for new subjects.

Table 4. Random Forest results for universal model in SHOAIB dataset.

Universal					
User	Accuracy	TP Rate	FP Rate	Precision	Recall	F-Measure
1	84.954	0.850	0.030	0.861	0.850	0.846
2	90.000	0.900	0.020	0.921	0.900	0.900
3	81.759	0.818	0.036	0.837	0.818	0.808
4	84.815	0.848	0.030	0.864	0.848	0.844
5	84.583	0.846	0.031	0.862	0.846	0.847
6	81.019	0.810	0.038	0.812	0.810	0.809
7	85.694	0.857	0.029	0.859	0.857	0.856
8	89.676	0.897	0.021	0.913	0.897	0.894
9	75.417	0.754	0.049	0.800	0.754	0.736
10	83.241	0.832	0.034	0.869	0.832	0.834
Mean	84.116	0.841	0.032	0.860	0.841	0.837
Std. Dev.	4.013	0.040	0.008	0.036	0.040	0.044

Table 5. Random Forest results for personalized model in SHOAIB dataset.

Personalized					
User	Accuracy	TP Rate	FP Rate	Precision	Recall	F-Measure
1	97.546	0.975	0.005	0.976	0.975	0.976
2	99.537	0.995	0.001	0.995	0.995	0.995
3	98.056	0.981	0.004	0.981	0.981	0.981
4	99.259	0.993	0.001	0.993	0.993	0.993
5	97.315	0.973	0.005	0.973	0.973	0.973
6	96.759	0.968	0.006	0.968	0.968	0.968
7	97.269	0.973	0.005	0.973	0.973	0.973
8	98.380	0.984	0.003	0.984	0.984	0.984
9	97.500	0.975	0.005	0.975	0.975	0.975
10	98.380	0.984	0.003	0.984	0.984	0.984
Mean	98.000	0.980	0.004	0.980	0.980	0.980
Std. Dev.	0.851	0.008	0.002	0.008	0.008	0.008

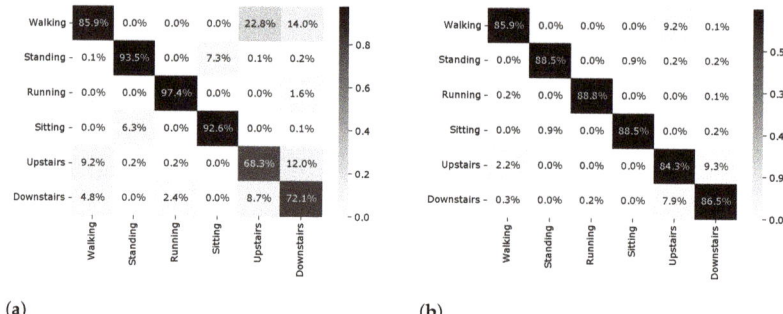

(a)   (b)

Figure 6. Confusion matrix of Random Forest algorithm results for universal model and personal model using the SHOAIB dataset. (**a**) Universal model. (**b**) Personalized model.

For methods whose goal is to generate a custom classification model, such as a personalized or hybrid model, k-CV will work very well. However, it may not be a good validation procedure for universal models. These results have shown the importance of a careful analysis of these different scenarios.

8.1. Global Explanations Using Shap Values

In this section, we showed through a summary plot [59,60] how validation methodologies affect feature importance and also discuss strategies to avoid potential issues in pre-processing data.

The summary plot combines feature importance with feature effects, considering the absolute average Shapley values along with all the classes. With a multi-classification problem, it shows the impact of each feature considering the different classes. The position on the y-axis is determined by the feature and on the x-axis by the Shapley value.

Figures 7 and 8 show that there are changes in the features that each model chose based on the validation methodology. This slightly different importance that the classification model gives for features when using different validations methodology causes a great boost in performance for cross-validation. Moreover, the CV has 17 features in common with holdout, a difference of 15%.

Given a feature, we also extract the importance proportion for each class. The results also show that the importance that each feature assigns to the classes is different according to the adopted methodology. By analyzing the contribution of each class for each feature, for example, Feature 53 (related with accelerometer gravity in x-axis) has a greater contribution to the class "walking upstairs" in the holdout methodology while it contributes more to the class "laying" when using the CV. Similar results can be observed in features 97, 57, 41 and many others.

When using cross-validation, the classifier already knows the individual attributes because its data can be shared in training and testing. Knowing the individual's pattern, the classifier can choose features that best suit the individual's behavior. Models trained using different training and test sets are more realistic because they reflect the approximate performance of what would happen in the real world, and thus it is possible to choose classifiers that select more generic features that better represent the population or group of individuals.

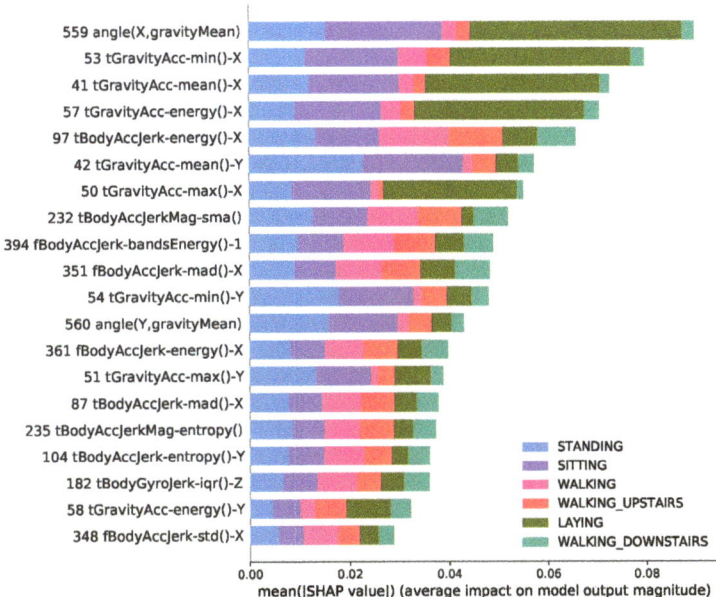

Figure 7. Summary plot for SHAP analysis using holdout methodology on UCI dataset. It shows the mean absolute SHAP value of 20 most important features for six activities.

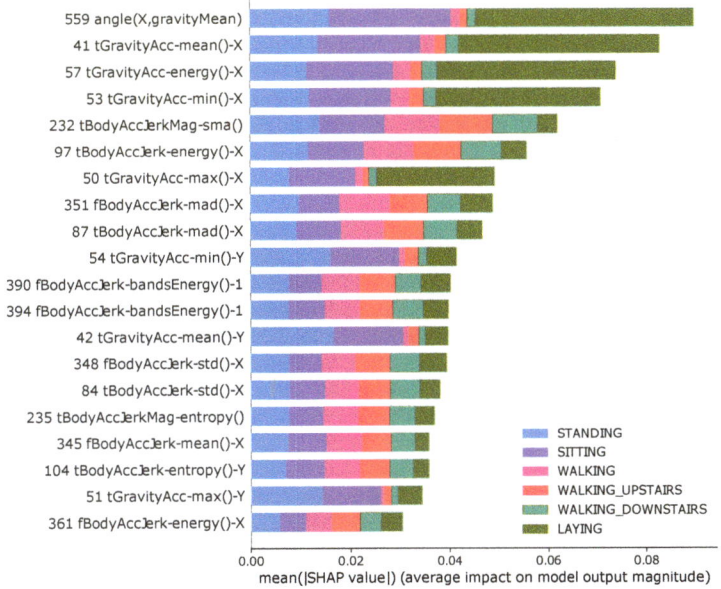

Figure 8. Summary plot for SHAP analysis using cross-validation on UCI dataset. It shows the mean absolute SHAP value of 20 most important features for six activities.

While the results presented are promising, in many situations, it is not trivial to find meanings in statistical features extracted from inertial sensors in HAR. However, our results show that the adopted methodology can significantly influence the selection of features to overestimate the results, not being appropriate for real-world applications.

8.2. Explaining Individual Predictions

In this section, we give a closer look at individual predictions to understand how validation influences at instance level. For this purpose, we present results based on shap force plot [60,64]. The force plot shows shap values contributions in generating the final prediction using an additive force layout. We can visualize feature attributions as "forces". The prediction starts from the baseline. The baseline for Shapley values is the average of all predictions. In the plot, each Shapley value is an arrow that pushes to increase with positive value (red) or decrease with negative value (blue) the prediction. These forces balance each other out at the actual prediction of the data instance.

We used data from subject 9 from the UCI database to conduct this experiment. For the walking activity, the model obtains high accuracy for cross-validation methodology. These results are expected and also confirm the results presented earlier in this section. For both methodologies, the top five features that contribute negatively to model prediction are the same. In addition, the model tends to give more importance to a set of different features according to the chosen methodology.

As shown in Figure 9b, half of the features (50%), if we look at the top 10 most important, are different for holdout and cross-validation. Feature number 70, based on the accelerometer, is ranked as one of the most important for the walking class. Features such as 393 and 508 are ranked as important when using holdout but do not appear in cross-validation. The cross-validation has features such as number 57, based on the accelerometer energy, which is top-rated by the model.

For non-stationary activities, such as walking and walking upstairs (Figure 10), the model shows a greater difference in prediction performance when compared to non-stationary activities. The model accuracy can achieve up to 10% higher when the cross-validation methodology is used. Moreover, the model can pick up to 50% different features to predict user activity when using each methodology.

Figure 10 show that the difference in the model accuracy can achieve up to 10%, showing that the classifier can overestimate the results when he knows patterns of an individual, choosing the features that best represent him. These results for the upstairs activity are similar to the walking activity. For the top 10 features, up to 50% can be different for holdout and cross-validation. Features like 71 are marked as relevant when using holdout for walking upstairs class, but they don't even appear in cross-validation.

Figures 11 and 12 showed that for stationary activities (e.g., stand activity) the model presents a similar performance in terms of accuracy in both methodologies, CV and holdout. However, there are differences between the selected features for decision making. For standing class, features such as 439 are marked as important when using cross-validation, but they do not appear in holdout (top 10).

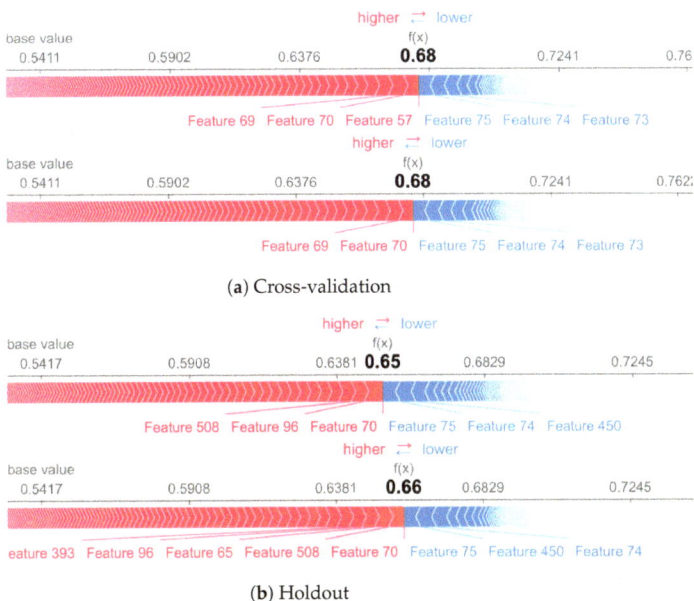

(**a**) Cross-validation

(**b**) Holdout

Figure 9. Walk activity for cross-validation (**a**) and holdout (**b**) validation methodology.

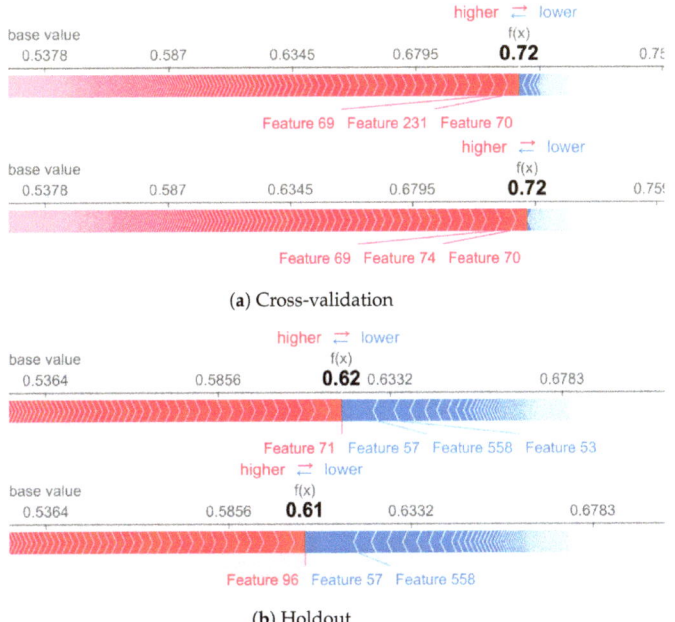

(**a**) Cross-validation

(**b**) Holdout

Figure 10. Walking upstairs activity for cross-validation (**a**) and holdout (**b**) validation methodology.

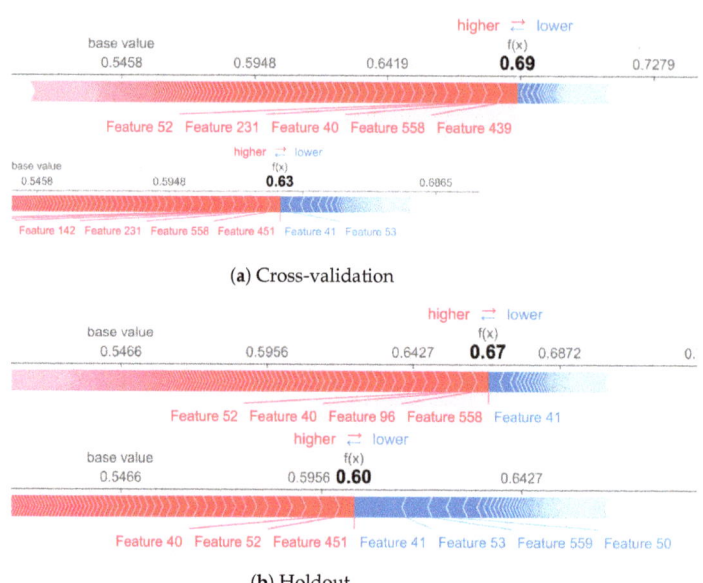

(a) Cross-validation

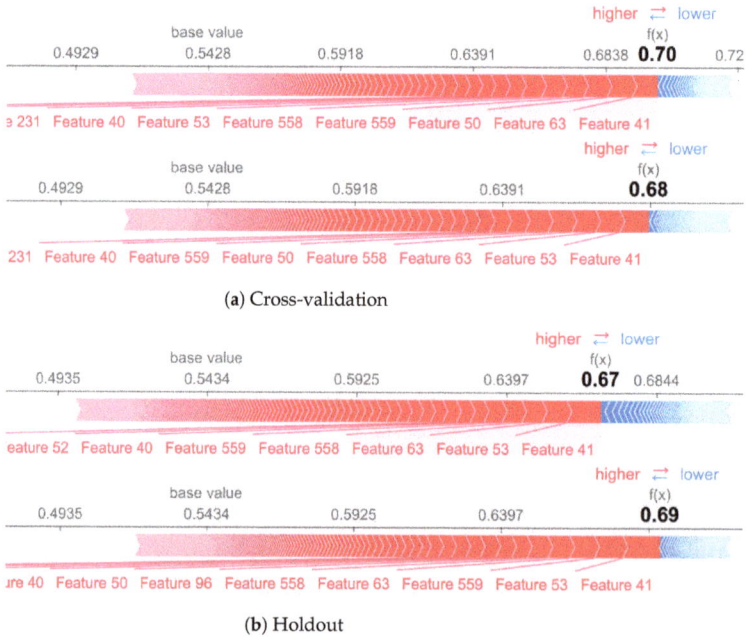

(b) Holdout

Figure 11. Standing activity for cross-validation (**a**) and holdout (**b**) validation methodology.

(a) Cross-validation

(b) Holdout

Figure 12. Sitting activity for cross-validation (**a**) and holdout (**b**) validation methodology.

We can observe in these studies that, when analyzing the predictions individually for a given class, the classifier can change the order of importance between the features, but we perceive these changes more drastically when holdout and cross-validation are compared.

9. Conclusions

In this paper, we present and discuss in detail the importance of a proper evaluation during the design and assessment of a HAR system with inertial sensors. We have conducted several experiments intending to exemplify the overall impact of the evaluation procedures on accuracy and fairness. We also illustrate how these procedures can be set up, showing how to reduce the accuracy overestimation. For this task, the tests were performed in three datasets (UCI-HAR, SHOAIB and WISDM) using k-fold cross-validation and leave-one-subject-out validation procedures. The main conclusions drawn from these results are summarized below.

The models that use k-CV in the data achieved 98% of accuracy. However, when considering individual information (i.e., the label associated to the subject), the accuracy achieves 85.37% in the best scenario. There is a 12% loss of accuracy when choosing a better evaluation method, that is, the initial result was overestimated by 12%.

The universal model performs poorly in the test phase and also has greater margins of error when compared with personalized models. This shows that the model will struggle to recognize new subjects. In general, the model may perform well in the training phase, but it has a degraded performance in the test set that leads to overfitting. To build a universal model, traditional k-CV is not the best solution. For this scenario, the recommended validation procedure would be LOSO or even Holdout when in scenarios were implement LOSO has a significant impact on training.

In personalized models, there is no problem if k-CV is used as a validation procedure since, for this type of application, the algorithm should aim at a model that fits the user. In this scenario, the classification algorithms have higher accuracy since the classification model was trained with instances that are very similar to those found in the test set. The very high accuracy values inductee that this is a suitable model for evaluating a customized application for a specific user. Besides, personal models can be trained with dramatically less data.

The hybrid model is used in many related works but they are not very suitable for real-world situations. Most of the commercial HAR applications have preferences for universal or personalized models. The results obtained from this model also present higher accuracy in the classification because some segments that belong to the same subject may be present in both the test set and training set, leading to an overoptimistic result. Again, this does not reflect the true accuracy.

We have shown how the SHAP framework presents itself as a tool that can provide graphical insights into how human activity recognition models manage to achieve their results. Our work has presented manners that can be explored by using explainable algorithms to improve the transparency of creating machine learning models. The SHAP results reinforce that the incorrect choice of validation methodology leads to changes in how attributes are used by models to improve their performance. This situation may cause poor prediction performance and can lead to unreliable results.

Our evaluations also reveal that while current XAI tools provide important functions for data and model analysis, they are still lacking when it comes to analyzing results in scenarios where it is not trivial to find meanings in statistical features extracted from sensors data.

Author Contributions: All authors (H.B., J.G.C., H.A.B.F.O. and E.S.) designed the study. H.B. and J.G.C. implemented and interpreted the experiments and wrote the manuscript. H.B., J.G.C., H.A.B.F.O. and E.S. reviewed and edited the article. J.G.C., H.A.B.F.O. and E.S. supervised the overall work and reviewed the experimental results. All the authors (H.B., J.G.C., H.A.B.F.O. and E.S.) contributed in discussing, reviewing, revising the article and approved the final manuscript. All authors have read and agreed to the published version of the manuscript.

Funding: This research, according to Article 48 of Decree n° 6.008/2006, was partially funded by Samsung Electronics of Amazonia Ltda, under the terms of Federal Law n° 8.387/1991, through agreement n° 003/2019, signed with ICOMP/UFAM and by the Coordenação de Aperfeiçoamento de Pessoal de Nível Superior—Brasil (CAPES)—Finance Code 001. The funding bodies played no role in the design of the study and collection, analysis and interpretation of data and in writing the manuscript.

Data Availability Statement: The WISDM can be found on http://www.cis.fordham.edu/wisdm/includes/datasets/latest/WISDM_ar_latest.tar.gz (accessed on 23 May 2019). The SHOAIB dataset can be found in the author's researchgate profile or https://www.researchgate.net/profile/Muhammad_Shoaib20/publication/266384007_Sensors_Activity_Recognition_DataSet/data/542e9d260cf277d58e8ec40c/Sensors-Activity-Recognition-DataSet-Shoaib.rar (accessed on 12 February 2020). The UCI-HAR dataset is avaliable on https://archive.ics.uci.edu/ml/machine-learning-databases/00240/UCI%20HAR%20Dataset.zip (accessed on 22 May 2019).

Conflicts of Interest: The authors declare that they have no competing interests. The funders had no role in the design of the study; in the collection, analyses or interpretation of data; in the writing of the manuscript or in the decision to publish the results.

Abbreviations

The following abbreviations are used in this manuscript:

ADL	Activity Daily Living
ARP	Activity Recognition Process
CNN	Convolutional Neural Networks
DL	Deep Learning
HAR	Human Activity Recognition
i.i.d.	Independent and Identically Distributed
k-CV	k-fold Cross-Validation
LOOCV	Leave-One-Out cross-Validation
LOOSO	Leave-One-Subject-Out
LSTM	Long-Short-Term Memory Recurrent
ML	Machine Learning
SHAP	Shapley additive explanations
XAI	Explainable Artificial Intelligence

References

1. Lara, O.D.; Labrador, M.A. A survey on human activity recognition using wearable sensors. *IEEE Commun. Surv. Tutor.* **2012**, *15*, 1192–1209. [CrossRef]
2. Shoaib, M.; Scholten, H.; Havinga, P.J. Towards physical activity recognition using smartphone sensors. In Proceedings of the 2013 IEEE 10th International Conference on Ubiquitous Intelligence and Computing and 2013 IEEE 10th International Conference on Autonomic and Trusted Computing, Vietri sul Mere, Italy, 8–21 December 2013; pp. 80–87.
3. Lathia, N.; Sandstrom, G.M.; Mascolo, C.; Rentfrow, P.J. Happier people live more active lives: Using smartphones to link happiness and physical activity. *PLoS ONE* **2017**, *12*, e0160589. [CrossRef] [PubMed]
4. Singh, D.; Merdivan, E.; Psychoula, I.; Kropf, J.; Hanke, S.; Geist, M.; Holzinger, A. Human activity recognition using recurrent neural networks. In Proceedings of the International Cross-Domain Conference for Machine Learning and Knowledge Extraction, Reggio, Italy, 15 May 2017; pp. 267–274.
5. Yang, S.; Gao, B.; Jiang, L.; Jin, J.; Gao, Z.; Ma, X.; Woo, W.L. IoT structured long-term wearable social sensing for mental wellbeing. *IEEE Internet Things J.* **2018**, *6*, 3652–3662. [CrossRef]
6. Nweke, H.F.; Teh, Y.W.; Al-Garadi, M.A.; Alo, U.R. Deep learning algorithms for human activity recognition using mobile and wearable sensor networks: State of the art and research challenges. *Expert Syst. Appl.* **2018**, *105*, 233–261. [CrossRef]
7. Ferrari, A.; Micucci, D.; Mobilio, M.; Napoletano, P. Trends in human activity recognition using smartphones. *J. Reliab. Intell. Environ.* **2021**, *7*, 189–213. [CrossRef]
8. Ferrari, A.; Micucci, D.; Mobilio, M.; Napoletano, P. Deep learning and model personalization in sensor-based human activity recognition. *J. Reliab. Intell. Environ.* **2022**, 1–13. [CrossRef]
9. Uddin, M.Z.; Soylu, A. Human activity recognition using wearable sensors, discriminant analysis, and long short-term memory-based neural structured learning. *Sci. Rep.* **2021**, *11*, 1–15. [CrossRef]
10. Harari, G.M.; Lane, N.D.; Wang, R.; Crosier, B.S.; Campbell, A.T.; Gosling, S.D. Using smartphones to collect behavioral data in psychological science: Opportunities, practical considerations, and challenges. *Perspect. Psychol. Sci.* **2016**, *11*, 838–854. [CrossRef]

11. Bragança, H.; Colonna, J.G.; Lima, W.S.; Souto, E. A Smartphone Lightweight Method for Human Activity Recognition Based on Information Theory. *Sensors* **2020**, *20*, 1856. [CrossRef]
12. Figo, D.; Diniz, P.C.; Ferreira, D.R.; Cardoso, J.M. Preprocessing techniques for context recognition from accelerometer data. *Pers. Ubiquitous Comput.* **2010**, *14*, 645–662. [CrossRef]
13. Shoaib, M.; Bosch, S.; Incel, O.D.; Scholten, H.; Havinga, P.J. A survey of online activity recognition using mobile phones. *Sensors* **2015**, *15*, 2059–2085. [CrossRef] [PubMed]
14. Li, F.; Shirahama, K.; Nisar, M.A.; Köping, L.; Grzegorzek, M. Comparison of feature learning methods for human activity recognition using wearable sensors. *Sensors* **2018**, *18*, 679. [CrossRef]
15. Bulling, A.; Blanke, U.; Schiele, B. A tutorial on human activity recognition using body-worn inertial sensors. *Acm Comput. Surv. (CSUR)* **2014**, *46*, 1–33. [CrossRef]
16. Arlot, S.; Celisse, A. A survey of cross-validation procedures for model selection. *Stat. Surv.* **2010**, *4*, 40–79. [CrossRef]
17. Varma, S.; Simon, R. Bias in error estimation when using cross-validation for model selection. *BMC Bioinform.* **2006**, *7*, 91. [CrossRef] [PubMed]
18. Kaufman, S.; Rosset, S.; Perlich, C.; Stitelman, O. Leakage in data mining: Formulation, detection, and avoidance. *Acm Trans. Knowl. Discov. Data (Tkdd)* **2012**, *6*, 1–21. [CrossRef]
19. Colonna, J.G.; Gama, J.; Nakamura, E.F. How to correctly evaluate an automatic bioacustics classification method. In Proceedings of the 17th Conference of the Spanish Association for Artificial Intelligence, Salamanca, Spain, 14–16 September 2016; pp. 37–47.
20. Saeb, S.; Lonini, L.; Jayaraman, A.; Mohr, D.C.; Kording, K.P. The need to approximate the use-case in clinical machine learning. *GigaScience* **2017**, *6*, 1–9. [CrossRef]
21. Little, M.A.; Varoquaux, G.; Saeb, S.; Lonini, L.; Jayaraman, A.; Mohr, D.C.; Kording, K.P. Using and understanding cross-validation strategies. Perspectives on Saeb et al. *GigaScience* **2017**, *6*, gix019. [CrossRef]
22. Widhalm, P.; Leodolter, M.; Brändle, N. Top in the lab, flop in the field? Evaluation of a sensor-based travel activity classifier with the SHL dataset. In Proceedings of the 2018 ACM International Joint Conference and 2018 International Symposium on Pervasive and Ubiquitous Computing and Wearable Computers, Singapore, 8–12 October 2018; pp. 1479–1487.
23. Bissoto, A.; Fornaciali, M.; Valle, E.; Avila, S. (De) Constructing Bias on Skin Lesion Datasets. In Proceedings of the IEEE Conference on Computer Vision and Pattern Recognition Workshops, Long Beach, CA, USA, 16–20 June 2019; pp. 1–9.
24. Veale, M.; Binns, R. Fairer machine learning in the real world: Mitigating discrimination without collecting sensitive data. *Big Data Soc.* **2017**, *4*, 2053951717743530. [CrossRef]
25. Kwapisz, J.R.; Weiss, G.M.; Moore, S.A. Activity recognition using cell phone accelerometers. *ACM Sigkdd Explor. Newsl.* **2011**, *12*, 74. [CrossRef]
26. Anguita, D.; Ghio, A.; Oneto, L.; Parra, X.; Reyes-Ortiz, J.L. A Public Domain Dataset for Human Activity Recognition Using Smartphones. In Proceedings of the European Symposium on Artificial Neural Networks, Computational Intelligence and Machine Learning, Bruges, Belgium, 24–26 April 2013; pp. 24–26.
27. Lima, W.S.; Bragança, H.L.S.; Quispe, K.G.M.; Souto, J.P. Human Activity Recognition based on Symbolic Representation Algorithms for Inertial Sensors. *Sensors* **2018**, *18*, 4045. [CrossRef] [PubMed]
28. Wang, J.; Chen, Y.; Hao, S.; Peng, X.; Hu, L. Deep learning for sensor-based activity recognition: A survey. *Pattern Recognit. Lett.* **2019**, *119*, 3–11. [CrossRef]
29. Dehghani, A.; Glatard, T.; Shihab, E. Subject cross validation in human activity recognition. *arXiv* **2019**, arXiv:1904.02666.
30. Dang, L.M.; Min, K.; Wang, H.; Piran, M.J.; Lee, C.H.; Moon, H. Sensor-based and vision-based human activity recognition: A comprehensive survey. *Pattern Recognit.* **2020**, *108*, 107561. [CrossRef]
31. Liu, H.; Hartmann, Y.; Schultz, T. A practical wearable sensor-based human activity recognition research pipeline. In Proceedings of the 5th International Conference on Health Informatics (HEALTHINF 2022), Vienna, Austria, 9–11 February 2022.
32. Chen, K.; Zhang, D.; Yao, L.; Guo, B.; Yu, Z.; Liu, Y. Deep learning for sensor-based human activity recognition: Overview, challenges, and opportunities. *ACM Comput. Surv. (CSUR)* **2021**, *54*, 1–40. [CrossRef]
33. Das, D.; Nishimura, Y.; Vivek, R.P.; Takeda, N.; Fish, S.T.; Ploetz, T.; Chernova, S. Explainable Activity Recognition for Smart Home Systems. *arXiv* **2021**, arXiv:2105.09787.
34. Bao, L.; Intille, S.S. Activity recognition from user-annotated acceleration data. In Proceedings of the International Conference on Pervasive Computing, Orlando, FL, USA, 14–17 March 2004; pp. 1–17.
35. Shoaib, M.; Bosch, S.; Incel, O.D.; Scholten, H.; Havinga, P.J. Fusion of smartphone motion sensors for physical activity recognition. *Sensors* **2014**, *14*, 10146–10176. [CrossRef] [PubMed]
36. Ravi, D.; Wong, C.; Lo, B.; Yang, G.Z. Deep learning for human activity recognition: A resource efficient implementation on low-power devices. In Proceedings of the 2016 IEEE 13th International Conference on Wearable and Implantable Body Sensor Networks (BSN), San Francisco, CA, USA, 14–17 June 2016; pp. 71–76.
37. Duda, R.O.; Hart, P.E.; Stork, D.G. *Pattern Classification*; John Wiley & Sons: Hoboken, NJ, USA, 2000; Volume 2, p. 688.
38. Ronao, C.A.; Cho, S.B. Human activity recognition with smartphone sensors using deep learning neural networks. *Expert Syst. Appl.* **2016**, *59*, 235–244. [CrossRef]
39. Ignatov, A. Real-time human activity recognition from accelerometer data using Convolutional Neural Networks. *Appl. Soft Comput.* **2018**, *62*, 915–922. [CrossRef]

40. Wong, T.T. Performance evaluation of classification algorithms by k-fold and leave-one-out cross validation. *Pattern Recognit.* **2015**, *48*, 2839–2846. [CrossRef]
41. Sousa Lima, W.; Souto, E.; El-Khatib, K.; Jalali, R.; Gama, J. Human activity recognition using inertial sensors in a smartphone: An overview. *Sensors* **2019**, *19*, 3213. [CrossRef] [PubMed]
42. Kohavi, R. A study of cross-validation and bootstrap for accuracy estimation and model selection. *Ijcai. Montr. Can.* **1995**, *14*, 1137–1145.
43. Hammerla, N.Y.; Plötz, T. Let's (not) stick together: pairwise similarity biases cross-validation in activity recognition. In Proceedings of the 2015 ACM International Joint Conference on Pervasive and Ubiquitous Computing, Osaka, Japan, 7–11 September 2015; pp. 1041–1051.
44. Banos, O.; Galvez, J.M.; Damas, M.; Pomares, H.; Rojas, I. Window size impact in human activity recognition. *Sensors* **2014**, *14*, 6474–6499. [CrossRef]
45. Gholamiangonabadi, D.; Kiselov, N.; Grolinger, K. Deep neural networks for human activity recognition with wearable sensors: Leave-one-subject-out cross-validation for model selection. *IEEE Access* **2020**, *8*, 133982–133994. [CrossRef]
46. Bettini, C.; Civitarese, G.; Fiori, M. Explainable Activity Recognition over Interpretable Models. In Proceedings of the 2021 IEEE International Conference on Pervasive Computing and Communications Workshops and other Affiliated Events (PerCom Workshops), Kassel, Germany, 22–26 March 2021; pp. 32–37.
47. Roy, C.; Nourani, M.; Honeycutt, D.R.; Block, J.E.; Rahman, T.; Ragan, E.D.; Ruozzi, N.; Gogate, V. Explainable activity recognition in videos: Lessons learned. *Appl. AI Lett.* **2021**, *2*, e59. [CrossRef]
48. Morales, J.; Akopian, D. Physical activity recognition by smartphones, a survey. *Biocybern. Biomed. Eng.* **2017**, *37*, 388–400. [CrossRef]
49. Lockhart, J.W.; Weiss, G.M. Limitations with activity recognition methodology & data sets. In Proceedings of the 2014 ACM International Joint Conference on Pervasive and Ubiquitous Computing, Seattle, WA, USA, 13–17 September 2014; pp. 747–756.
50. Ferrari, A.; Micucci, D.; Mobilio, M.; Napoletano, P. On the personalization of classification models for human activity recognition. *IEEE Access* **2020**, *8*, 32066–32079. [CrossRef]
51. Siirtola, P.; Koskimäki, H.; Huikari, V.; Laurinen, P.; Röning, J. Improving the classification accuracy of streaming data using SAX similarity features. *Pattern Recognit. Lett.* **2011**, *32*, 1659–1668. [CrossRef]
52. Weiss, G.M.; Lockhart, J. The impact of personalization on smartphone-based activity recognition. In Proceedings of the Workshops at the Twenty-Sixth AAAI Conference on Artificial Intelligence, Toronto, ON, Canada, 22–26 July 2012.
53. Linardatos, P.; Papastefanopoulos, V.; Kotsiantis, S. Explainable ai: A review of machine learning interpretability methods. *Entropy* **2021**, *23*, 18. [CrossRef] [PubMed]
54. Yin, M.; Wortman Vaughan, J.; Wallach, H. Understanding the effect of accuracy on trust in machine learning models. In Proceedings of the 2019 chi Conference on Human Factors in Computing Systems, Glasgow, UK, 4–9 May 2019; pp. 1–12.
55. Toreini, E.; Aitken, M.; Coopamootoo, K.; Elliott, K.; Zelaya, C.G.; Van Moorsel, A. The relationship between trust in AI and trustworthy machine learning technologies. In Proceedings of the 2020 Conference on Fairness, Accountability, and Transparency, Barcelona, Spain, 27–30 January 2020; pp. 272–283.
56. Alikhademi, K.; Richardson, B.; Drobina, E.; Gilbert, J.E. Can Explainable AI Explain Unfairness? A Framework for Evaluating Explainable AI. *arXiv* **2021**, arXiv:2106.07483.
57. Ribeiro, M.T.; Singh, S.; Guestrin, C. Model-agnostic interpretability of machine learning. *arXiv* **2016**, arXiv:1606.05386.
58. Shrikumar, A.; Greenside, P.; Kundaje, A. Learning important features through propagating activation differences. In Proceedings of the International Conference on Machine Learning, PMLR, Sydney, Australia, 6–11 August 2017; pp. 3145–3153.
59. Lundberg, S.M.; Lee, S.I. A unified approach to interpreting model predictions. In Proceedings of the 31st International Conference on Neural Information Processing Systems, Long Beach, CA, USA, 4–9 December 2017; pp. 4768–4777.
60. Molnar, C. *Interpretable Machine Learning*; Lulu: Morrisville, NC, USA, 2020.
61. Ibrahim, M.; Louie, M.; Modarres, C.; Paisley, J. Global explanations of neural networks: Mapping the landscape of predictions. In Proceedings of the 2019 AAAI/ACM Conference on AI, Ethics, and Society, Honolulu, HI, USA, 27–28 January 2019; pp. 279–287.
62. Lundberg, S.M.; Erion, G.; Chen, H.; DeGrave, A.; Prutkin, J.M.; Nair, B.; Katz, R.; Himmelfarb, J.; Bansal, N.; Lee, S.I. From local explanations to global understanding with explainable AI for trees. *Nat. Mach. Intell.* **2020**, *2*, 2522–5839. [CrossRef] [PubMed]
63. Witten, I.H.; Frank, E. Data mining: practical machine learning tools and techniques with Java implementations. *Acm Sigmod Rec.* **2002**, *31*, 76–77. [CrossRef]
64. Lundberg, S.M.; Nair, B.; Vavilala, M.S.; Horibe, M.; Eisses, M.J.; Adams, T.; Liston, D.E.; Low, D.K.W.; Newman, S.F.; Kim, J.; et al. Explainable machine-learning predictions for the prevention of hypoxaemia during surgery. *Nat. Biomed. Eng.* **2018**, *2*, 749. [CrossRef] [PubMed]

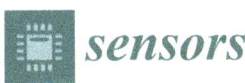

sensors

MDPI

Article

Gated Recurrent Unit Network for Psychological Stress Classification Using Electrocardiograms from Wearable Devices

Jun Zhong [1,2], Yongfeng Liu [1,2], Xiankai Cheng [1,2], Liming Cai [2], Weidong Cui [2] and Dong Hai [2,*]

1 School of Biomedical Engineering (Suzhou), University of Science and Technology of China, Hefei 230026, China
2 Suzhou Institute of Biomedical Engineering and Technology, Chinese Academy of Sciences, Suzhou 215163, China
* Correspondence: haid@sibet.ac.cn; Tel.: +86-0512-6958-8055

Abstract: In recent years, research on human psychological stress using wearable devices has gradually attracted attention. However, the physical and psychological differences among individuals and the high cost of data collection are the main challenges for further research on this problem. In this work, our aim is to build a model to detect subjects' psychological stress in different states through electrocardiogram (ECG) signals. Therefore, we design a VR high-altitude experiment to induce psychological stress for the subject to obtain the ECG signal dataset. In the experiment, participants wear smart ECG T-shirts with embedded sensors to complete different tasks so as to record their ECG signals synchronously. Considering the temporal continuity of individual psychological stress, a deep, gated recurrent unit (GRU) neural network is developed to capture the mapping relationship between subjects' ECG signals and stress in different states through heart rate variability features at different moments, so as to build a neural network model from the ECG signal to psychological stress detection. The experimental results show that compared with all comparison methods, our method has the best classification performance on the four stress states of resting, VR scene adaptation, VR task and recovery, and it can be a remote stress monitoring solution for some special industries.

Keywords: psychological stress; electrocardiogram; heart rate variability; gated recurrent unit; VR high-altitude experiment; wearable devices

Citation: Zhong , J.; Liu, Y.; Cheng, X.; Cai, L.; Cui, W.; Hai, D. Gated Recurrent Unit Network for Psychological Stress Classification Using Electrocardiograms from Wearable Devices. *Sensors* **2022**, *22*, 8664. https://doi.org/10.3390/s22228664

Academic Editors: Hugo Gamboa, Tanja Schultz and Hui Liu

Received: 28 September 2022
Accepted: 3 November 2022
Published: 10 November 2022

Publisher's Note: MDPI stays neutral with regard to jurisdictional claims in published maps and institutional affiliations.

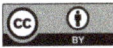
1. Introduction

When one's ability cannot match the requirements of the external environment, psychological stress will appear, such as too difficult a work task or too heavy a financial burden [1]. In fact, we all live under stress, and moderate stress can keep us competitive. However, chronically living under high stress will increase the risk of physical and psychological disease [2], including severe cardiac arrhythmias, high blood pressure, stroke, gastric ulcers, cancer and depression [3,4]. If people could get their stress situation in a low-cost and convenient way and manage it appropriately, it would not only reduce people's risk of disease but also improve people's efficiency, creativity and security at work, especially for special industry practitioners, such as military personnel, pilots, firefighters and high-speed rail drivers. Therefore, it is of great value and of social significance to develop a non-invasive stress estimation system to monitor people's stress changes in their daily work.

At present, the main basis for psychological stress assessment includes social media information and physiological signals. For the former, it is easy to understand that people's psychological stress can be roughly estimated by multimodal fusion and analysis of information such as texts, images, and videos posted on social media, and many methods have been proposed in this research direction [5,6]. Further, it is easier for people to obtain social media data than physiological signals. However, the accuracy of its stress assessment depends on how active users are on social media, and it seems difficult to make accurate stress assessments for users who are less active on social media. In addition, because of psychological defense mechanisms, people are likely to deliberately disguise their real stress situations in their behavioral performance. Compared with social media data, physiological signals can provide more objective and reliable information for psychological stress assessment [7]. Physiological signals used for stress assessment mainly include electroencephalogram (EEG), electrodermal activity (EDA), photoplethysmographic (PPG) and electrocardiogram (ECG). Although EEG can provide useful information for psychological stress analysis with high temporal resolution [8], the wearing process of its collection equipment is cumbersome and requires the help of professionals. Moreover, the EEG signal is easily disturbed by movements during the collection process. Therefore, EEG is not suitable for daily monitoring of human psychological stress. Compared with EEG, the acquisition equipment for PPG and EDA is portable, and the acquisition process is simple. However, after being interfered with by body movements, the signal is prone to a large degree of distortion, which will increase the difficulty of subsequent feature extraction and analysis. ECG offers advantages over PPG in terms of stability and reliability and is by far the most widely used cardiac monitoring method in healthcare. In recent years, with the development of wearable devices, many wearable ECG devices with both comfort and anti-interference have been developed, including vests, bracelets and chest belts [9–11]. The development of these non-invasive ECG devices is the basis for research on the daily monitoring of people's psychological stress. Wearable physiological parameter monitoring equipment has also been widely used in the field of human action recognition, which has some implications for our research [12–15].

Compared with psychological stress detection methods based on scales or social media data, the use of wearable devices to collect ECG signals and detect psychological stress obviously has more advantages in real-time and flexibility of usage scenarios. In practical applications, we can use this solution to monitor the psychological stress state of police, firefighters, pilots and other special industry workers during the execution of tasks in real-time and even give real-time psychological intervention at the right time to relieve their anxiety. This not only can improve their work efficiency but also probably play an important role in keeping them safe. In addition, this solution can also be used in the recruitment and selection of workers in special industries.

When changes in the external environment make people feel tense or anxious, it will also cause a physiological response in the body. At this time, the parasympathetic branch of the human autonomic nervous system (ANS) is temporarily suppressed, and the sympathetic branch is activated, which causes a rapid increase in heart rate, cardiac contractility, blood pressure and respiration, and promotes hormone release [16]. It puts the body in a state of hyperactivity to cope with the upcoming challenge. The changes in the ANS associated with psychological stress can be obtained by recording the ECG signal of the subject. Specifically, these ANS changes can be obtained by HRV (Heart Rate Variability) analysis [17].

In this field, previous studies have mostly used classical machine learning methods to detect psychological stress through HRV features, namely, binary classification of stressed and unstressed [18–24]. First of all, such a binary classification is not completely consistent with people's stress experience in real life, and it is more and more necessary to study the evaluation methods of human stress in different states. Secondly, deep learning methods have achieved good results in many fields, such as image recognition, natural language processing and signal processing, so the powerful representation ability of deep learning methods can achieve good results in the multi-classification of psychological stress is a problem worth studying. Furthermore, the generation of psychological stress is not instantaneous, and whether its temporal features can be used to improve the accuracy of psychological stress classification is also an interesting problem.

To this end, in this paper, we introduce an ECG dataset collected under four stress states and propose to introduce the concept of time series into psychological stress assessment in order to improve the classification accuracy. Specifically, by constructing a continuous HRV time series, we use a multi-layer GRU network to extract multi-level features related to psychological stress and finally obtain the results through a classification network composed of multi-layer perceptrons. The contributions of this paper are mainly in two aspects. The first is that we propose the concept of time series in the classification of psychological stress states and introduce a recurrent neural network into the classification of psychological stress to obtain the representation of psychological stress in continuous HRV sequences to improve the classification accuracy. The second is that we conducted a psychological stress data collection experiment with 80 participants, designed and developed a stress-induced VR high-altitude scene and collected ECG signals from the subjects during four stress states, including resting, VR scene adaptation, VR high-altitude task and recovery. The purpose is to construct a dataset that can be used to study the mapping relationship between ECG signals and psychological stress in various states. After data cleaning and elimination, this dataset finally contains the ECG data and corresponding status labels of 63 subjects.

2. Related Works

Compared with the subjective scales used in the past, psychological stress assessment based on physiological signals has advantages in objectivity and reliability. In the field of psychological stress or emotion estimation based on physiological signals, many methods have been proposed, and some scholars have put forward their insights and analysis on the relationship between physiological signals and psychological stress.

Classical machine learning methods are widely used to classify psychological stress or emotions. Ref. [18] uses Principal Component Analysis (PCA) to verify the HRV time domain, frequency domain and statistical features and then classify two emotions and five emotions by Support Vector Machines. Ref. [21] selects robust HRV features through the mRMR method, reduces the differences in physiological parameters between individuals through baseline data to improve the classification accuracy, and finally, classifies psychological stress in relaxation and task states through a variety of machine learning methods. In the study of driver stress detection, ref. [25] proposes the use of an enhanced random forest classifier to monitor driver stress by combining ECG waveform features and HRV features. Ref. [23] tries to use various machine learning algorithms, including KNN and multi-layer perceptron (MLP), to classify the psychology stress level using the HRV obtained from the ECG signal, and achieved good classification results through the MLP method. Ref. [26] uses the multi-scale analysis method to evaluate the stress of pilots flying at night by fusing the area of the heart rate curve and constructing the functional relationship between the stress intensity and the training frequency, which effectively improved the effect of high-altitude training. Some researchers use genetic algorithm, artificial bee colony algorithm and improved particle optimization algorithm to optimize multi-kernel support vector machine, which improves the accuracy of stress detection [22].

At the same time, there are also studies that use biochemical indicators as a reference in the experiment and apply a variety of physiological signals to the detection of psychological stress. Ref. [27] proves that some indicators of HRV (e.g., HF, LF) have a strong correlation with some features of the EEG signal (e.g., LAPFpl) for stress estimation by analyzing the linear correlation between the HRV features of the ECG signal and the EEG signal features. Based on the above study, the authors propose that combining EEG with HRV can improve the accuracy of psychological stress detection. Ref. [19] develops a wearable multiphysiological parameter system to measure human stress and collect salivary cortisol as a reference. Specifically, the MAST (Maastricht Acute Stress Test) experiment is used to induce the generation of psychological stress, PCA and statistical methods are used to select and reduce the dimensionality of the features extracted from the recorded ECG, EDA and EEG signals, and finally, the SVM is used to classify psychological stress during the experimental period and the relaxation period. In addition, the experimental results in the paper show that salivary cortisol levels are highly correlated with HRV features. Some researchers also propose the detection of rest and task states of the human body by combining HRV features and PPG waveform features. A wrapping method based on ensemble learning is designed for feature selection, and a decision tree-based bagging model is developed for final state classification [20]. In [28], the salivary amylase and salivary cortisol concentrations are used to label the stress of subjects in TSST experiments into three levels, and the fuzzy ARTMAP method and voting integration method optimized by genetic algorithms have been used to establish a predictive model from subject HRV to psychological stress level, and good accuracy rates have been obtained.

In recent years, the use of deep learning methods to classify psychological stress has gradually emerged. Ref. [24] uses a one-dimensional convolutional neural network to extract the complex features of the RR intervals, thereby building an end-to-end neural network model to detect stress states through ECG signals. The RR interval is the time interval between two adjacent R waves in the ECG signal; that is, the time interval between two heartbeats. Ref. [29] proposes the use of a Gabor wavelet transform and discrete Fourier transform to convert the ECG signal into pictures in the time-frequency domain and frequency domain, respectively, and fuse the original signal, time-frequency domain and frequency domain information through a convolutional neural network to classify five levels of stress. Ref. [30] designs a deep convolutional neural network with a transformer mechanism to detect psychological stress using the location information of R-waves in ECG signals and achieves good performance through the fine-tuned network. Ref. [31] proposes the concept of real-time monitoring of psychological stress, and a convolutional neural network is used for the real-time recognition of acute cognitive stress from ECG signals with a 10-s window, which reduces the detection error rate compared to traditional methods. In previous studies, we used a multi-layer GRU network for the heartbeat classification of ballistocardiogram (BCG) signals and a bidirectional LSTM method for end-to-end heart rate estimation of BCG signals in a regression way, which achieved the best results compared to previous algorithms [32,33]. The successful application of a recurrent neural network in heartbeat detection also inspires and helps us in this work.

3. Materials

In this section, the wearable ECG signal collection device, VR scene, the process of the experiment and the dataset will be introduced in detail.

3.1. Smart ECG T-Shirt

Figure 1 is the smart ECG T-shirt designed and developed in our laboratory, which can simultaneously record various human physiological signals such as ECG, respiration and electrodermal activity [34]. The left and right of Figure 1a show the front lining and the front of the smart ECG T-shirt, respectively. In the experiment, it is used to record the ECG signals of subjects under different stress states. The sensor system of the smart ECG T-shirt is shown in the left half of Figure 1a, which consists of five flexible electrodes. The right half of Figure 1a shows the signal processing module of the smart ECG T-shirt, which can collect and store three lead ECG signals at a sampling rate of 250 Hz and provide power for the entire system through the built-in lithium battery. Figure 1b shows a subject wearing the smart ECG T-shirt. Figure 2 shows the three-lead ECG signal collected by this device. Each prominently raised peak in Figure 2 represents a heartbeat, and the heartbeat location is consistent across each lead. The recording of three-lead ECG signals can guarantee the signal quality of ECG to a large extent and improve the tolerance of our ECG acquisition equipment to motion or noise interference.

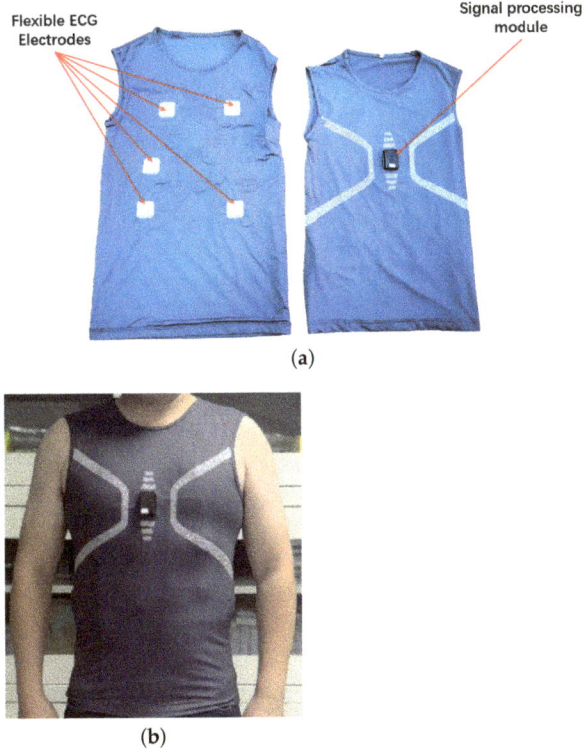

Figure 1. The smart ECG T-shirt. (**a**) The main modules of the smart ECG T-shirt. (**b**) A subject wearing the smart ECG T-shirt.

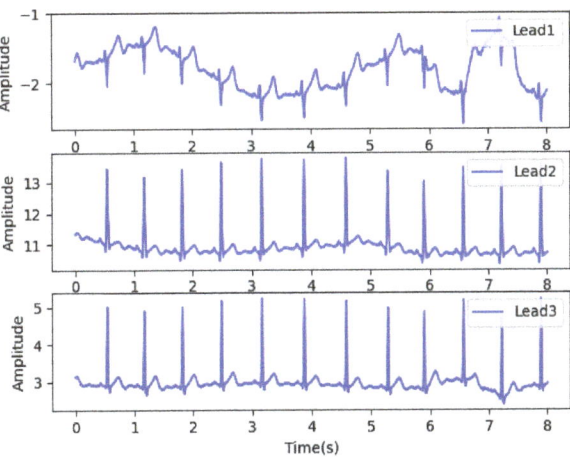

Figure 2. Three-lead ECG signal collected by smart ECG T-shirt.

3.2. *VR Scenarios and Tasks*

Figure 3 visualizes the VR experiment. The left of Figure 3a shows the experimental scene, and the right shows the VR scene seen by the subjects (in which the curves of various physiological parameters will not be seen). The positions and sizes of key objects in the experimental scene are consistent with the VR scene. During the experiment, the subjects need to wear a VR helmet to enter the virtual high-altitude scene and complete the following three tasks on the board in this scene, as shown in Figure 3b. These three tasks are described in detail as follows:

Task 1 : Go to the end of the board to pick up the tennis ball from basket B and put it in basket A. Basket A and basket B are shown in the left of Figure 3a.

Task 2: Go back to the end of the board to pick up the prop snake from basket C and put it in basket A. Basket A and basket C are shown in the left of Figure 3a.

Task 3: Go to the end of the board and jump to the square board shown in the right of Figure 3a.

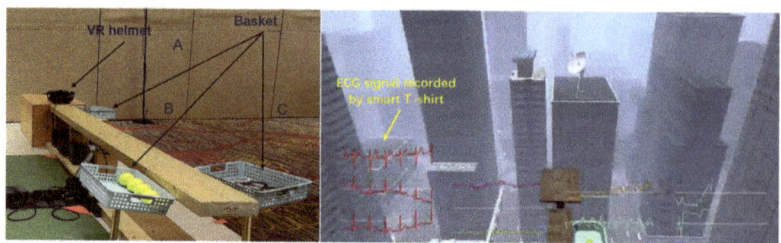

The real scene   The virtual scene

(**a**)

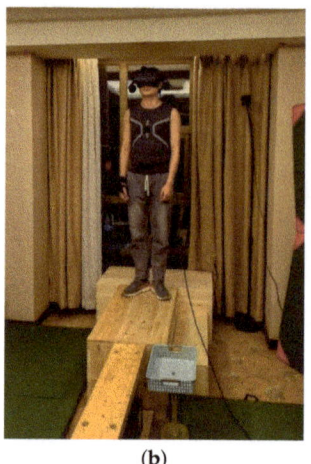

(**b**)

Figure 3. VR experiment. (**a**) Experimental scene and VR scene. (**b**) A subject performing the VR task.

3.3. Experimental Procedure and Dataset

The experiment consisted of four phases: resting, VR scene adaptation, VR task and recovery. The ECG signals were recorded synchronously in each phase of the experiment. Each of these phases is described in detail as follows:

Phase 1—Resting (5 min) : Sit calmly in a chair. This phase lasts 5 min.

Phase 2—VR scene adaptation (2 min): Wear VR equipment to enter the VR high-altitude scene, and adapt to the scene. This phase lasts 2 min.

Phase 3—VR task: Complete the tennis ball and prop snake transport and jump to the board in the VR high-altitude scene. The duration of this phase depends on how fast the subject is performing the task.

Phase 4—Recovery (5 min): After the VR task, stay calm and sit back in the chair. This phase lasts 5 min.

The above four experimental phases correspond to the four stress states of the subjects. This experiment collects the ECG signals of 63 healthy male subjects with an average age of 17.89 ± 0.45. Considering the adaptability of the subjects and the possible duration of each stress state, we select the subjects' ECG data in the first 70 s in the VR scene adaptation and recovery states and the subjects' data in the last 70 s in the resting and VR task states as the stress state classification dataset. Different stress states are the stress classification labels of the corresponding ECG signals so that we can obtain a stress state classification dataset consisting of the ECG data of 63 subjects and four labels. By summarizing the intuitive feelings of each subject in the experiment, we found that the stress level during resting is the lowest, the stress during the VR task is the highest, and the stress during recovery is greater than that in the VR scene adaptation.

4. Proposed Method

The purpose of our proposed deep GRU network is to perform the classification of four stress states through ECG signals collected by smart ECG T-shirts. In the HRV feature extraction stage, first, the R waves are detected, and the RR intervals are extracted from the ECG signal, and then the RR interval data under each stress state is divided into fixed-length data segments and arranged in time series. Finally, multiple HRV features, including time domain, frequency domain and entropy information, are extracted from the RR interval data of each segment. In the data preprocessing stage, considering the different physical meanings and numerical dimensions of each HRV feature, the time series relationship between the same HRV feature and the requirements of the input and optimization of the recurrent neural network, we standardize each feature of a single sample at each time by calculating the maximum and minimum values of each HRV feature of all samples at each moment. In the stage of deep feature extraction and stress classification, we design a deep feature extraction model composed of a multi-layer GRU network and a classifier composed of a multi-layer, fully connected network for time series feature extraction and classification of four stress states. The overall process of the proposed deep classification method is shown in Figure 4, and each of these processes is elaborated as follows. Figure 5 is a flow chart of the proposed method, which can make the process of each stage in Figure 4 easier to understand.

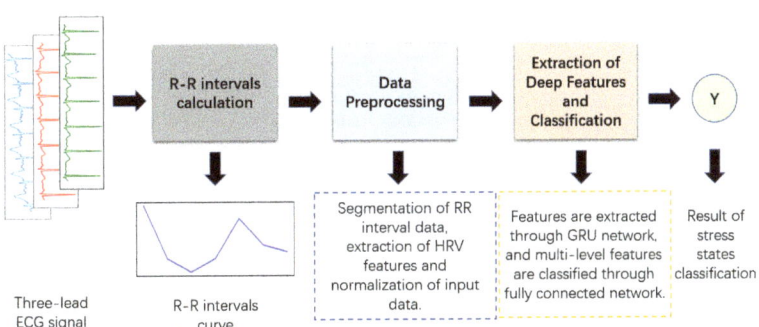

Figure 4. The overall process of the deep classification method based on the GRU network proposed in this paper.

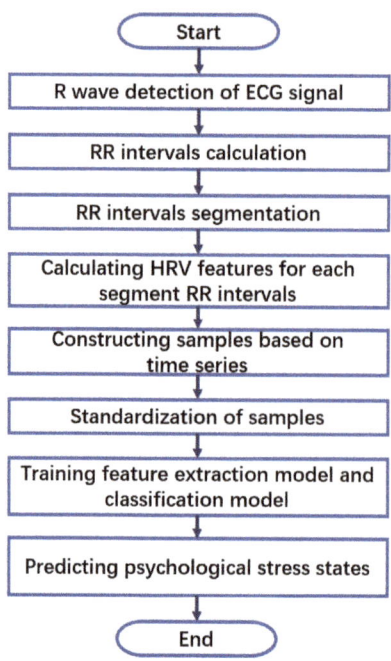

Figure 5. The flow chart of the proposed method.

4.1. HRV Feature Extraction

In this section, we first use a fourth-order Butterworth bandpass filter with a cutoff frequency of 10–35 Hz to filter out high-frequency noise and low-frequency perturbations generated by limb movements in each subject's ECG signal. Then, the locations of the R waves in the ECG signal are detected, and the RR intervals are calculated for each subject in each stress state. Finally, after the analysis and comparison of previous studies on the classification of psychological stress [18–21], we select seven HRV features to represent the information of ECG signals, namely, mRR and SDNN containing their time domain information, HFn, LFn and LF/HF containing RR intervals frequency domain information, ApEn containing their entropy information and their nonlinear feature SD1/SD2. The description of each feature is shown in Table 1.

Table 1. HRV features and their descriptions in the paper.

Feature	Description
mRR	The mean value of the RR interval (time between adjacent heartbeats) sequence.
SDNN	The standard deviation of RR intervals (time series of adjacent heartbeat intervals).
HFn	Normalized spectral energy of heart rate variability from 0.15 to 0.4 Hz.
LFn	Normalized spectral energy of heart rate variability from 0.04 to 0.15 Hz.
LF/HF	The ratio of low-frequency to high-frequency power for heart rate variability.
ApEn	The approximate entropy of the RR interval sequence, which is used to measure the complexity of the sequence.
SD1/SD2	In the point cloud data of the poincare plots drawn with the RR intervals, the variance of the distribution along the longer axis is SD2, and the variance of the distribution along the shorter axis is SD1. SD1/SD2 is the ratio of SD1 and SD2.

4.2. Data Preprocessing

In this section, sample construction and feature standardization processing of ECG signals are elaborated. The complete process is shown in Figure 6. The left of Figure 6 shows the sample construction process, and the right shows the sample standardization method. In the process of sample construction, we first intercept N RR interval segments of length L from the RR interval sequence with sliding step d according to the time series and calculate the HRV features corresponding to each segment. Finally, the HRV features of the RR interval segments are arranged in the sample matrix shown in Figure 6, where t_n represents the moment corresponding to the n-th segment of the RR interval sequence. In this paper, we take L as 30 s, sliding step d as 2 s and N as 20. It should be noted that the physical meanings of the HRV features in the constructed samples are different, and there is a temporal relationship between the HRV feature sequences. Therefore, we use the min-max standardization method to standardize each feature at each moment in each sample based on the time series characteristics. The specific process is shown on the right of Figure 6. f_1 and f_2 represent different HRV features, and M represents the total number of samples. The final standardized samples can be obtained by processing the feature sequence composed of each feature at each moment in all samples. The calculation formula of the minimum and maximum standardization is shown in Equation (1):

$$\hat{f}_{i,j} = \frac{f_{i,j} - \min(F_{i,j})}{\max(F_{i,j}) - \min(F_{i,j})},$$
(1)

where $f_{i,j}$ is the HRV feature of the i-th row and the j-th column in the sample (its physical meaning is the j-th feature in the HRV feature sequence at the i-th moment), $i = 1, 2, \ldots, N$, and $j = 1, 2, \ldots, 7$; $\max(F_{i,j})$ and $\min(F_{i,j})$ are the maximum and minimum values of HRV features in row i and column j in training samples; $\hat{f}_{i,j}$ is the standardized HRV feature.

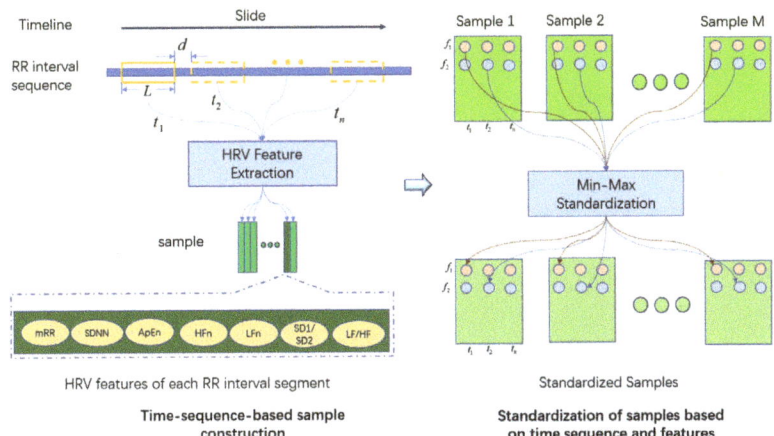

Figure 6. Sample construction and standardization.

4.3. GRU Model

GRU is a kind of recurrent neural network (RNN). GRU and Long Short-Term Memory (LSTM) are both proposed to solve the problem of gradient disappearance in the long-term dependence of learning time series in traditional RNN [35,36]. The performance of GRU and LSTM on many deep learning tasks is similar [37], but GRU has fewer parameters and less computation, so it has advantages in reducing the consumption of computing resources and the risk of overfitting. The structure of the GRU model is shown in Figure 7. Where the circles and ellipses with a blue background represent operators, the boxes with a green background represent functions and the boxes with a gray background represent inputs. There are two important gate functions in the GRU model: the update gate and reset gate. The function of the reset gate is to determine how much of the hidden state information of the previous moment will be added to the candidate state according to the current input and the hidden state of the previous moment, thereby generating the candidate state of the current moment. The function of the update gate is to determine which historical information in the hidden state at the previous moment can be forgotten and which information in the candidate state at the current moment can be added to the new hidden state, thereby generating the hidden state at the current moment. Equations (2) and (3) are the calculation formulas for the weights of the reset gate and the update gate, and the update formulas of the candidate state and the hidden state are shown in Equations (4) and (5) [37].

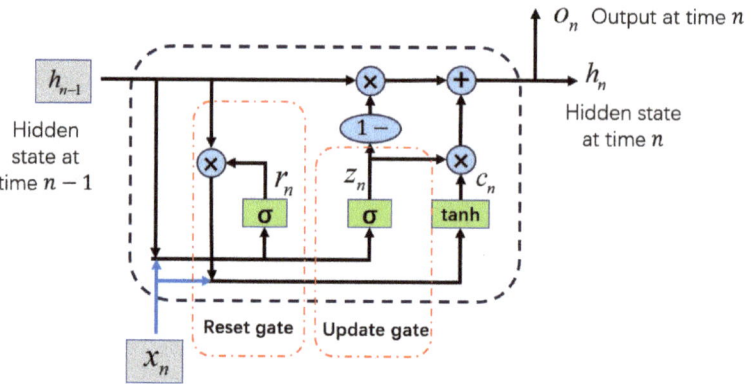

Figure 7. The GRU model structure.

$$r_n = \sigma(W_{ir}x_n + W_{hr}h_{n-1}), \tag{2}$$

$$z_n = \sigma(W_{iz}x_n + W_{hz}h_{n-1}), \tag{3}$$

$$c_n = \tanh(W_{ic}x_n + W_{hc}(r_n \odot h_{n-1})), \tag{4}$$

$$h_n = o_n = (1 - z_n)\odot c_n + z_n \odot h_{n-1}, \tag{5}$$

where x_n is the input at the n-th moment, and h_{n-1} is the hidden state at the $n-1$-th moment, W_{ir} and W_{hr} are the weight matrices of the reset gate input layer and the hidden state layer, W_{iz} and W_{hz} are the weight matrices of the update gate input layer and the hidden state layer, W_{ic} and W_{hc} are the input layer weight matrices and the hidden state layer weight matrices in the candidate state calculation, the bias matrices are all included by the weight matrices. c_n is the candidate state at the n-th moment, and h_n and o_n are the hidden state and output at the n-th moment. Operator $\odot$ is an element-wise multiplication. σ and tanh are activation functions, and their calculation formulas are $\sigma(x) = \frac{1}{1+e^{-x}}$ and $\tanh(x) = \frac{e^x - e^{-x}}{e^x + e^{-x}}$, respectively. They can improve the nonlinear capabilities of the model.

4.4. Psychological Stress Classification Model

The proposed psychological stress classification model consists of two sub-models, deep feature extraction and psychological stress classification, and its overall structure is shown in Figure 8. The deep feature extraction model is composed of two cascaded GRU blocks, and the output of each moment of the first block is input to the second block in the same order. The content in the green dotted box in Figure 8 shows the structure diagram of each GRU block expanded by time steps. Each GRU block is composed of K layers of the GRU network, and each layer of the GRU network contains N time step inputs, where x_n and o_n represent the input and output of the n-th moment, and the structure of each GRU model is shown in Figure 7. Considering that the output of the GRU network at the last moment contains the information of the entire sequence, the multi-level deep features composed of the outputs of the last moment of the two GRU blocks are used as the input of the psychological stress classification model. The psychological stress classification model consists of a multi-layer, fully connected network and a SoftMax classifier. As shown in the blue dotted box in Figure 8, there is a batch normalization layer between each layer of fully connected networks to standardize the distribution of neural network output, and ReLU is used as the activation function. The numbers in the FC block in Figure 8 are the number of neurons in each layer of the neural network.

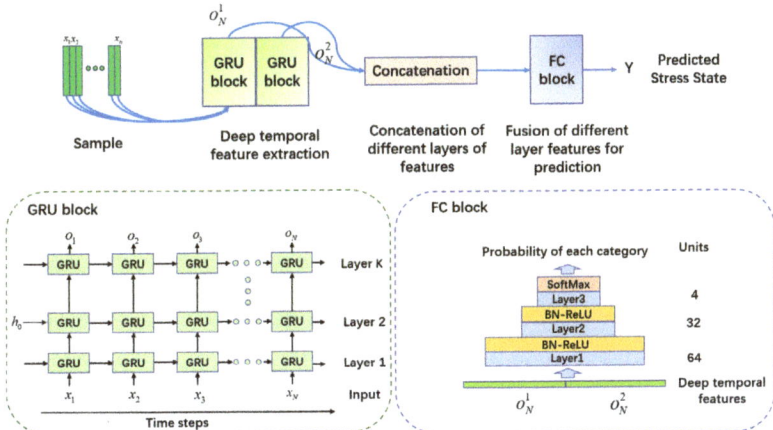

Figure 8. Psychological stress classification model.

The loss function used in the proposed method is shown in Equation (6), which consists of cross entropy loss and L2 regular loss. Cross entropy loss is used to measure the classification error of the model, and L2 loss is used to measure the complexity of the model to reduce the risk of overfitting. In training, the deep network model is optimized by minimizing the loss function.

$$loss(y, \hat{y}) = -\frac{1}{M}\left(\sum_{i=1}^{M}\sum_{k=1}^{K} y_i^{(k)} log\hat{y}_i^k\right) + \gamma\|\mathbf{W}\|_2, \qquad (6)$$

where M is the number of each batch sample in the training process, K is the total number of categories and y and $\hat{y}$ are the real labels and prediction probabilities of samples, respectively. γ is the hyperparameter of L2 loss, which controls the participation of L2 loss.

4.5. Evaluation Indicators

Since the number of samples under the four classes (psychological stress states) in this dataset is equal, the accuracy rate is used as an evaluation index to measure the performance of the methods. The accuracy of classification is the ratio of the number of correctly classified samples to the total number of samples, and its calculation formula is shown in Equation (7). When the number of samples in each category is balanced, the accuracy rate can objectively and intuitively show the classification accuracy of the algorithms. The higher the accuracy rate, the higher the classification performance of the algorithm.

$$Accuracy = \frac{T_1 + T_2 + T_3 + T_4}{M}, \tag{7}$$

where M is the total number of samples, and $T_1 \sim T_4$ are the number of correctly predicted samples of category $1 \sim 4$, respectively.

5. Experiments and Results

5.1. Experimental Setting and Parameters

The proposed method is built and evaluated on the dataset mentioned in Section 3.3. In order to be more consistent with the actual applications, the cross-subject test method is used to verify the estimated performance of the method. In this paper, the training set consists of ECG data on 47 subjects, in which 8 subjects' ECG data are randomly selected as the validation set, and the remaining 16 subjects' ECG data are the test set. In data processing, each subject's ECG signal under each stress state is broken into 20 ECG signal segments with a length of 30 s, and the interception interval is 2 s. These 20 signal segments correspond to the time steps of the GRU network inputs.

In the deep feature extraction model, each GRU block is formed by stacking 5 layers of the GRU network, each layer of the GRU network has 256 neurons, and the length of the input sequence is 20 time steps. The classification model is composed of three layers of fully connected networks stacked, and the number of neurons from the bottom layer to the top layer is 64, 32 and 4. During the training process, the L2 regularization coefficient γ is 0.002, the learning rate is 0.0002, the batch size is 52, the model is optimized by Adam and the number of epochs is about 80. The training ends when the accuracy of the training set and the validation set is high, and the accuracy of the validation set is stable. During validation and testing, the validation and test sets are standardized using the parameters in the training set. In order to evaluate the performance of the model more objectively, we conduct five independent repeated experiments and take the average of its accuracy as the final evaluation index.

5.2. Experimental Platform

The hardware configuration of the workstation for this experiment is Intel i7-11700F CPU with 16GB RAM, and NVIDIA 1060Ti GPU. The software platform is Python 3.7.11, Pytorch 1.10.0 and CUDA 11.3.

5.3. Results and Analysis

In this section, the psychological stress state estimation performance of the proposed method is presented and discussed from different perspectives. First, different numbers of HRV features are tried to train deep models to observe the contribution of different features to the estimation performance of the proposed method, and the results are shown in Table 2. When only mRR and ApEn features are used, the classification accuracy of the model is only 0.51. As more HRV features are added to the training of the model, its classification accuracy keeps rising and eventually reaching 0.73 when all HRV features are used. In addition, it can be seen that compared with the HRV features, for except mRR and ApEn, SDNN has a higher contribution to stress state classification performance. Then, Figure 9 shows the training set accuracy and validation set accuracy curves of the proposed algorithm during training. It can be seen that as the number of epochs increases, the estimated accuracy of the model in both the training set and the validation set keeps rising steadily. It should be noted that the gap between the accuracy of the training set and the accuracy of the validation set continues to increase as the training progresses, and the risk of overfitting the model will increase if the training continues. Therefore, the model with the iteration number of 80 epochs is selected for performance evaluation on the test set.

Table 2. Classification accuracy of the proposed method in stress state with different HRV features. In this sub-experiment, 28 subjects are randomly selected from the training set described in Section 5.1 to train the model, and 15 subjects are randomly selected from the remaining data for validation. The accuracy in the table is the average accuracy of three independent repeated experiments on the validation set. The number in bold represents the best result.

Features	Accuracy
mRR, ApEn	0.51
mRR, ApEn, SD1/SD2	0.56
mRR, ApEn, SD1/SD2, SDNN	0.68
mRR, ApEn, SD1/SD2, SDNN, HFn	0.67
mRR, ApEn, SD1/SD2, SDNN, HFn, LFn	0.71
mRR, ApEn, SD1/SD2, SDNN, HFn, LFn, LF/HF	**0.73**

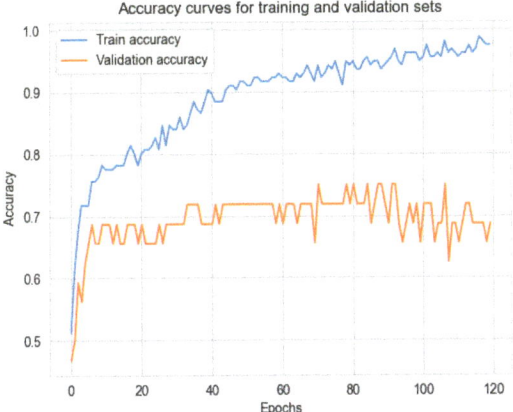

Figure 9. Accuracy curves of training set and validation set during training.

The classification performance of the proposed method and the comparison algorithms are presented in Table 3; the number in bold is the best result. Among them, comparison algorithms include the traditional machine learning algorithm KNN, ensemble learning method XGBoost [38], deep learning method MLP [23] and one-dimensional CNN (CNN-1D) network. KNN has been widely used in the study of psychological stress classification. XGBoost, as a state of art ensemble learning method, has been applied in many machine learning fields. In [23], a good psychological stress classification result is obtained by using the MLP method. At present, a one-dimensional CNN network is also widely used in the field of physiological signal processing and has achieved good results [39,40]. GRU-b1, GRU-b2 and GRU-b3 in Table 3 are the methods proposed in this paper, which represent the deep time series feature extraction model composed of one GRU block, two GRU blocks and three GRU blocks, respectively. It can be seen that the classification accuracy of psychological stress obtained by our methods is better than all comparison algorithms. When using two GRU blocks to extract deep features, the classification accuracy of psychological stress is the highest among all methods, reaching 0.78. We believe that this is because the long-short-term memory network may be able to capture longer-term dependencies between time series than other machine learning methods, thereby obtaining more global and robust characteristics of psychological stress. In addition, with the increase in GRU blocks, the classification performance of the model tends to increase first and then maintain or slightly decrease. This is because when there are fewer model parameters, the risk of model underfitting is high. When there are too many model parameters, it is easy for the model to fall into overfitting, which will reduce the classification performance of the model on the test set.

Table 3. Psychological stress state classification accuracy of the proposed algorithm and comparison algorithms on the test set. The number in bold represents the best result.

Algorithms	KNN	XGBoost	MLP [23]	CNN-1D	GRU-b1	GRU-b2	GRU-b3
Accuracy	0.65	0.69	0.71	0.7	0.73	**0.78**	0.77

We also perform some exploration on the impact of other model hyperparameters on model performance; Tables 4 and 5 show the estimated performance of the proposed algorithm under different model parameters. Table 4 shows the impact of GRU networks with different numbers of neurons on the model estimation performance, and Table 5 shows the impact of different numbers of GRU network layers on the model estimation performance. It can be seen that with the increasing number of neurons and network layers in the network, the classification accuracy of the model shows a trend of rising first and then declining under the influence of the risk of underfitting and overfitting. When the number of neurons is 256 and the number of network layers is 5, the classification accuracy of the model is the highest. Furthermore, it can be seen that the depth of the GRU network significantly affects the classification accuracy of the model. This is because, compared with the shallow network, the deep network can extract more essential features from HRV data. These features represent the common characteristics of physiological data of different subjects under the same stress state, and they can affect the generalization performance of the model.

Table 4. The classification accuracy of the psychological stress of the GRU network of the proposed method under different numbers of neural units. The number in bold represents the best result.

The number of GRU units	64	128	256	512
Accuracy	0.75	0.75	**0.78**	0.73

Table 5. The classification accuracy of the psychological stress of the GRU block of the proposed method under different numbers of neural network layers. The number in bold represents the best result.

The number of layers of GRU block	1	3	5	7
Accuracy	0.67	0.7	**0.78**	0.76

In addition, we also explore the classification performance of the model in each class. Labels and classes 1, 2, 3 and 4 in Table 6 and Figure 10 represent four stress states, namely, resting, VR task, recovery and VR scene adaptation. Table 6 is the confusion matrix for the classification of the proposed method on the test set, and the data in the table is the proportion of the number of samples predicted to be in this class among all the samples in this class. It can be seen that the model has the lowest classification accuracy for class 1 (resting state), 38% of the samples are wrongly classified into class 4 (the state of adapting to the VR scene), and 13% of the samples in class 4 are also wrongly classified into class 1. This is because, in the process of adapting to the VR scene, the subjects only need to keep standing to observe and become familiar with the VR high-altitude scene, which induces less psychological stress so that the physiological parameters of the subjects at this time are very close to those at rest. This results in a lower classification accuracy of the model in class 1 compared to other classes. As shown in Figure 10, we also use the t-distributed Stochastic Neighbor-Embedding (T-SNE) [41] method to reduce the dimensionality and visualize the deep feature output by the CNN-1D and proposed method, respectively, where the dots with different colors represent the class to which the feature belongs. The position of each dot represents the distribution characteristics of the deep features extracted from a sample in the two-dimensional feature space. It can be seen from Figure 10a that the classification boundaries between the features of each class extracted by the CNN-1D model are relatively blurred, and the feature distribution of each category of samples is loose. The extracted features using the proposed deep model are shown in Figure 10b. It can be seen that compared with the CNN-1D model, the classification boundaries between the various categories of features extracted by our method are more obvious, and the distribution of sample features of each category is also more concentrated. Furthermore, we can see that the method proposed by us can also improve the separability between class 1 and class 4 samples to a certain extent, which indicates that our method extracts more essential psychological stress features from HRV data. Although our method has some improvement in feature extraction compared to the CNN-1D method, the classification boundaries of deep features of class 1 and class 4 are still blurred, which is consistent with the results in the confusion matrix. The identification of this weak-intensity stress is a difficult problem in the current research field of psychological stress estimation, and it will be also the focus of our future research.

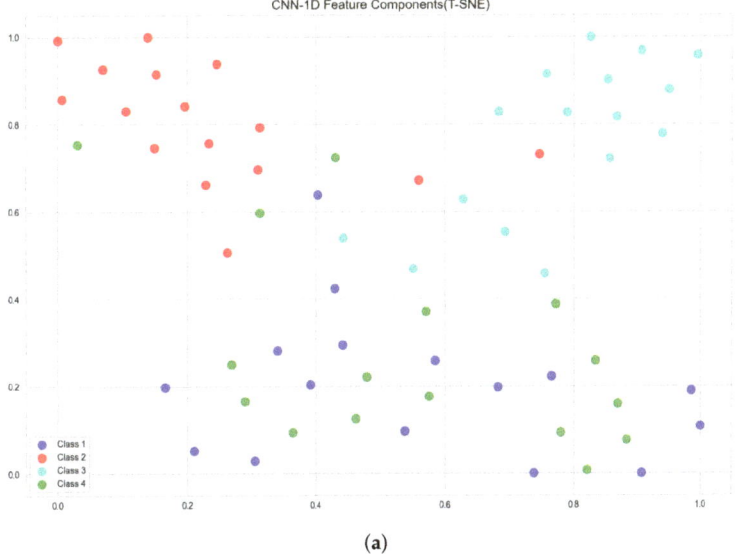

(a)

Figure 10. *Cont.*

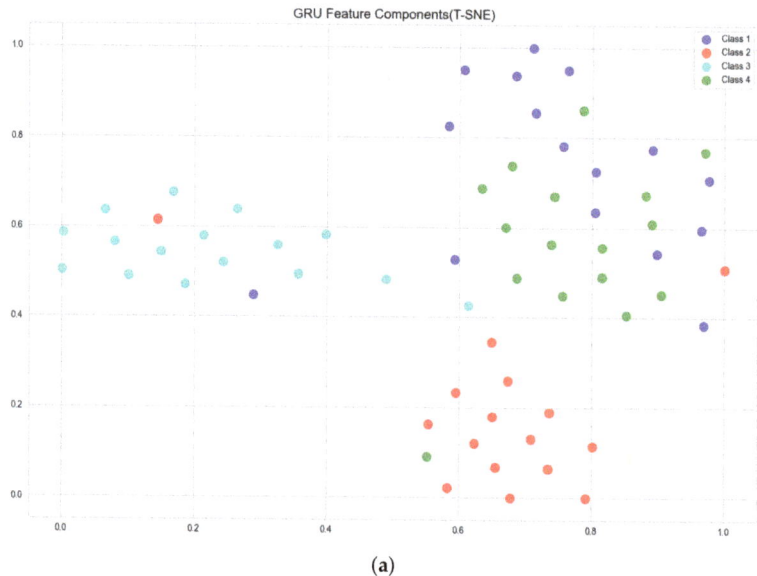

(a)

Figure 10. Feature extraction results of CNN-1D and the proposed method on subject HRV data. (**a**) The distribution of the features output by the CNN-1D model after T-SNE dimensionality reduction. (**b**) The distribution of the features output by the proposed method after dimensionality reduction by T-SNE.

Table 6. The classification confusion matrix of the proposed method for psychological stress states. The data in the table is the proportion of the number of samples predicted to be this label in all samples of this label.

Proportion	Predict Labels			
	1	2	3	4
True Labels				
1	0.56	0.06	0	0.38
2	0	0.88	0.06	0.06
3	0.06	0	0.94	0
4	0.13	0.06	0	0.81

6. Conclusions

This paper proposes a deep psychological stress classification method based on ECG signals. First, HRV feature samples containing the timing information of ECG signals are constructed. Deep GRU networks are then used to extract deep features from HRV feature samples that have more essential and general connections to psychological stress states. Finally, a multi-layer, fully connected network is used to fuse the deep and shallow features of the GRU network to predict the psychological stress state. The experimental results show that the proposed method is a robust psychological stress estimation scheme, and its estimation accuracy in this dataset is 0.78 better than other mainstream methods.

However, we noticed that the classification accuracy is not very high. In future work, we will try to further improve the accuracy of psychological stress classification from the following aspects. The first is that the amount of information input to the classification model can be increased by introducing other physiological signals besides ECG, such as

EEG and EDA, or extracting more valuable features from ECG signals, thereby improving the performance of stress classification. Secondly, we can also consider reducing the differences in physiological signals between individuals to improve the classification accuracy of psychological stress. Specifically, domain adaptation methods in transfer learning have achieved good results in many image datasets with large distribution differences, and in recent years, this method has achieved high performance in EEG-based cross-subject emotion recognition accuracy [42,43]. Therefore, we will consider introducing a transfer learning method to further improve the classification accuracy of psychological stress states. Furthermore, high-level feature design and feature space applicable reduction to multidimensional wearable sensors, such as referable approaches for wearable-based HAR, are also worthy of further experimentation [14,44].

Author Contributions: All of the authors made significant contributions to this work. J.Z. and D.H. designed the psychological stress experiment, developed the algorithm and wrote the manuscript. Y.L. and L.C. developed the ECG collection equipment and organized the experiment. X.C. and W.C. developed the VR equipment and experimental scenarios. All authors have read and agreed to the published version of the manuscript.

Funding: This research was supported by the Key Deployment Project of the Chinese Academy of Sciences (Psychophysiological Intelligence Monitoring Technology for Small Group Target Figures, No. KGFZD-145-21-09-01) and Jiangsu Province Industrial Foresight and the Key Core Technology Project (Research and Development of Key Technologies for Demonstration and Application of Multi-scenario Brain-Computer Interaction System for Smart Elderly Care, No. BE2022064-2).

Institutional Review Board Statement: The research was conducted according to the guidelines of the Declaration of Helsinki, and approved by the Institutional Review Board the Suzhou Institute of Biomedical Engineering and Technology, Chinese Academy of Sciences.

Informed Consent Statement: Informed consent was obtained from all subjects involved in the study.

Data Availability Statement: The data are not publicly available due to the relevant project regulations.

Conflicts of Interest: The authors declare no conflict of interest.

References

1. Blaug, R.; Kenyon, A.; Lekhi, R. Stress at Work: A Report Prepared for The Work Foundation's Principal Partners. Project Report. The Work Foundation, London. 2007. Available online: https://www.researchgate.net/publication/274040847_Structural_Equation_Modeling_of_Occupational_Stress_in_the_Construction_Industry (accessed on 2 November 2022).
2. Cohen, S.; Kessler, R.; Gordon, L.G. Strategies for measuring stress in studies of psychiatric and physical disorder. *Meas. Stress. Guide Health Soc. Sci.* **1995**, *141*, 3–26.
3. McEwen, B.S. Central effects of stress hormones in health and disease: Understanding the protective and damaging effects of stress and stress mediators. *Eur. J. Pharmacol.* **2008**, *583*, 174–185. [CrossRef] [PubMed]
4. Duman, R.S. Neurobiology of stress, depression, and rapid acting antidepressants: Remodeling synaptic connections. *Depress. Anxiety* **2014**, *31*, 291–296. [CrossRef] [PubMed]
5. Lin, H.; Jia, J.; Guo, Q.; Xue, Y.; Huang, J.; Cai, L.; Feng, L. Psychological stress detection from cross-media microblog data using Deep Sparse Neural Network. In Proceedings of the 2014 IEEE International Conference on Multimedia and Expo (ICME), Chengdu, China, 14–18 July 2014; pp. 1–6. [CrossRef]
6. Tajuddin, M.; Kabeer, M.; Misbahuddin, M. Analysis of Social Media for Psychological Stress Detection using Ontologies. In Proceedings of the 2020 Fourth International Conference on Inventive Systems and Control (ICISC), Coimbatore, India, 8–10 January 2020; pp. 181–185. [CrossRef]
7. Giannakakis, G.; Grigoriadis, D.; Giannakaki, K.; Simantiraki, O.; Roniotis, A.; Tsiknakis, M. Review on Psychological Stress Detection Using Biosignals. *IEEE Trans. Affect. Comput.* **2022**, *13*, 440–460. [CrossRef]
8. He, B.; Yang, L.; Wilke, C.; Yuan, H. Electrophysiological Imaging of Brain Activity and Connectivity—Challenges and Opportunities. *IEEE Trans. Biomed. Eng.* **2011**, *58*, 1918–1931. [CrossRef]
9. Curone, D.; Secco, E.L.; Tognetti, A.; Loriga, G.; Dudnik, G.; Risatti, M.; Whyte, R.; Bonfiglio, A.; Magenes, G. Smart Garments for Emergency Operators: The ProeTEX Project. *IEEE Trans. Inf. Technol. Biomed.* **2010**, *14*, 694–701. [CrossRef]
10. Lee, Y.D.; Chung, W.Y. Wireless sensor network based wearable smart shirt for ubiquitous health and activity monitoring. *Sens. Actuators Chem.* **2009**, *140*, 390–395. [CrossRef]
11. Chen, C.C.; Lin, S.Y.; Chang, W.Y. Novel Stable Capacitive Electrocardiogram Measurement System. *Sensors* **2021**, *21*, 3668. [CrossRef]

12. Liu, H.; Hartmann, Y.; Schultz, T. A Practical Wearable Sensor-Based Human Activity Recognition Research Pipeline. In Proceedings of the 15th International Joint Conference on Biomedical Engineering Systems and Technologies—Volume 5: HEALTHINF, Online, 9–11 February 2022; pp. 847–856. [CrossRef]

13. Liu, H.; Hartmann, Y.; Schultz, T. CSL-SHARE: A Multimodal Wearable Sensor-Based Human Activity Dataset. *Front. Comput. Sci.* **2021**, *3*, 90. [CrossRef]

14. Hartmann, Y.; Liu, H.; Schultz, T. Interactive and Interpretable Online Human Activity Recognition. In Proceedings of the PERCOM 2022—20th IEEE International Conference on Pervasive Computing and Communications Workshops and Other Affiliated Events (PerCom Workshops), Pisa, Italy, 21–25 March 2022; pp. 109–111. [CrossRef]

15. Hartmann, Y.; Liu, H.; Lahrberg, S.; Schultz, T. Interpretable High-Level Features for Human Activity Recognition. In Proceedings of the 15th International Joint Conference on Biomedical Engineering Systems and Technologies—Volume 4: BIOSIGNALS, Online, 9–11 February 2022; pp. 40–49. [CrossRef]

16. Smeets, T.; Cornelisse, S.; Quaedflieg, C.W.E.M.; Meyer, T.; Jelicic, M.; Merckelbach, H. Introducing the Maastricht Acute Stress Test (MAST): A quick and non-invasive approach to elicit robust autonomic and glucocorticoid stress responses. *Psychoneuroendocrinology* **2012**, *37*, 1998–2008. [CrossRef]

17. Nitzan, M.; Babchenko, A.; Khanokh, B.; Landau, D. The variability of the photoplethysmographic signal—A potential method for the evaluation of the autonomic nervous system. *Physiol. Meas.* **1998**, *19*, 93–102. [CrossRef] [PubMed]

18. Guo, H.W.; Huang, Y.S.; Lin, C.H.; Chien, J.C.; Haraikawa, K.; Shieh, J.S. Heart Rate Variability Signal Features for Emotion Recognition by Using Principal Component Analysis and Support Vectors Machine. In Proceedings of the 2016 IEEE 16th International Conference on Bioinformatics and Bioengineering (BIBE), Taichung, Taiwan, 31 October–2 November 2016; pp. 274–277. [CrossRef]

19. Betti, S.; Lova, R.M.; Rovini, E.; Acerbi, G.; Santarelli, L.; Cabiati, M.; Ry, S.D.; Cavallo, F. Evaluation of an Integrated System of Wearable Physiological Sensors for Stress Monitoring in Working Environments by Using Biological Markers. *IEEE Trans. Biomed. Eng.* **2018**, *65*, 1748–1758. [CrossRef] [PubMed]

20. Peláez, M.D.C.; Albalate, M.T.L.; Sanz, A.H.; Vallés, M.A.; Gil, E. Photoplethysmographic Waveform Versus Heart Rate Variability to Identify Low-Stress States: Attention Test. *IEEE J. Biomed. Health Inform.* **2019**, *23*, 1940–1951. [CrossRef]

21. Giannakakis, G.; Marias, K.; Tsiknakis, M. A stress recognition system using HRV parameters and machine learning techniques. In Proceedings of the 2019 8th International Conference on Affective Computing and Intelligent Interaction Workshops and Demos (ACIIW), Cambridge, UK, 3–6 September 2019; pp. 269–272. [CrossRef]

22. Malhotra, V.; Sandhu, M. Improved ECG based Stress Prediction using Optimization and Machine Learning Techniques. *ICST Trans. Scalable Inf. Syst.* **2021**, *8*, 169175. [CrossRef]

23. Dalmeida, K.; Masala, G. HRV Features as Viable Physiological Markers for Stress Detection Using Wearable Devices. *Sensors* **2021**, *21*, 2873. [CrossRef]

24. Giannakakis, G.; Trivizakis, E.; Tsiknakis, M.; Marias, K. A novel multi-kernel 1D convolutional neural network for stress recognition from ECG. In Proceedings of the 2019 8th International Conference on Affective Computing and Intelligent Interaction Workshops and Demos (ACIIW), Cambridge, UK, 3–6 September 2019; pp. 1–4. [CrossRef]

25. Nita, S.; Bitam, S.; Mellouk, A. A Body Area Network for Ubiquitous Driver Stress Monitoring based on ECG Signal. In Proceedings of the 2019 International Conference on Wireless and Mobile Computing, Networking and Communications (WiMob), Barcelona, Spain, 21–23 October 2019; pp. 1–6. [CrossRef]

26. Shao, S.; Zhou, Q.; Liu, Z. A New Assessment Method of the Pilot Stress Using ECG Signals During Complex Special Flight Operation. *IEEE Access* **2019**, *7*, 185360–185368. [CrossRef]

27. Attar, E.T.; Balasubramanian, V.; Subasi, E.; Kaya, M. Stress Analysis Based on Simultaneous Heart Rate Variability and EEG Monitoring. *IEEE J. Transl. Eng. Health Med.* **2021**, *9*, 1–7. [CrossRef]

28. Liew, W.S.; Seera, M.; Loo, C.K.; Lim, E.; Kubota, N. Classifying Stress From Heart Rate Variability Using Salivary Biomarkers as Reference. *IEEE Trans. Neural Netw. Learn. Syst.* **2016**, *27*, 2035–2046. [CrossRef]

29. Ahmad, Z.; Khan, N.M. Multi-level Stress Assessment Using Multi-domain Fusion of ECG Signal. In Proceedings of the 2020 42nd Annual International Conference of the IEEE Engineering in Medicine and Biology Society (EMBC), Virtual, 20–24 July 2020; pp. 4518–4521. [CrossRef]

30. Behinaein, B.; Bhatti, A.; Rodenburg, D.; Hungler, P.; Etemad, A. A transformer architecture for stress detection from ecg. In Proceedings of the 2021 International Symposium on Wearable Computers, Virtual, 21–26 September 2021; pp. 132–134.

31. He, J.; Li, K.; Liao, X.; Zhang, P.; Jiang, N. Real-Time Detection of Acute Cognitive Stress Using a Convolutional Neural Network From Electrocardiographic Signal. *IEEE Access* **2019**, *7*, 42710–42717. [CrossRef]

32. Hai, D.; Chen, C.; Yi, R.; Gou, S.; Yu Su, B.; Jiao, C.; Skubic, M. Heartbeat Detection and Rate Estimation from Ballistocardiograms using the Gated Recurrent Unit Network. In Proceedings of the 2020 42nd Annual International Conference of the IEEE Engineering in Medicine and Biology Society (EMBC), Montreal, QC, Canada, 20–24 July 2020; pp. 451–454. [CrossRef]

33. Jiao, C.; Chen, C.; Gou, S.; Hai, D.; Su, B.Y.; Skubic, M.; Jiao, L.; Zare, A.; Ho, K.C. Non-Invasive Heart Rate Estimation From Ballistocardiograms Using Bidirectional LSTM Regression. *IEEE J. Biomed. Health Inform.* **2021**, *25*, 3396–3407. [CrossRef]

34. Zhong, J.; Zhou, H.; Liu, Y.; Cheng, X.; Cai, L.; Zhu, W.; Liu, L. Integrated Design Of Physiological Multi-Parameter Sensors On A Smart Garment By Ultra-Elastic E-Textile. *J. Mech. Med. Biol.* **2021**, *21*, 2140037. [CrossRef]

35. Chung, J.; Gulcehre, C.; Cho, K.; Bengio, Y. Gated Feedback Recurrent Neural Networks. In Proceedings of the International conference on machine learning, Lille, France, 6–11 July 2015; pp. 2067–2075.
36. Graves, A. Supervised Sequence Labelling. In *Supervised Sequence Labelling with Recurrent Neural Networks*; Springer: Berlin/Heidelberg, Germany, 2012; pp. 5–13. [CrossRef]
37. Chung, J.; Gulcehre, C.; Cho, K.; Bengio, Y. Empirical Evaluation of Gated Recurrent Neural Networks on Sequence Modeling. In Proceedings of the NIPS 2014 Workshop on Deep Learning, Montreal, QC, Canada, 8–13 December 2014.
38. Chen, T.; Guestrin, C. Xgboost: A Scalable Tree Boosting System. In Proceedings of the 22nd ACM Sigkdd International Conference on Knowledge Discovery and Data Mining, San Francisco, CA, USA, 13–17 August 2016; pp. 785–794.
39. Vijayvargiya, A.; Khimraj; Kumar, R.; Dey, N. Voting-based 1D CNN model for human lower limb activity recognition using sEMG signal. *Phys. Eng. Sci. Med.* **2021**, *44*, 1297–1309. [CrossRef] [PubMed]
40. Wu, B.; Yang, G.; Yang, L.; Yin, Y. Robust ECG Biometrics Using Two-Stage Model. In Proceedings of the 2018 24th International Conference on Pattern Recognition (ICPR), Beijing, China, 20–24 August 2018; pp. 1062–1067. [CrossRef]
41. Hinton, G.E. Visualizing High-Dimensional Data Using t-SNE. *Vigiliae Christ.* **2008**, *9*, 2579–2605.
42. Saito, K.; Watanabe, K.; Ushiku, Y.; Harada, T. Maximum Classifier Discrepancy for Unsupervised Domain Adaptation. In Proceedings of the 2018 IEEE/CVF Conference on Computer Vision and Pattern Recognition, Salt Lake City, UT, USA, 18–23 June 2018; pp. 3723–3732. [CrossRef]
43. Zhao, L.M.; Yan, X.; Lu, B.L. Plug-and-play domain adaptation for cross-subject EEG-based emotion recognition. In Proceedings of the AAAI Conference on Artificial Intelligence, Virtually, 2–9 February 2021; Volume 35, pp. 863–870. [CrossRef]
44. Hartmann, Y.; Liu, H.; Schultz, T. Feature Space Reduction for Human Activity Recognition based on Multi-channel Biosignals. In Proceedings of the 14th International Joint Conference on Biomedical Engineering Systems and Technologies, Vienna, Austria, 11–13 February 2021; pp. 215–222. [CrossRef]

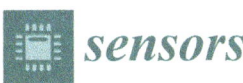

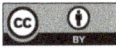

sensors

MDPI

Systematic Review

Research and Development of Ankle–Foot Orthoses: A Review

Congcong Zhou [1,2], Zhao Yang [2], Kaitai Li [2] and Xuesong Ye [2,*]

1 Sir Run Run Shaw Hospital, School of Medicine, Zhejiang University, 3 East Qingchun Road, Hangzhou 310016, China
2 Key Laboratory for Biomedical Engineering of Education Ministry, Department of Biomedical Engineering, Zhejiang University, Hangzhou 310027, China
* Correspondence: yexuesong@zju.edu.cn

Abstract: The ankle joint is one of the important joints of the human body to maintain the ability to walk. Diseases such as stroke and ankle osteoarthritis could weaken the body's ability to control joints, causing people's gait to be out of balance. Ankle–foot orthoses can assist users with neuro/muscular or ankle injuries to restore their natural gait. Currently, passive ankle–foot orthoses are mostly designed to fix the ankle joint and provide support for walking. With the development of materials, sensing, and control science, semi-active orthoses that release mechanical energy to assist walking when needed and can store the energy generated by body movement in elastic units, as well as active ankle–foot orthoses that use external energy to transmit enhanced torque to the ankle, have received increasing attention. This article reviews the development process of ankle–foot orthoses and proposes that the integration of new ankle–foot orthoses with rehabilitation technologies such as monitoring or myoelectric stimulation will play an important role in reducing the walking energy consumption of patients in the study of human-in-the-loop models and promoting neuro/muscular rehabilitation.

Keywords: ankle–foot orthoses; energy consumption; functional electrical stimulation; human in the loop

Citation: Zhou, C.; Yang, Z.; Li, K.; Ye, X. Research and Development of Ankle–Foot Orthoses: A Review. *Sensors* **2022**, *22*, 6596. https://doi.org/10.3390/s22176596

Academic Editor: Antonio Fernández-Caballero

Received: 27 June 2022
Accepted: 29 August 2022
Published: 1 September 2022

Publisher's Note: MDPI stays neutral with regard to jurisdictional claims in published maps and institutional affiliations.

Copyright: © 2022 by the authors. Licensee MDPI, Basel, Switzerland. This article is an open access article distributed under the terms and conditions of the Creative Commons Attribution (CC BY) license (https://creativecommons.org/licenses/by/4.0/).

1. Introduction

Ankle joint injury is mainly caused by external forces or nervous system diseases such as hemiplegia. Particularly, stroke has the highest morbidity and fatality rate, there are 16 million people worldwide who suffer from strokes yearly and 6 million patients die from the disease [1]. Stroke patients with foot drop often exhibit a pattern of motion compensation that causes the slowing down of swing rhythm. At the same time, due to the shortened standing phase on the affected side, the energy consumption (EC) of walking is increased [2]. Ankle osteoarthritis (AO) affects more than 1% of the global population, and 70–80% of AO cases are caused by traumatic injury [3], which leads to long-term joint pain and decreased quality of life [4]. Severe ankle motor dysfunction could affect the patient's lower limb motor ability, and increase the burden on family and society [5].

An ankle–foot orthosis (AFO) is applied to the ankle joint to improve walking ability, prevent or correct ankle–foot deformities, maintain the stability of lower limb joints, and enhance the load-bearing capacity of lower limbs [6]. It can also compensate for ankle–foot functions and promote the functional recovery of lower limbs through elastic materials or external forces [7]. In the case of muscle weakness, AFO provides auxiliary torques for dorsiflexion and plantarflexion. While in the case of muscle spasms, AFO provides limiting torques [8]. Appropriate orthotic design directly promotes the patient's rehabilitation process, especially in restoring natural gait patterns [9]. AFO has attracted extensive attention from researchers since the 1970s. With more than 40 years of development, researchers have carried out a large number of targeted and innovative designs on the AFOs aiming at promoting lower limb rehabilitation. This review analyzes the design and development of

AFOs from the perspective of improving walking ability and reducing walking EC, and it is concluded that the fusion of new AFO design and other rehabilitation technologies such as functional electrical stimulation (FES) may be expected to play a more important role in reducing EC in human in the loop and promoting neuromuscular rehabilitation.

2. The Design and Development of AFOs

2.1. Literature Review Strategy

The systematic review protocol was developed in accordance with the Preferred Reporting Items for Systematic Reviews and Meta-Analyses (PRISMA) statement.

2.1.1. Search Strategy

Electronic database searches were performed from March 2022 to June 2022, conducted in Web of Science, IEEE Xplore, and PubMed Central according to search terms related to AFOs categories (Ankle Foot Orthosis*, Static ankle-foot orthoses*, fixed ankle-foot orthoses*, dynamic ankle-foot orthoses*, articulating ankle-foot orthoses*, non-articulating ankle-foot orthoses*, semi-active ankle-foot orthoses*) combined with lower extremity rehabilitation-related vocabulary (stroke*, foot drop*, foot inversion*, foot valgus*, gait cycle*, walking energy*, muscle activation*).

2.1.2. Eligibility Criteria, Research Options, and Data Extraction

Studies of human participants of any sample size were eligible, and there were no age, gender, cultural, or ethnic restrictions. Studies must have investigated the use of any type of ankle–foot orthosis (static ankle–foot orthosis, fixed ankle–foot orthosis, dynamic ankle–foot orthosis, articulating ankle–foot orthosis, non-articulating ankle-foot orthosis, semiactive ankle–foot orthosis) on outcomes related to walking ability or biomechanical function, mechanical properties, patient comfort, pain, and disability. Any other type of orthoses (orthoses for ankle joints, hip and knee joints) or orthoses not used for walking (such as massage therapy) were excluded. Unpublished data and data from studies that were not fully published were excluded.

After duplicates were removed, two authors (C.Z.) and (Z.Y.) screened titles and abstracts from the search results using predetermined eligibility criteria. Full-text articles were searched and independently reviewed for inclusion by two authors (X.Y. and K.L.). Data extraction and evaluation of the remaining articles were then independently completed by two authors (C.Z. and Z.Y.). Data extraction included study design, design features, and experimental effects.

2.1.3. Description of Included Studies

The initial electronic database search retrieved a total of 2126 articles, leaving 689 articles after deduplication. After completing the title and abstract screening, 83 articles were selected for possible inclusion in this review. After full-text screening, 52 studies met the inclusion criteria and were included in this review [10–61]. A flowchart of the search history and selection process is shown in Figure 1.

AFOs are usually designed from the shank to the sole of the foot and can maintain proper movement of the ankle joint. AFOs act on the shank and foot through the action of force to prevent foot drop, eversion, and inversion. The benefits of using AFOs are to help patients relieve physical pain and improve their self-care ability and quality of life. Scholars have also paid attention to utilizing AFOs to improve walking ability and reduce walking EC. Currently, new AFOs design mainly focus on the manufacture and combination with elastic materials or external dynamics.

Sensors **2022**, 22, 6596

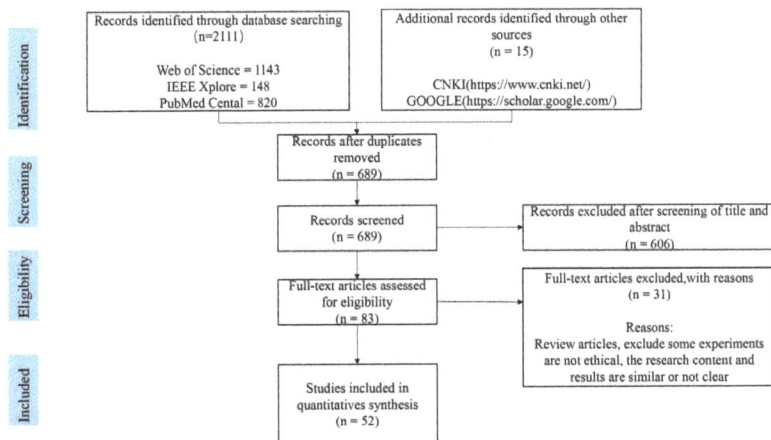

Figure 1. Flow diagram of the literature review process.

2.2. Classification and Development

There are many types of orthoses at present. In 1992, the International Standardization Organization (ISO) defined AFOs with the nomenclature of orthosis assembly parts into ankle–foot orthoses (AFOs), knee-ankle–foot orthoses (KAFOs), and hip-knee-ankle–foot orthoses (HKAFOs) [62]. According to the different functional structures, AFOs can be divided into static AFOs, dynamic AFOs, and custom AFOs [63]. Recently, AFOs are divided into passive ankle–foot orthoses (PAFOs), semi-active ankle–foot orthoses (SAFOs), and active ankle–foot orthoses (AAFOs) according to whether the devices can directly provide power for walking [10,11].

This review will describe the detailed research and development process based on how the AFOs provide power. As shown in Figure 2, this includes: (1) PAFOs, which include static ankle–foot orthosis, partial hinged ankle–foot orthosis, and dynamic ankle–foot orthosis. The PAFOs proposed in this review are not comprised of electrical/electronic elements or power sources. They are usually comprised of mechanical elements such as dampers or springs; (2) SAFOs, which use brakes as control elements, such as active clutches and adaptive dampers. SAFOs can adaptively adjust joint impedance or recycle walking energy, but do not provide additional power for walking directly; (3) AAFOs, which are usually composed of a power supply, control system, sensors, and actuators. AAFOs can provide extra power directly for walking. Generally, PAFOs usually have a relatively simple structure and production process. They are mainly applied to limit the movement of the ankle joint, while PAFOs can store part of the energy generated by body movement in linear or spring elements, then release energy when needed to assist walking. The structure, utilizations, and control strategies of AFOs are shown in Figure 3. SAFOs and AAFOs can provide assistance for patients to walk by controlling actuators, and improve the ankle joint movement of patients with dysfunction caused by various injuries and neurological diseases. In recent years, researchers focus on how to improve walking ability and reduce walking EC by proper system design.

2.3. General Research and Development Processes of AFOs

The design and manufactural processes of different AFOs categories are mainly consistent. In this section, this review summarizes and analyzes the general design and production processes of AFOs. As shown in Figure 4, the processes flow includes functional design, structural design, model design, motion simulation, production inspection [64,65], and clinical research [66]. Within these processes, structural design, model design, and motion simulation play significant and important roles in achieving reliable function and reaching the standards of clinical research. The detail design contents are concluded as follows.

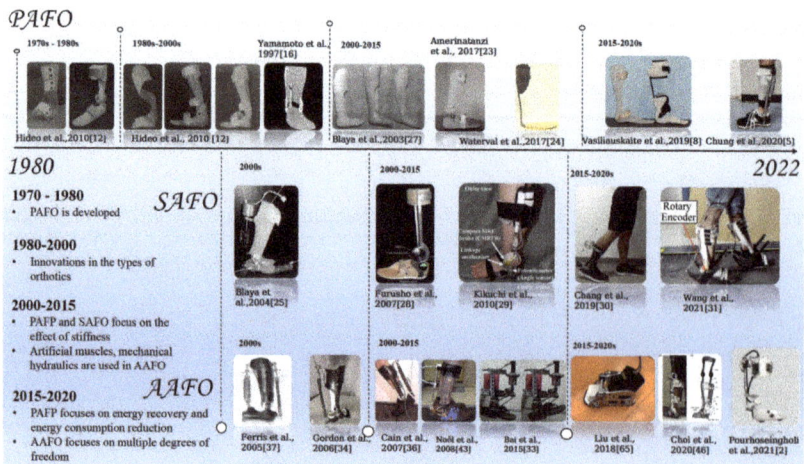

Figure 2. Classification and development trends of AFOs.

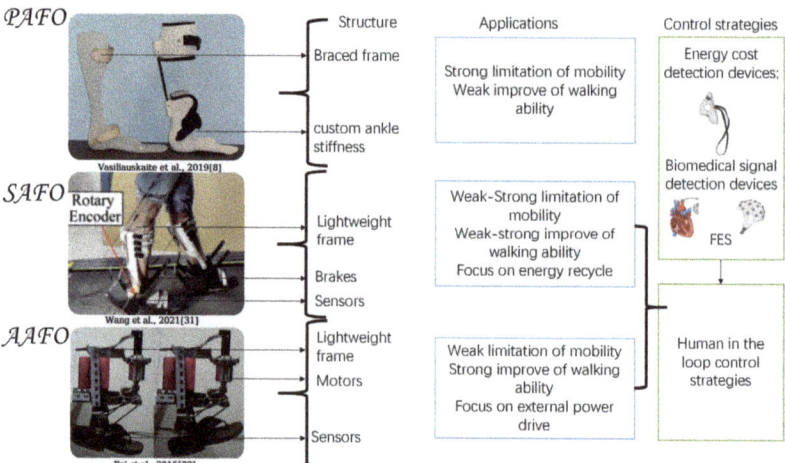

Figure 3. Structure, utilizations, and control strategies of AFOs.

(1) Functional design: Functional design process includes requirements analysis. The requirements analysis mainly focuses on understanding, analyzing, and sorting out the basic demands of the user. It can be divided into physical needs and psychological needs. The functional design of AFOs are carried out on the basis of requirements analysis.

(2) Structural design: Structural design mainly refers to the determination of the overall structure of the AFOs. The overall structure may be divided into fixed type and active type. The fixed type generally plays the role of support, protection, fixation, and load relief. The active type could increase the range of motion of the ankle joint and assist the movement.

(3) Model design: The model design includes model establishment and material selection. The model establishment is mainly to obtain human body data through direct measurement or three-dimensional scanning, and then generate ankle models on the

computer. Material selection is based on the function of each structure. The main materials are carbon fiber and synthetic plastics, occasionally alloys, foams, ceramics, and so forth.

(4) Motion simulation: It is important for the orthosis to work according to the functional design. Finite element analysis of the assembly, which provides the analysis of static structural strength and stiffness, should be performed. If the analysis results meet the strength and stiffness requirements, the product could be processed and produced. Otherwise, if the analysis results are not satisfactory, the structural design of the AFOs need to be re-carried out.

(5) Production inspection: Production inspection includes device fabrication and experimental inspection. The traditional fabrication method of AFOs adopts the method of injection molding, which uses a plate with a constant thickness that normally has a long production cycle. This method is difficult to iteratively optimize in the future [67,68]. On the other hand, 3D printing technology is based on intelligent digital models, it uses metal, plastic, and other adhesive materials to construct objects with layer-by-layer printing. It can be directly formed or customized and has great potential in the production of AFOs. After the production process, the orthosis is tested through material experiments which focus on evaluating the mechanical properties of the orthosis. The structural design needs to be re-carried out if it does not meet the standards.

(6) Clinical research: Clinical research usually recruits healthy volunteers or patients as experimental subjects to analyze the impact of AFOs on human walking ability, biomechanics, and walking EC through 3D motion capture equipment, EMG sensors, EC testers, and other instruments [69,70]. In addition, some studies have shown that AFOs combined with rehabilitation methods such as botulinum toxin and FES may have better effects on rehabilitation [71,72]. Some authors utilized botulinum toxin type A injection combined with an ankle–foot orthosis to improve the rehabilitation process of patients with post-stroke lower limb spasticity.

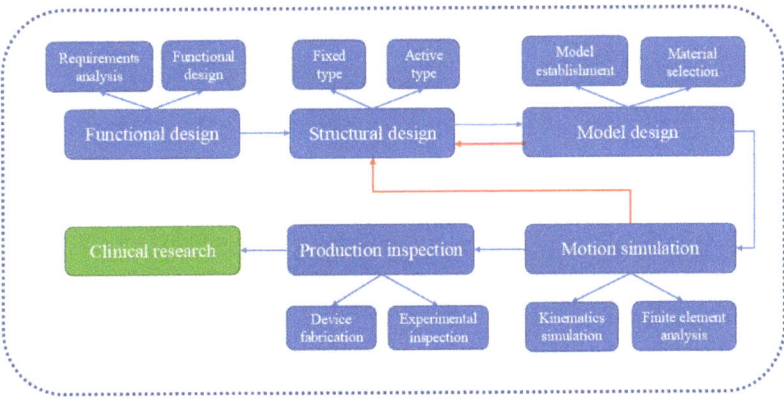

Figure 4. Design and manufactural processes of AFOs.

2.3.1. Passive Ankle–Foot Orthoses (PAFOs)

As analyzed previously, PAFOs do not have any electronic control elements to control ankle motion during gait other than mechanical elements such as springs or shock absorbers. PAFOs can be subdivided into articulated devices and nonarticulated devices [10]. Passive non-articulating ankle–foot orthoses (PNAAFOs) are usually one piece that holds the ankle completely in one position. Passive articulating ankle–foot orthoses (PAAFOs) are designed to combine a lightweight thermoplastic or carbon composite shell with an articulating joint that allows a range of motion in the ankle joint. Articulated joints come in different designs with various hinges, flexion stops, and stiffness control elements such as springs, oil dampers, one-way friction clutches, and so forth.

Primevally, a large number of PNAAFOs were studied [12]. They were mainly designed to hold the ankle in one position and limit the mobility of plantarflexion thoroughly. However, the materials of the orthoses were stiff, which might result in excessive knee flexion moments during load response which resulted in unsteady walking. With the advancement of material science, the design of PNAAFOs gradually evolved from rigid to elastic. The characteristics of these orthoses mainly depended on the material and geometry [11,13,14]. Rear leaf spring orthoses were semi-rigid plastic orthoses that assisted toe flexion and prevented falls during the pre-swing period. Carbon fiber orthoses are another typical semi-rigid orthoses that can significantly improve pathological gait by storing energy during deformation and increasing thrust during the pre-swing period. Researchers have shown that carbon fiber orthoses can reduce energy expenditure in impaired patients [15].

PAAFOs appeared in large numbers in the 1980s and 1990s. The Okawa Ankle-Foot Orthosis was developed by Okawa Hara in 1981 [12] and provided some lateral stability through its lateral joints. Since then, articulated orthoses of different joint styles have sprung up one after another. At the beginning of the 21st century, articulated orthoses were continuously improved. In 1997, Yamamoto et al. [16] improved articulated orthosis with dorsiflexion assistance. A traditional AFO along with the Klenzak ankle joint was modified to prevent falls during walking. Their modified design added a spring to the rear of the orthotic tibia, which might create plantarflexion resistance when the heel touches the ground and prevent the foot from slipping. In 2002, Kawamura et al. [17] developed a passive mechanical element with variable elasticity and viscosity. The material was soft and light, and the element itself was small in size. The mechanical impedance of the element could be changed by adjusting the vacuum pressure applied to it. These characteristics made passive pneumatic components more convenient than active components of the wearable robot, such as electromagnetic, magnetorheological, or electrorheological brakes. Before the advent of oil dampers, orthoses were more likely to use spring dampers. In 2005, Yamamoto et al. [18] developed a small, lightweight hydraulic oil damper to provide torque resistance to plantarflexion. The oil damper absorbed the shock of heel impact and provided damping during load response.

Researchers have also studied the interaction between AFOs and the human body. Geboers et al. [19] studied ankle fixation and its effect on dorsiflexor strength, and their results showed that the use of AFO after nerve injury may lead to reduced dorsiflexor strength in a short period of time. Studies have shown that AFOs should provide horizontal resistance to flexion of the digits to simulate eccentric contraction of the dorsiflexors, thereby allowing a limited amount of loading response to act on plantarflexion [20]. A study by Hesse et al. [21] found that reduced dorsiflexor activity may lead to disuse atrophy and long-term dependence on orthoses. These studies suggested that insufficient orthotic stiffness may result in insufficient biomechanical control of ankle motion and excessive knee extension during gait, which in turn might lead to a stiff walking gait cycle, lower muscle activity, and muscle atrophy. Therefore, ankle-fixed AFOs, including PNNAFOs, might delay recovery in patients with neurological impairment.

In view of this, researchers have developed innovative AFOs with the motive of designing AFOs with predetermined stiffness or variable stiffness that meet the individual needs of patients. In 2015, Mataee et al. [22] proposed two technical solutions for the design of variable stiffness orthosis based on the mechanical and structural stiffness control of shape memory alloys. These designs could improve gait abnormalities in patients with foot drop for different walking conditions (e.g., different walking speeds). The first design modulated the torsional stiffness by controlling the axial load with the superelastic rod, and the other modulated the bending stiffness of the element by adjusting the effective length of the superelastic hinge. Although Mataee's study effectively solved the problem of variable stiffness, it was difficult to control the shape-memory alloy components during cooling. Amirhesam et al. [23] found that the hyperelastic NiTi spring had nonlinear characteristics in elongation and compression. They hypothesized that the hinge could make the stiffness of the ankle more similar to that of a healthy person, which could help patients walk more naturally. On this basis, they focused on the performance of the hyperelastic NiTi spring and the transmission stainless steel spring and found that the NiTi spring could provide a wider range of motion and increased torque level. In addition to exploring the effect on gait, some studies also showed that the reduction in walking energy was related to the stiffness of the orthosis. Niels et al. [24] produced an AFO with adjustable stiffness using carbon fiber plate springs. For each patient, they assessed the walking energy costs, gait biomechanics, and walking speed of five AFOs with different stiffness. The results were used to determine the optimal stiffness for each patient.

In conclusion, PNAAFOs and PAAFOs are mainly distinguished by the degree of wrapping of the ankle and the structural design, as shown in Table 1. There are various types of PNAAFOs, and their main functions are to limit the movement of the ankle joint and provide support for the patient to walk. Although PNAAFOs can improve pathological gait to a certain extent and reduce walking EC, they limit the normal motion of the ankle joint. On the basis of the PNAAFOs, the PAAFOs provide a certain range of motion for the ankle joint through structural design. Both of PNAAFOs and PAAFOs can improve foot biomechanics and walking ability, reduce walking EC by adjusting joint stiffness, and enable patients to have a near-normal gait.

Table 1. Comparison of features and functions between PNAAFOs and PAAFOs.

Category	Device Name/Author	Design Features	Effects	Ref.
PNAAFOs	Ortholen drop foot brace	Half wrap ankle	1. Fix ankle 2. Provide lateral stability	[12]
	Ortop AFO LH	No wrap ankle	1. Limit plantarflexion 2. Provide lateral stability	[12]
	Finer AFO	Full wrap ankle	1. Fix ankle 2. Provide lateral stability	[12]
PAAFOs	Okawa, H	Simple hinge	1. Promote dorsiflexion 2. Limit plantarflexion 3. Provide lateral stability	[12]
	Yamamoto, S	Spring	1. Reduce knee hyperextension 2. Increase walking speed 3. Adjust the dorsiflexion auxiliary moment	[16]
	Yamamoto, S	Oil Damper	1. Promote dorsiflexion 2. Correct varus/valgus 3. Adjust orthosis stiffness	[18]
	Mataee, M	Shape Memory Alloys	1. Improve biomechanics 2. Promote normal plantarflexion	[22]
	Amerinatanzi, A	Superelastic NiTi Spring	1. Greater range of motion 2. Promote normal plantarflexion	[23]
	Waterval, N	Customed spring	1. Reduce walking EC 2. Improve biomechanics 3. Increase walking speed	[24]

2.3.2. Semi-Active Ankle–Foot Orthoses (SAFOs)

The motor control of PAFOs is limited by passive components as discussed while SAFOs and AAFOs have the ability to interact with the walking environment. SAFOs consist of electronic control systems, actuators, tethered or untethered powertrains, and stiffness control elements such as magnetorheological (MR) fluid brakes. Normal control systems typically include components such as force sensors, accelerometers, and microprocessors. Blaaya et al. [25–27] developed a SAFO with variable impedance based on elastic brakes. The elastic brake consists of a direct current motor, a mechanical connecting rod, and a torsion spring which could actively adjust the joint impedance of the ankle. The developed actuator weighed 2.6 Kg and required a bulky battery as a power supply. Furusho et al. [28,29] proposed installing an MR fluid brake at the ankle joint. The device could control the brake force by changing the intensity of the applied magnetic field, and it could provide a maximum resisting torque of 11.8 N·m. In addition, the authors applied the connecting rod mechanism to amplify the torque which was up to 24 N·m. Kikuchi et al. [29] further developed a more compact MR fluid brake. Compared with the previous prototypes, the proposed orthosis had a lighter weight, a more sensitive control system, and could assist ankle plantarflexion. SAFOs were further applied to recover gait energy during walking, provided assistance, and reduced walking EC. Chang et al. [30] developed an energy recovery system composed of a torsion spring and two actively controlled clutches to control the accurate time point of energy recovery and energy release. Wang et al. [31] developed a novel, lightweight heel strike energy storage mechanism including a clutch. They applied a series of springs that helped users reduce walking EC.

Table 2 demonstrates the comparison of SAFOs in mass and effects. The power assist control units within SAFOs are evolving in the direction of lightness and precise control. The weights of SAFOs are gradually reduced from 2.6 Kg to nearly 1 Kg, or even less than 800 g. This is a clear advantage of SAFOs over AAFOs. In terms of the assisting effects provided by SAFOs, the range of resistance torque that the device could provide should be studied first. Then, the benefits of SAFOs on human walking might be studied in the form of muscle activation during walking by myoelectric sensors and EC testing instruments directly.

Table 2. Comparison of SAFOs in mass and effect.

Author	Motion Control Elements	Mass	Effect	Ref.
Blaya, J	Series Elastic Actuator	2.6 Kg	——	[25]
Furusho, J	Magnetorheological Fluid	1.6 Kg	Provide 24 N·m resistance torque	[28]
Kikuchi, T	Magnetorheological Fluid	0.99 Kg	Provide 10 N·m resistance torque	[29]
Chang, Y	Spring Clutch	0.9 Kg	10–20% decrease in gastrocnemius muscle activation	[30]
Wang, C	Spring Clutch	0.754 Kg	6% reduction in metabolic cost	[31]

2.3.3. Active Ankle–Foot Orthoses (AAFOs)

Torque can be transmitted to the ankle by AAFOs using external energy and power units, while the orthosis may be adjusted by computer control to give the users a more natural gait [32]. Pneumatic muscles are characterized by light weight and high power, and are gradually being applied in the development of AAFOs [33]. As a typical representative, Ferris et al. [34–37] proposed an AAFO that could provide the torque required for toe flexion and dorsiflexion through two artificial pneumatic muscles. The device was relatively lightweight (1.6 Kg), and the user's peak plantarflexion torque was reduced by 64% and the peak dorsiflexion torque was increased by 23% after wearing it. The experiment required an onboard power supply and computer assistance, which was suitable for laboratory research and rehabilitation. In view of the above-mentioned limits, Alex et al. [38] proposed a kind of pneumatic driven orthosis that might be used daily in the household. The device had a bidirectional rotating air motor at the ankle and a CO_2 bottle with a regulator at the waist. The power supply was separated from the actuator to minimize the weight of the ankle. The experimental results showed that the system had an obvious auxiliary effect on functional plantarflexion. However, since the system could only provide 9 N·m of torque at rated power, it was mainly suitable for auxiliary plantarflexion.

With the deepening of research, hydraulic technology has also emerged in this research area. Compared with electromechanical systems, hydraulic technology has the advantages of high power and is only limited by the pressure of the working fluid [39,40]. Studies have shown that compared with the equivalent electromechanical system above 500 pounds per square inch (psi), the overall weight of the 100-watt hydraulic system is lighter [41]. Compared to electric motors, hydraulic systems have higher responsiveness and greater stiffness, enabling faster start-up and stops along with small position errors [39,42]. Brett et al. [32] designed a hydraulic AAFO which consisted of a hydraulic power source at the waist and a hydraulic brake at the ankle, connected by a pair of hoses. The weight of the ankle actuator and the power supply met the design requirements of 1.0 Kg for the ankle and 3.5 Kg for the waist. Although the total weight of the system was similar to the weight of the electromechanical system, lightweight hydraulic actuators could significantly decrease the ankle weight compared with the electromechanical system. Martin et al. [43] combined the characteristics of the electric and hydraulic systems, and designed an electro-hydraulic AAFO that could provide forward rotation of the ankle joint. Kim et al. [44] proposed a completely unconstrained pneumatic AAFO powered by a custom compressor, which miniaturized the compressor by optimizing the air compression rate to help foot-fall patients.

Studies have shown that the range of motion (ROM) of the ankle valgus is highly correlated with walking stability [45]. The ankle valgus maintains the center of pressure (COP) of the supporting foot and prevents the body from tilting to one side. Specifically, when the body is tilted, the misalignment between the projection of the center of gravity and the COP causes the tilting moment, and the subtalar joint could be rotated around the front surface to maintain the balance of the body. This move, known as the foot tilting strategy (FTS), produces stabilizing moments and returns the unstable body to a balanced position. Most studies of AAFOs have focused on sagittal motion, and they are useful in assisting with dorsiflexion, but not in valgus ROM. Choi et al. [46] designed a 2-DOF (degree of freedom) AFO by simulating the ankle joint and subtalar joint, and verified the performance of artificial pneumatic muscles used for balance training.

As demonstrated in Table 3, AAFOs and SAFOs have obvious differences in the way of providing walking assistance. SAFOs commonly use spring clutches, elastic actuators, and MR fluid as brakes. They provide assistance for walking by changing the stiffness of the ankle joint or recovering energy instead of providing assistance for plantarflexion and dorsiflexion directly. AAFOs usually use pneumatic artificial muscles, mechanical electric drives, and hydraulic methods to provide the torque of plantarflexion and dorsiflexion for human walking directly. The weight gradually decreases as a split design is usually applied to reduce the load-bearing of the ankle joint.

Table 3. Comparison of AAFOs in mass and effect.

Author	Motion Control Elements	Mass	Effect	Ref.
Neubauer, B	Hydraulic boost	1 Kg at the ankle, 1.5 Kg at the Waist	Maximum 60 N·m auxiliary torque	[32]
Ferris, D	Artificial Pneumatic Muscle	Total weight 1.7 Kg	64% reduction in peak plantarflexion torque and 23% increase in peak dorsiflexion torque	[35]
Cain, S	Artificial Pneumatic Muscle	――	53% reduction in peak plantarflexion torque	[36]
Shorter, K	Bidirectional pneumatic rotary actuator	1.9 Kg at the ankle, total weight 3.1 Kg	Provides 9 N·m plantarflexion torque	[38]
Noel, M	Electro-hydraulic system	Total weight 1.7 Kg	Provide 20 N·m auxiliary torque	[43]
Kim, S	Pneumatic components	0.5 Kg at the ankle, total weight 2.6 Kg	Provide 9.8 N·m plantarflexion torque	[44]
Choi, H	Artificial Pneumatic Muscle	1.44 Kg at the ankle, total weight 2.14 Kg	――	[46]

3. Discussion

The motion control units and potential effects of the discussed three types of AFOs are shown in Tables 1–3. PAFOs are widely applied in the field of ankle and foot rehabilitation because of their simple structural design and production process. However, PNAAFOs limit the movement of the ankle joint and are more effective in fixing the ankle and providing support for patients to walk, which have limitations when applied. Compared with non-articulating orthoses, articulated ankle–foot orthoses can adjust ankle stiffness by controlling springs, oil dampers, and magnetorheological fluid brakes, further improving biomechanics and promoting patient recovery. SAFOs and AAFOs can directly or indirectly assist patients in walking through electronic control systems, and they have advantages in improving walking ability and reducing walking energy consumption.

The development of orthoses, on the basis of the above-summarized structures and efforts, draws more attention to the integration with other rehabilitation technologies such as FES technology. Another development trend is as a part of walking assistance devices which are used for the study of walking ability and walking EC in human-in-the-loop models, and to explore new motion control strategies to further promote the motion recovery of single and multi-joint lower limbs.

3.1. Combined Study of AFOs and FES

For individuals with stroke or hemiplegia, walking ability is one of the most important indicators to evaluate the recovery of motor function. During the rehabilitation process, the joint movement pattern of the extensor muscles may cause abnormal gait such as foot drop, which affects walking efficiency and increases the risk of falling [47]. Studies have shown that the combination of AFOs and FES has a better effect on foot drop caused by upper motor neuron palsy, by installing electrodes locally on the AFOs and applying FES during walking. During this process, AFOs can control the joint mobility of the ankle joint to a certain extent, which helps to improve walking stability, while it may limit the plantarflexion of the ankle joint when the foot is off the ground and affect the walking speed [48,49]. FES can enhance the input stimulation of nerves and accelerate the establishment of cerebral collateral circulation without affecting the ankle plantarflexion when off the ground, which promotes the establishment of normal movement patterns [50,51]. The establishment of cerebral collateral circulation could reflect the rehabilitation status of patients with cerebral palsy. Early ankle dorsiflexion training and toe stimulation of peripheral sensory muscles can regulate the excitability of neurons in the neural reflex circuit, as well as promote the establishment of ankle dorsiflexion muscle responses. These rehabilitation strategies can improve the contractile load and muscle tension of related muscle groups and inhibit pathological gait such as foot drop [52].

Pagnussat et al. [53] assessed the effect of FES on the peroneal nerve on walking speed, ankle dorsiflexion range of motion, balance, and functional range of motion. Results showed that FES could improve ankle dorsiflexion, balance, and functional mobility. Nevisipour's team [54] investigated: (1) the underlying biomechanical mechanisms of falls in chronic stroke patients using AFOs and FES for a long time; (2) the effects of AFOs and FES devices on the occurrence of falls in chronic stroke patients. The results showed that the AFOs/FES devices had a positive effect on static balance (balance ability during static motion) and could reduce the occurrence of falling events. It is necessary to explore methods and devices to enhance the establishment of dynamic balance (balance ability during dynamic motion) in the future. Khaghani's team [55] compared the improvement of balance and walking ability in patients with multiple sclerosis (MS), a chronic progressive nervous disorder, by using FES alone and FES combined with AFOs. The results showed that under the condition of the AFOs equipped with the FES system, the patient's postural response when walking back and forth was better than that of the FES system alone. In their study, only PNAAFO is used, while PAAFO, SAFO, and AAFO are expected to show better results in comparative studies in terms of rehabilitation.

Some other researchers focused on comparing the effects of AFOs and FES as separate rehabilitation methods on the establishment of static and dynamic balance, and comparing the advantages and disadvantages of the two methods in reducing walking EC and improving walking ability [56,57]. There was also research comparing the improvement of walking ability between FES alone and FES with PNAAFO, and the preliminary results verified that the fusion of the above two technologies could help improve the rehabilitation effect. However, there is still a lack of assessment and discussion on how FES and AFOs can be integrated, and the exploration of the sequence and method of FES application still needs to be further developed to reduce the occurrence of falls caused by long-term use [54].

3.2. Research on AFOs in Human in the Loop

In recent years, AFOs have played an important role in the study of human-in-the-loop control strategies. Prof. Collins' team [58] designed an underactuated ankle exoskeleton. The device used a spring to simulate the Achilles tendon of the human body, which realized the energy storage and release at each stage of the human walking process and reduced the walking EC by 7.2%. Based on the idea of human in the loop, the assist torque was corrected through EC detection, and the target ankle joint assist curve was parameterized. By detecting the metabolic consumption of the human body, their team used the covariance matrix adaptive evolution strategy to adjust the parameters of the assist curve and iteratively generate the optimal assist curve, so that the metabolic consumption of the human body under the assistance of the exoskeleton was the lowest. The metabolic consumption was 24.2 ± 7.4% lower than that of the zero assist torque. Zhang's team [59] presented 10 kinds of ankle walking-assist exoskeleton assist curves, and used the particle swarm algorithm to solve a set of optimal weight coefficient combinations of the activation degrees of different muscles as an evaluation function of the human in the loop.

The related research results showed that the use of the new evaluation function to optimize the power assist curve in the loop control of the human body could further reduce the degree of muscle activation during walking. Zachary's team designed a real-time adaptive ankle exoskeleton controller capable of accurately assisting in a variety of walking conditions without the need for walking condition classification or real-time assessment of muscle activity, which provided the foundation for the application of AAFO in free-living situation [60]. However, the muscle coordination mode of the human body during walking can be changed to a certain extent affected by AFO, and then result in the compensatory phenomenon of some muscle groups. It is necessary for researchers to further study the theory of physical–physiological integration of human–computer interaction [61]. The problem of how to reasonably select the activation degree and weight of the lower limb muscles is still unsolved. A strategy that ensures the optimal labor saving achieved under the condition of AFOs assistance and maintains the original muscle coordination mode as much as possible should be studied in future work. To conclude, firstly, there are a series of studies focusing on how to map kinematics or kinetics parameters such as joint angles and torques from 'superior' bio-parameters such as located EEG signals and muscle synergies. These 'superior' bio-parameters can be obtained by a series of processing methods, such as blind source separation methods and over complete dictionary methods on collected EEG signals and sEMG signals to obtain sparsity features or features in other domains for data dimension reduction or a more accurate and robust mapping result. These features contain physiological factors so that, on one hand, they have a better real-time ability and a more compliant man-machine control strategy. On the other hand, they are closer to the physiological background of motion control strategies so they are normally appropriate for research on neural rehabilitation. Secondly, energy consumption during human activities such as walking has been fully researched in recent years. However, energy consumption relies on real-time dynamics gas component analysis techniques and devices which are commonly difficult to be used in real environments. More convenient energy consumption evaluation methods need to be further researched in the future.

4. Conclusions

In conclusion, this paper reviews the recent literature on the innovative design of AFOs, and discusses the development of PAFOs, SAFOs, and AAFOs. PAFOs have attracted attention since the 1980s and scholars have studied continuous designs for the shape and ankle joint styles of AFOs. With the advancement of clinical rehabilitation technology and the in-depth study of human walking gait, the further development of AFOs has been promoted from shape and style to material properties and muscle group responses. SAFOs and AAFOs have been studied since the early 21st century. Scholars focused on how to reduce the weight of the overall device and increase the portability and wearing experience of the device through different technical methods firstly, and then mainly focus on the role in the field of rehabilitation recently. In addition, it is also important to pay attention to the impact of joint movements other than the ankle so as to provide a new way for clinical rehabilitation training. However, the fundamental research on AFOs is still facing problems such as most experiments on AFOs focusing on the motion angle of the ankle joint, the moment of plantarflexion, and dorsiflexion while the muscle state and in-depth physiological indicators are rarely assessed accurately. Some studies have carried out experiments on the combination of AFOs, botulinum toxin, and FES while most of them are mechanical combinations, and the discussions on the mechanism are rare. In order to achieve smooth and labor-saving walking assistance, it is urgent to focus on breakthroughs in the AFOs elastic drive design and human-in-the-loop assist control technology to carry out theoretical research on the integration of human–computer interaction and physics–physiology integration theory. In addition to studying detailed materials and mechanical properties, innovative AFOs also need to be combined with other clinical rehabilitation methods to provide new ideas and methods for patient rehabilitation.

Author Contributions: Conceptualization, C.Z. and X.Y.; Data curation and Formal analysis, Z.Y. and C.Z.; Funding acquisition, C.Z.; Investigation, Z.Y., K.L. and C.Z.; Methodology, Z.Y. and C.Z. Resources, C.Z. and X.Y.; Writing—original draft, Z.Y. and C.Z.; Writing—review and editing, C.Z., Z.Y., K.L. and X.Y. All authors have read and agreed to the published version of the manuscript.

Funding: This research was supported by Zhejiang Provincial Natural Science Foundation of China under Grant No. LY22H180006, No. LY21E050020.

Institutional Review Board Statement: Not applicable.

Informed Consent Statement: Not applicable.

Data Availability Statement: Not applicable.

Acknowledgments: The authors would like to thank the related researchers in this area. We also would like to thank Heng Liao, Heyuan Wang, Xuqing Dai, Hangqin Ni, and Qi Zhou for their kind help.

Conflicts of Interest: The authors declare no conflict of interest.

Abbreviations

The following abbreviations are used in this manuscript:

AO	Ankle osteoarthritis
AFO	Ankle–foot orthosis
FES	Functional electrical stimulation
EC	Energy consumption
PAFO	Passive ankle–foot orthosis
SAFO	Semi-active ankle–foot orthosis
AAFO	Active ankle–foot orthosis
PNAAFO	Passive non-articulating ankle–foot orthosis
PAAFO	Passive articulating ankle–foot orthosis
ROM	Range of motion
COP	Center of pressure
FTS	Foot tilting strategy
DOF	Degree of freedom

References

1. Pitchai, B.; Khin, M.; Gowraganahalli, J. Prevalence and prevention of cardiovascular disease and diabetes mellitus. *Pharmacol. Res.* **2016**, *113*, 600–609.
2. Pourhoseingholi, E.; Saeedi, H. Role of the newly designed Ankle Foot Orthosis on balance related parametersin drop foot post stroke patients. *J. Bodyw. Mov. Ther.* **2021**, *26*, 501–504. [CrossRef]

3. Barg, A.; Pagenstert, G.I.; Hügle, T.; Gloyer, M.; Wiewiorski, M.; Henninger, H.B.; Valderrabano, V. Ankle osteoarthritis: Etiology, diagnostics, and classification. *Foot Ankle Clin.* **2013**, *18*, 411–426. [CrossRef]
4. Brockett, C.L.; Chapman, G.J. Biomechanics of the ankle. *Orthop. Trauma* **2016**, *30*, 232–238. [CrossRef]
5. Chung, C.L.; DiAngelo, D.J.; Powell, D.W.; Paquette, M.R. Biomechanical comparison of a new dynamic ankle orthosis to a standard ankle-foot orthosis during walking. *J. Biomech. Eng.* **2020**, *142*, 051003–051010. [CrossRef]
6. Tang, Y.M.; Shu, B. Application and improvement of ankle-foot orthosis in cerebral palsy treatment. *Chin. J. Tissue Eng. Res.* **2008**, *39*, 7703–7706.
7. Li, W.; Wu, D.Y. Research Progress in Application of Ankle Foot Orthosis in Sports Rehabilitation of Children with Cerebral Palsy. *J. Fujian Norm. Univ.* **2017**, *33*, 102–108.
8. Vasiliauskaite, E.; Ielapi, A.; De Beule, M.; Van Paepegem, W.; Deckers, J.P.; Vermandel, M.; Forward, M.; Plasschaert, F. A study on the efficacy of AFO stiffness prescription. *Disabil. Rehabil.-Assit.* **2019**, *1*, 27–39. [CrossRef]
9. Ielapi, A.; Forward, M.; De Beule, M. Computational and experimental evaluation of the mechanical properties of ankle foot orthoses: A literature review. *Prosthet. Orthot. Int.* **2019**, *43*, 339–348. [CrossRef]
10. Alam, M.; Choudhury, I.A.; Mamat, A.B. Mechanism and design analysis of articulated ankle foot orthoses for drop-foot. *Sci. World J.* **2014**, *2014*, 867869. [CrossRef]
11. Daryabor, A.; Arazpour, M.; Aminian, G. Effect of different designs of ankle-foot orthoses on gait in patients with stroke: A systematic review. *Gait Posture* **2018**, *62*, 268–279. [CrossRef] [PubMed]
12. Hideo, W. *Lower Limb Braces for Stroke Patients*; Hochitw: Beijing, China, 2010; pp. 1–191.
13. Mulroy, S.J.; Eberly, V.J.; Gronely, J.K.; Weiss, W.; Newsam, C.J. Effect of AFO design on walking after stroke: Impact of ankle plantar flexion contracture. *Prosthet. Orthot. Int.* **2010**, *34*, 277–292. [CrossRef] [PubMed]
14. Ramsey, J.A. Development of a method for fabricating polypropylene non-articulated dorsiflexion assist ankle foot orthoses with predetermined stiffness. *Prosthet. Orthot. Int.* **2011**, *35*, 54–69. [CrossRef] [PubMed]
15. Bregman, D.J.J.; Harlaar, J.; Meskers, C.G.M.; De Groot, V. Spring-like Ankle Foot Orthoses reduce the energy cost of walking by taking over ankle work. *Gait Posture* **2012**, *35*, 148–153. [CrossRef]
16. Yamamoto, S.; Ebina, M.; Miyazaki, S.; Kawai, H.; Kubota, T. Development of a new ankle-foot orthosis with dorsiflexion assist, part 1: Desirable characteristics of ankle-foot orthoses for hemiplegic patients. *JPO J. Prosthetics Orthot.* **1997**, *9*, 174–179.
17. Kawamura, S.; Yamamoto, T.; Ishida, D.; Ogata, T.; Nakayama, Y.; Tabata, O.; Sugiyama, S. Development of passive elements with variable mechanical impedance for wearable robots. In Proceedings of the 2002 IEEE International Conference on Robotics and Automation (Cat. No. 02CH37292), Washington, DC, USA, 11–15 May 2002.
18. Yamamoto, S.; Hagiwara, A.; Mizobe, T.; Yokoyama, O.; Yasui, T. Development of an ankle–foot orthosis with an oil damper. *Prosthet. Orthot. Int.* **2005**, *29*, 209–219. [CrossRef]
19. Geboers, J.F.; Tuijl, J.V.; Seelen, H.A.M.; Drost, M.R. Effect of immobilization on ankle dorsiflexion strength. *Scand. J. Rehabil. Med.* **2000**, *32*, 66–71.
20. Ounpuu, S.; Bell, K.J.; Davis, R.B., III; DeLuca, P.A. An evaluation of the posterior leaf spring orthosis using joint kinematics and kinetics. *Prosthet. Orthot. Int.* **1996**, *16*, 378–384.
21. Hesse, S.; Werner, C.; Matthias, K.; Stephen, K.; Berteanu, M. Non–velocity-related effects of a rigid double-stopped ankle-foot orthosis on gait and lower limb muscle activity of hemiparetic subjects with an equinovarus deformity. *Stroke* **1999**, *30*, 1855–1861. [CrossRef]
22. Mataee, M.G.; Andani, M.T.; Elahinia, M. Adaptive ankle–foot orthoses based on superelasticity of shape memory alloys. *J. Intell. Mater. Syst. Struct.* **2015**, *26*, 639–651. [CrossRef]
23. Amerinatanzi, A.; Zamanian, H.; Shayesteh Moghaddam, N.; Jahadakbar, A.; Elahinia, M. Application of the superelastic NiTi spring in ankle foot orthosis (AFO) to create normal ankle joint behavior. *Bioengineering* **2017**, *4*, 95. [CrossRef] [PubMed]
24. Waterval, N.F.; Nollet, F.; Harlaar, J.; Brehm, M.A. Precision orthotics: Optimising ankle foot orthoses to improve gait in patients with neuromuscular diseases; protocol of the PROOF-AFO study, a prospective intervention study. *BMJ Open* **2017**, *7*, e013342. [CrossRef] [PubMed]
25. Blaya, J.A.; Herr, H. Adaptive control of a variable-impedance ankle-foot orthosis to assist drop-foot gait. *IEEE Trans. Neural Syst. Rehabil. Eng.* **2004**, *12*, 24–31. [CrossRef]
26. Blaya, J.A.; Newman, D.; Herr, H. *Active Ankle Foot Orthoses (AAFO)*; Artificial Intelligence Laboratory, Massachusetts Institute of Technology: Cambridge, MA, USA, 2002; pp. 275–277.
27. Blaya, J.A. Force-Controllable Ankle Foot Orthosis (AFO) to Assist Drop Foot Gait. Doctoral Dissertation, Massachusetts Institute of Technology, Cambridge, MA, USA, 2003.
28. Furusho, J.; Kikuchi, T.; Tokuda, M.; Kakehashi, T.; Ikeda, K.; Morimoto, S.; Hashimoto, Y.; Tomiyama, H.; Nakagawa, A.; Akazawa, Y. Development of shear type compact MR brake for the intelligent ankle-foot orthosis and its control; research and development in NEDO for practical application of human support robot. In Proceedings of the 2007 IEEE 10th International Conference on Rehabilitation Robotics, Noordwijk, The Netherlands, 13–15 June 2007.
29. Kikuchi, T.; Tanida, S.; Otsuki, K.; Yasuda, T.; Furusho, J. Development of Third-Generation Intelligently Controllable Ankle-Foot Orthosis with Compact MR Fluid Brake. In Proceedings of the 2010 IEEE International Conference on Robotics and Automation, Anchorage, AK, USA, 3–8 May 2010.

30. Chang, Y.; Zhang, J.; Chen, K.; Fu, C. Design and preliminary evaluation of a clutch-spring lower limb exoskeleton. In Proceedings of the 2019 5th International Conference on Control, Automation and Robotics (ICCAR), Beijing, China, 19–22 April 2019.
31. Wang, C.; Dai, L.; Shen, D.; Wu, J.; Wang, X.; Tian, M.; Shi, Y.; Su, C. Design of an Ankle Exoskeleton that Recycles Energy to Assist Propulsion during Human Walking. *IEEE Trans. Biomed. Eng.* **2021**, *69*, 1212–1224. [CrossRef] [PubMed]
32. Neubauer, B.; Durfee, W. Preliminary design and engineering evaluation of a hydraulic ankle–foot orthosis. *J. Med. Devices* **2016**, *10*, 041002–0410011. [CrossRef]
33. Bai, Y.; Gao, X.; Zhao, J.; Jin, F.; Dai, F.; Lv, Y. A portable ankle-foot rehabilitation orthosis powered by electric motor. *Open Mech. Eng. J.* **2015**, *9*, 982–991. [CrossRef]
34. Gordon, K.E.; Sawicki, G.S.; Ferris, D.P. Mechanical performance of artificial pneumatic muscles to power an ankle–foot orthosis. *IEEE J. Biomech.* **2006**, *39*, 1832–1841. [CrossRef]
35. Ferris, D.P.; Gordon, K.E.; Sawicki, G.S.; Peethambaran, A. An improved powered ankle–foot orthosis using proportional myoelectric control. *Gait Posture* **2006**, *23*, 425–428. [CrossRef]
36. Cain, S.M.; Gordon, K.E.; Ferris, D.P. Locomotor adaptation to a powered ankle-foot orthosis depends on control method. *IEEE J. Neuroeng. Rehabil.* **2007**, *4*, 1–13. [CrossRef]
37. Ferris, D.P.; Czerniecki, J.M.; Hannaford, B. An ankle-foot orthosis powered by artificial pneumatic muscles. *J. Appl. Biomech.* **2005**, *21*, 189–197. [CrossRef]
38. Shorter, K.A.; Kogler, G.F.; Loth, E.; Durfee, W.K.; Hsiao-Wecksler, E.T. A portable powered ankle-foot orthosis for rehabilitation. *J. Rehabil. Res. Dev.* **2011**, *48*, 459–472. [CrossRef] [PubMed]
39. Akers, A.; Gassman, M.; Smith, R. *Hydraulic Power System Analysis*; CRC Press: Boca Raton, FL, USA, 2006; pp. 100–400.
40. Durfee, W.; Sun, Z.; Van de Ven, J. *Fluid Power System Dynamics*; Center for Compact and Efficient Fluid Power: Minneapolis, MN, USA, 2009.
41. Xia, J.; Durfee, W.K. Analysis of small-scale hydraulic actuation systems. *J. Mech. Des.* **2013**, *135*, 091001–091012. [CrossRef]
42. Manring, N.D.; Fales, R.C. *Hydraulic Control Systems*, 2nd ed.; John Wiley & Sons: Chichester, UK, 2019; pp. 87–300.
43. Noël, M.; Cantin, B.; Lambert, S.; Gosselin, C.M.; Bouyer, L.J. An electrohydraulic actuated ankle foot orthosis to generate force fields and to test proprioceptive reflexes during human walking. *IEEE Trans. Neural Syst. Rehabil. Eng.* **2008**, *16*, 390–399. [CrossRef] [PubMed]
44. Kim, S.J.; Na, Y.; Lee, D.Y.; Chang, H.; Kim, J. Pneumatic AFO powered by a miniature custom compressor for drop foot correction. *IEEE Trans. Neural Syst. Rehabil. Eng.* **2020**, *28*, 1781–1789. [CrossRef] [PubMed]
45. Bok, S.K.; Lee, T.H.; Lee, S.S. The effects of changes of ankle strength and range of motion according to aging on balance. *Ann. Rehabil. Med.* **2013**, *37*, 10–16. [CrossRef] [PubMed]
46. Choi, H.S.; Lee, C.H.; Baek, Y.S. Design and validation of a two-degree-of-freedom powered ankle-foot orthosis with two pneumatic artificial muscles. *Mechatronics* **2020**, *72*, 102469–102482. [CrossRef]
47. Alnajjar, F.; Zaier, R.; Khalid, S.; Gochoo, M. Trends and technologies in rehabilitation of foot drop: A systematic review. *Expert Rev. Med. Devices* **2021**, *18*, 31–46. [CrossRef]
48. Daryabor, A.; Kobayashi, T.; Yamamoto, S.; Lyons, S.M.; Orendurff, M.; Akbarzadeh Baghban, A. Effect of ankle-foot orthoses on functional outcome measurements in individuals with stroke: A systematic review and meta-analysis. *Disabil. Rehabil.* **2021**, 1–16. [CrossRef]
49. Vlad, C.V. The Comparison of Utilizing Functional Electrical Stimulation Device Versus Ankle Foot Orthosis Brace and the Effect on Participants' Activities of Daily Living After a Cerebrovascular Accident. Master's Thesis, Cynthia Victoria Vlad, Montclair State University, Montclair, NJ, USA, May 2020.
50. Zahradka, N.; Behboodi, A.; Sansare, A.; Lee, S.C. Evaluation of individualized functional electrical stimulation-induced acute changes during walking: A case series in children with cerebral palsy. *Sensors* **2021**, *21*, 4452. [CrossRef]
51. Moll, I.; Marcellis, R.G.; Coenen, M.L.; Fleuren, S.M.; Willems, P.J.; Speth, L.A.; Witlox, M.A.; Meijer, K.; Vermeulen, R.J. A randomized crossover study of functional electrical stimulation during walking in spastic cerebral palsy: The FES on participation (FESPa) trial. *BMC Pediatr.* **2022**, *22*, 37. [CrossRef]
52. Smith, A.D.; Prokopiusova, T.; Jones, R.; Burge, T.; Rasova, K. Functional electrical stimulation for foot drop in people with multiple sclerosis: The relevance and importance of addressing quality of movement. *Mult. Scler. J.* **2021**, *5*, 653–660. [CrossRef] [PubMed]
53. da Cunha, M.J.; Rech, K.D.; Salazar, A.P.; Pagnussat, A.S. Functional electrical stimulation of the peroneal nerve improves post-stroke gait speed when combined with physiotherapy. A systematic review and meta-analysis. *Ann. Phys. Rehabil. Med.* **2021**, *64*, 101388. [CrossRef] [PubMed]
54. Nevisipour, M.; Honeycutt, C.F. Investigating the underlying biomechanical mechanisms leading to falls in long-term ankle-foot orthosis and functional electrical stimulator users with chronic stroke. *Gait Posture* **2022**, *92*, 144–152. [CrossRef] [PubMed]
55. Aslani, P.; Khaghani, A.; Babaee, T. Comparing the Effects of Functional Electrical Stimulation With and Without Ankle-foot Orthosis on the Balance and Walking Ability of Patients with Multiple Sclerosis. *Iran. Rehabil. J.* **2021**, *19*, 307–314. [CrossRef]
56. Renfrew, L.; Lord, A.C.; McFadyen, A.K.; Rafferty, D.; Hunter, R.; Bowers, R.; Mattison, P.; Moseley, O.; Paul, L. A comparison of the initial orthotic effects of functional electrical stimulation and ankle-foot orthoses on the speed and oxygen cost of gait in multiple sclerosis. *J. Rehabil. Assist. Technol. Eng.* **2018**, *5*, 2055668318755071.

57. Renfrew, L.; Paul, L.; McFadyen, A.; Rafferty, D.; Moseley, O.; Lord, A.C.; Bowers, R.; Mattison, P. The clinical-and cost-effectiveness of functional electrical stimulation and ankle-foot orthoses for foot drop in Multiple Sclerosis: A multicentre randomized trial. *Clin. Rehabil.* **2019**, *33*, 1150–1162. [CrossRef]
58. Collins, S.H.; Wiggin, M.B.; Sawicki, G.S. Reducing the energy cost of human walking using an unpowered exoskeleton. *Nature* **2015**, *522*, 212–215. [CrossRef]
59. Zhang, J.; Fiers, P.; Witte, K.A.; Jackson, R.W.; Poggensee, K.L.; Atkeson, C.G.; Collins, S.H. Human-in-the-loop optimization of exoskeleton assistance during walking. *Science* **2015**, *356*, 1280–1284. [CrossRef]
60. Bishe, S.S.P.A.; Nguyen, T.; Fang, Y.; Lerner, Z.F. Adaptive ankle exoskeleton control: Validation across diverse walking conditions. *IEEE Trans. Med. Robot. Bionics* **2021**, *3*, 801–812. [CrossRef]
61. Han, H.; Wang, W.; Zhang, F.; Li, X.; Chen, J.; Han, J.; Zhang, J. Selection of muscle-activity-based cost function in human-in-the-loop optimization of multi-gait ankle exoskeleton assistance. *IEEE Trans. Neural Syst. Rehabil. Eng.* **2021**, *29*, 944–952. [CrossRef]
62. Zhang, X.Y. Advances in Intelligent Technology of Paraplegic Walking Orthotics. *Sci. Technol. Rev.* **2019**, *37*, 51–59.
63. Fang, X. Analysis on Medical Device Supervision of Orthoses. *Chin. J. Rehabil. Theory Pract.* **2016**, *22*, 737–740.
64. Shao, J.J.; Tao, Y.B.; Pan, L.; Li, P. Application Status of Design and Materials of Rehabilitation Orthotics. *Prog. Mod. Biomed.* **2019**, *19*, 794–797.
65. Liu, Y.X.; Zang, X.Z.; Zhang, N.S.; Wu, M. Design and evaluation of a wearable powered foot orthosis with metatarsophalangeal joint. *Appl. Bionics Biomech.* **2018**, *2018*, 9289505. [CrossRef] [PubMed]
66. Waterval, N.F.; Nollet, F.; Harlaar, J.; Brehm, M.A. Modifying ankle foot orthosis stiffness in patients with calf muscle weakness: Gait responses on group and individual level. *J. Neuroeng. Rehabil.* **2019**, *16*, 1–9. [CrossRef]
67. Liu, Z. Research on Digital Design, Material Optimization and Intelligent Manufacturing of Rehabilitation Aids Based on 3D Printing Technology. Doctoral Dissertatation, Southern Medical University, Guangzhou, China, 10 June 2020.
68. Abdalsadah, F.H.; Hasan, F.; Murtaza, Q.; Khan, A.A. Design and manufacture of a custom ankle-foot orthoses using traditional manufacturing and fused deposition modeling. *Prog. Addit. Manuf.* **2021**, *6*, 555–570. [CrossRef]
69. Kesikburun, S.; Yavuz, F.; Güzelküçük, Ü.; Yaşar, E.; Balaban, B. Effect of ankle foot orthosis on gait parameters and functional ambulation in patients with stroke. *Turk. J. Phys. Med. Rehabil.* **2017**, *63*, 143–148. [CrossRef]
70. de Sèze, M.P.; Bonhomme, C.; Daviet, J.C.; Burguete, E.; Machat, H.; Rousseaux, M.; Mazaux, J.M. Effect of early compensation of distal motor deficiency by the Chignon ankle-foot orthosis on gait in hemiplegic patients: A randomized pilot study. *Clin. Rehabil.* **2011**, *25*, 989–998. [CrossRef]
71. Berenpas, F.; Geurts, A.C.; den Boer, J.; van Swigchem, R.; Nollet, F.; Weerdesteyn, V. Surplus value of implanted peroneal functional electrical stimulation over ankle-foot orthosis for gait adaptability in people with foot drop after stroke. *Gait Posture* **2019**, *71*, 157–162. [CrossRef]
72. Ding, X.D.; Chen, H.X.; Wang, W.; Wang, H.; Huang, L. The effect of botulinum toxin type A injection with ankle-foot orthosis on patients with post-stroke lower limb spasticity. *Chin. J. Phys. Med. Rehabil.* **2014**, *12*, 349–352.

MDPI

St. Alban-Anlage 66

4052 Basel

Switzerland

Tel. +41 61 683 77 34

Fax +41 61 302 89 18

www.mdpi.com

Sensors Editorial Office

E-mail: sensors@mdpi.com

www.mdpi.com/journal/sensors

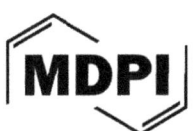

www.ingramcontent.com/pod-product-compliance
Lightning Source LLC
LaVergne TN
LVHW070358100526
838202LV00014B/1339